Promoting Healthy Behaviour

There is ever growing recognition by governments and healthcare professionals of the need to respond to the challenges of preventable diseases, especially so-called 'lifestyle diseases', and of the influence that social class, gender, ethnicity, as well as individual differences play in health. This text explores the fundamental importance of psychology in the development of these lifestyle diseases, and how an understanding of psychological models is essential for the healthcare practitioner to predict behaviours and develop evidence-based interventions.

This thoroughly updated edition includes new chapters looking at health inequalities, health promotion, working with special populations and understanding the role of social and psychological factors in some common conditions. These four additional chapters will enable the reader to better understand the place of lifestyle change within wider society. Beginning with an introduction to healthy behaviour and the context that health practitioners work in, the book goes on to look at issues, including:

- The role of psychology in lifestyle change
- Diet, alcohol, smoking and active lifestyles
- Sexual behaviour
- Chronic illness and vulnerable populations.

Each chapter includes key features including learning objectives, case studies, key points and discussion questions, as well as how to apply the various research and theories to practice. *Promoting Healthy Behaviour* is a practical and informative guide for your practice both now and in the future, and is invaluable reading for healthcare professionals at any stage of their careers.

Dominic Upton is Professor of Health Psychology at the University of Worcester, UK.

Katie Thirlaway is Head of Applied Psychology at Cardiff Metropolitan University, UK.

Promoting Healthy Behaviour

A Practical Guide

Second edition

Dominic Upton and Katie Thirlaway

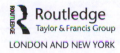
Routledge
Taylor & Francis Group

LONDON AND NEW YORK

First published 2010 by Pearson Education Limited
Edinburgh Gate, Harlow, Essex, CM20 2JE

This edition published 2014 by Routledge
2 Park Square, Milton Park, Abingdon, Oxon, OX14 4RN

and by Routledge
270 Madison Avenue, New York, NY 10016

Routledge is an imprint of the Taylor & Francis Group, an informa business

British Library Cataloguing in Publication Data
A catalogue record for this book is available from the British Library

Library of Congress Cataloging-in-Publication Data
Upton, Dominic, author.
Promoting healthy behaviour : a practical guide / Dominic Upton and Katie
Thirlaway. -- Second edition.
p. ; cm.
Includes bibliographical references and index.
ISBN 978-0-415-73386-1 (hardback) -- ISBN 978-1-4479-2136-3 (pbk.) --
ISBN 978-1-315-81910-5 (ebook)
I. Thirlaway, Kathryn, author. II. Title.
[DNLM: 1. Health Behavior. 2. Health Promotion--methods.
3. Life Style. W 85]
RA427.8
613--dc23
2013030251

ISBN13: 978-0-415-73386-1 (hbk)
ISBN13: 978-1-447-92136-3 (pbk)
ISBN13: 978-1-315-81910-5 (ebk)

Typeset in Bembo by
Saxon Graphics Ltd, Derby

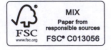

Printed and bound in Great Britain by
TJ International Ltd, Padstow, Cornwall

For Penney (DU)
For Mark (KT)

Contents

List of figures and tables

Figures

Tables

Preface

Background to this book

In 2010 the first edition of this text was published in response to the growing recognition that health practitioners needed to respond to the challenges of preventable disease with more than just education and advice. During the three years between editions there have been concerted efforts by governments and practitioners to encourage healthy lifestyles and prevent or delay the onset of so called 'lifestyle diseases'. Some initiatives have shown promise whilst others have been less successful but the real benefits of our efforts to improve our lifestyles are unlikely to be seen at a population level for at least a decade. Nevertheless, it was clearly time to update and reflect on what we have learnt during the three years since the first edition of the book. In addition to updating all the original chapters we have included four additional chapters on healthy inequalities, health promotion, working with special conditions and working with special populations. We hope that these four additional chapters will enable the reader to better understand the place of lifestyle change within wider society.

The rationale for this book remains the same as the first edition: 'lifestyle diseases' are one of the major challenges facing the NHS. This is not a supposition put forward by us exclusively but by many others, including not least the former prime minister, Tony Blair (Blair, 2006). Of course, politicians are not the only ones to have entered the debate. Opinion formers, academics and leader writers have all contributed to the debate, with increasing attention given to these diseases, whether this be within academia, social policy or the media. We and many others have long recognised the importance of psychology in the development of these lifestyle diseases and we wanted to ensure that appropriate psychological theory and practice were discussed and disseminated for use as part of the armoury available for healthcare professionals.

It has been appreciated for some time that poor lifestyles are associated with increasing health risk – at both an individual and a population level. Of course, such diseases are not distributed evenly across the population; there are certain sections of society that may suffer more than others. Hence, the influence of social class, gender and ethnicity should not be overlooked. It is essential that all healthcare professionals take into account these variables when discussing some of the approaches in this text. Furthermore, it is obvious that cognisance has to be taken of the individual differences when in a clinical situation; the personal characteristics and situation of the individual client can have a significant bearing on an individual's health and lifestyle. These characteristics may be related to their current situation or may be related to more cultural aspects. Moreover, there are differences between the individual countries of the UK, with certain behaviours and health and illnesses more prominent in some areas compared to others. There are also psychological variables that may be described as either 'risk' factors or 'protective' factors – 'personality' variables, self-efficacy or mood, for example.

Psychological models have attempted to integrate all of these social, demographic and psychological variables to predict behaviours and develop theoretically based interventions. This has been the fundamental foundation of this text. We have tried to demonstrate the value of these psychological models and how they can be used practically by healthcare professionals.

We see the role of psychology in lifestyle as of significant, if not of primary, importance. Similarly, we see the role of lifestyle in health and in illness as predominating and likely to become ever more important to the NHS in the coming decades. Indeed, the Foresight report described the 'obesity epidemic' as a problem comparable to climate change (Jones *et al.*, 2007). Obviously, how these issues are going to be addressed is a matter of debate and potential solutions range from the theoretically driven to the more light-hearted. Lifestyle is an issue about which every commentator feels confident to express an opinion. For example, the stigmatisation of obese people (albeit in, one would assume, a humorous article) is not uncommon: 'Most obesity is a consequence of stupidity and indolence and not of some genetic affliction. It is a lifestyle choice which people would be less inclined to adopt if they knew we all hated them for it' (Liddle, 2008). In this text, we review some of the more serious and theoretically driven approaches, debate their value and discuss the potential ways that healthcare professionals can use these for the benefit of their patients and clients.

Overall, we hope that you find this book useful and informative and a guide for your practice both now and in the future. It is geared towards healthcare professionals at any stage of their careers: those wishing to enter a health education/promotion, health (or social) care profession, those new to their particular role and those who have been engaged in professional practice for a number of years but wish to enhance their practice. It is not a manual of tips or a series of laws that have to be followed by all. There are some methods and guiding principles that we hope you will find useful, but this text is intended to be a series of thought-provoking chapters that will intrigue, stimulate and provoke, and hopefully enhance your practice for the benefit of your patients and clients.

The content of this book

We thought for some time about the content of this book – what should we include and what should be excluded? We also had advice from others who suggested additional material, but then others suggested other forms of behaviour that could be included. For example, should we include sleeping? After all, it is a behaviour and can affect health either positively or negatively. Similarly, others considered that we should include stress, which can impact on both mental and physical health and contributes significant mortality through accidents. In the first book we included a chapter on drug taking but for the second edition decided to concentrate on the five main behaviours that are the focus of the majority of health promotion activities.

We also knew the psychology that needed to be included. So what was the cause of our consternation? Why did we spend so much time discussing the content over well-brewed coffee (other than the obvious)? We appreciated at the outset that there was a possibility of considerable repetition within this text. Many of the behaviours discussed are underpinned by similar psychological variables and have been investigated within similar theoretical modes. After writing the first couple of chapters we recognised this and re-jigged the book to include the chapter on psychological concepts, which presents the information in a more coherent and sensible manner. We hope that this has removed considerable overlap, although we recognise that there are key psychological principles and models which will play a central part in many of the behaviours we discuss. For the second edition we have included new chapters that consider more carefully who is responsible for promoting lifestyle change, how we address inequalities and the implications of lifestyle change in different groups of people.

We should emphasise at the outset that this is not a book about smoking or obesity or psychological concepts *alone*. It is a book that attempts to cover a range of topics in an integrating framework. Hence, there are sections on social support, for example, that some may consider skimpy, and there are psychological factors and models that could have been included in many more chapters than currently presented. We have done this on purpose – we have not written a book that is dedicated to any one behaviour or any one approach. We obviously cannot compete with more narrowly focused texts for specific behaviours or models. However, we present an overview with a thematic connection between the chapters which we hope readers will find interesting, thought provoking and, most importantly, of practical use.

Chapter 1: Introduction to healthy behaviour

In this opening chapter we set the context within which health practitioners are working and individuals are making choices about how they behave. We look historically at the socio-cultural climate in which we all operate, considering how and why lifestyle diseases and related behaviours have become so pertinent for us in the twenty-first century. We also consider the political imperative to encourage individual responsibility for long-term health and we reflect on the environmental influences over twenty-first century lifestyles.

Chapter 2: Health promotion

In this chapter we introduce the concept of health promotion, health education and health literacy and where these various activities sit within public health. The chapter considers who is responsible for health promotion and how the health promotion priorities for a community are established.

Chapter 3: Health and health inequalities

Inequalities in health are apparent in practically all societies across the world. In the developed world, and in the UK in particular, these inequalities can be significant. This chapter explores these inequalities with a particular focus on socio-economic differences in health. Prior to this, however, a brief overview is provided on defining health, measuring health and measuring socio-economic status and deprivation.

Chapter 4: Psychology in practice

In this chapter we describe a number of key psychological concepts that are of relevance to the topic of lifestyle and lifestyle change. There are a great many theories of behavioural change, many of which include similar psychological concepts in different theoretical frameworks. The decision not to introduce specific theories but rather to introduce the key concepts that have consistently proved relevant for behavioural change is an attempt to bridge the gap between theory and practice. It is intended to make identifying the key aspects of research relevant to practice simpler. However, this is in no way intended to undermine the importance of theory, and the chapter highlights further reading that will enable interested readers to gain greater insight into the psychological theory that underpins these concepts. The existence of a large number of theories of behavioural change has been beneficial to our understanding of how and why people change their behaviour. It has enabled us to identify and understand those factors we might have expected to be important but are not, and those factors that are important in behavioural choices. However, it does make exploring the psychological research into behavioural change somewhat daunting for non-psychologists, so this chapter hopes to make the key psychological concepts to date easier to identify.

Chapter 5: Eating well

In this chapter we explore eating and diet. The problems in providing a clear message of a 'healthy diet' are stressed, as are the issues surrounding the social environment impact on diet. The governmental approaches to the 'obesity epidemic' are outlined and the role of psychological models in the development of appropriate interventions is stressed – ultimately, what the healthcare professional can do to promote healthy eating in those who are currently overweight, and how healthy eating can be promoted in the young.

Chapter 6: Being active

In this chapter we consider the predominance of sedentary lifestyles in the population. Physical activity is the output side of the input–output energy equation and so is a key factor in the rising levels of obesity. The role of the obesogenic environment and how psychological interventions can work in such adverse environmental conditions are explored.

Chapter 7: Sensible drinking

Drinking is a popular component of many aspects of leisure in Britain. Drinking has adverse consequences for social and physical well-being. The changing nature of drinking patterns in the UK and in particular in women is described and discussed. Government policies to establish healthy drinking patterns in the young and promote healthy drinking in adults are outlined and the role of psychological interventions to support healthy drinking and deter deleterious drinking is evaluated.

Chapter 8: Smoking

The health consequences of smoking are well established and well known throughout the population – smoking can have a significant impact on morbidity and mortality. However, approximately a quarter of the population still smokes and this has a significant impact on both the individual and the country's health. Given the significant impact that smoking has on the health of the nation, there has been extensive research into smoking and much of this has a psychological nature. In this chapter, the psychological variables and models that have been applied to smoking and, more importantly, how they can be used to promote smoking cessation are discussed.

Chapter 9: Sexual activity

The safe sex message is being promoted in order to reduce the spread of sexually transmitted diseases. Sexual behaviours are not simply a consequence of physiological drives, but there are social, emotional and cultural (to name but three) variables that influence such behaviour. Within these broader influences the psychological factors have to be appreciated and developed. These psychological models and how they can be applied to promote safer sex are discussed. Importantly, safer sex is discussed within a pleasure-promoting context rather than a fear-inducing one.

Chapter 10: Special conditions

Increasingly it is acknowledged that healthy lifestyles are as relevant (if not more so in some cases) for individuals diagnosed with chronic conditions as they are for individuals with no diagnosed condition. Recommending and supporting lifestyle change for individuals with a chronic condition requires health practitioners to consider any particular risks and associated amendments to standard advice that different conditions indicate. For some conditions there are specialist lifestyle support courses available.

This chapter considers four different chronic conditions: type 2 diabetes; coronary heart disease; mental health; and chronic obstructive pulmonary disease.

Chapter 11: Special populations

Although approaches to lifestyle behaviour change are common across all the population, there are specific groups that require targeted interventions. These groups are numerous across the population but this chapter will explore three specific groups: those with a learning difficulty, those in prison and the elderly. To a large degree, these were selected at random but are there to exemplify the skills, attributes and targeted interventions required to alter unhealthy health behaviours.

Chapter 12: Conclusion

This final chapter attempts to draw together the diverse behaviours discussed in the previous chapters and identify the key similarities and differences in the various behaviours we have considered. It is crucial for health practitioners to recognise which psychological techniques are effective across all behaviours in order to enable them to deal more effectively with the various prevention and promotion targets they are required to meet. This final chapter also tries to look ahead and identify what else we need to know to make our interventions more effective.

For each of these chapters we have included a selection of the following features:

- *Learning objectives:* what you will find in this book, so that you can navigate your way through the text and know what to expect and what you can achieve.
- *Case study:* We provide a brief case study that highlights some key principles to be discussed later in the chapter. In some of these you are asked to take the role of the individual practitioner dealing with the client and we hope that this will highlight issues that you may face in practice (or have faced), whether this be as a qualified or student healthcare professional. We hope that the case study will raise questions and issues that we address later in the chapter.
- *Introduction:* the introduction follows the case study – we hope that the case study has whetted your appetite and you will begin to appreciate during the chapter the importance of the case study and how it relates to the chapter content.
- *Applying this to ...:* at stages throughout the chapter a box highlights how the principles discussed in the text can be applied to the case study.
- *Applying research in practice:* in the chapter, empirical research studies are presented throughout to demonstrate the evidence base of the suggested techniques. More detail on a couple of these is provided in these boxes.
- *Working with others:* each chapter will consider the other professionals who may also be involved with or could support you in your health promotion activities.
- *Key points:* at the end of chapter the key points will be summarised.
- *Discussion points:* these act as points for discussion – they relate either to all of the chapter content or to the case study highlighted at the outset.

We hope you are interested and engaged in this book and that it leads to an enhancement of your personal and professional skills. Overall, we hope that it leads to an improvement in healthy behaviours in your client group and goes some way to reducing the immense health problems associated with a poor lifestyle currently evident in the UK today.

References

Blair, T. (2006). Speech on healthy living. *Guardian*, 26 July. Available at: http://www.guardian.co.uk/society/2006/jul/26/health.politics (accessed 30 November 2009).

Jones, A., Bentham, G., Foster, C., Hillsdon, M. and Panter, J. (2007). *Tackling Obesities: Future Choices – Obesogenic Environments – Evidence Review*. London: United Kingdom Government Foresight Programme, Office of Science and Innovation.

Liddle, R. (2008). Laugh at the lard butts – but just remember Fatty Fritz lives longer. *Sunday Times*, 27 January.

Acknowledgements

Both of us have spent considerable time on this project, collating, reading and reviewing research articles and textbooks before trying to develop the material into a series of practical chapters that could assist and develop an individual professional's practice. The material we have read has not only been presented by psychologists but also by those from the wider academic community, including those from healthcare, medicine, sociology, philosophy and policy developments. We have tried to encompass the literature from both an academic and a practitioner basis. We thank the researchers, clinicians and policy makers for all this work and the contributions they have made to the current knowledge base.

On a more personal level, several key colleagues have acted as researchers and reviewers for us and have contributed their time, effort and opinions with vigour and a frankness that was as refreshing as it was useful. Particular mention should go to Helena Darby (for DU) and Lindsey Davies (for KT) who made a significant contribution to the new chapters in this second edition ensuring it is not only completely updated but also a more wide-reaching and comprehensive text. Thanks also to Helen Campling for her essential work on the figures and diagrams (KT).

Many thanks also to the Publishers for helping us through this project. Finally, we also thank those involved in the production of this text – the designers and production editors – for enhancing the text with some excellent features, which we hope will provide guidance, direction and added value to all readers.

We must also offer thanks and acknowledgements to those who have provided support for us both at work and at home. We also thank our colleagues (for DU) at the University of Worcester and (for KT) at the Cardiff Metropolitan University for their help, advice, friendship and practical guidance.

Finally, we would like to thank our family and friends for bringing us sustenance and calming us down during our manic periods. In particular, our children: Dominic's children – Francesca, Rosie and Gabriel and Katie's children – Anna, Hetty and Keir. As always, Katie would not have been able to complete the book without the support of Mark, Megan and Vicky.

<table>
<tr><td>

1

</td><td>

Introduction to healthy behaviour

</td></tr>
</table>

Learning objectives

At the end of this chapter you will:
- recognise how the concepts of lifestyle diseases and lifestyle behaviours have arisen
- understand the health behaviours central to the development and progression of chronic diseases
- recognise why lifestyle change is so complex and difficult
- recognise the multiple influences on lifestyle choice
- understand the challenges for health professionals involved in health promotion.

Health professionals and particularly primary care practitioners have health promotion and disease prevention as a central aspect of their role. This book is about this central element of a healthcare professional's role. Although lifestyle change should be a key part of *all* health professionals' role, and this has been recognised for many decades, in recent years its importance has moved higher up the policy hierarchy. For example, the then prime minister of the UK, Tony Blair, in 2006 called for 'lifestyle change' to relieve the pressure on the National Health Service (BBC News, 2006): the prime minister suggested that 'failure to address bad lifestyles was putting an "increasing strain" on the health service'. The impact of this key message, the role of lifestyle in health, has been significant. Many health professionals now provide the patients and clients who come into their clinics with expert advice about lifestyle behaviours and health. The frustration and disillusionment that are felt when advice is ignored and patients go on to develop chronic diseases that could probably have been avoided are among the motivating factors for this book. This frustration is frequently articulated by health professionals involved in treating the major lifestyle diseases of the twentieth century. In 2009, Professor Wiseman, medical and scientific adviser for the World Cancer Research Fund, said:

This means that we are now more sure than ever before that by limiting the amount of alcohol they drink, maintaining a healthy weight and being physically active women can make a significant difference to their risk. We estimate over 40% of breast cancer cases in the UK could be prevented just by making these relatively straightforward changes.

Wiseman (2009)

Lifestyle change is a tantalising solution to the chronic ill health that is the scourge of modern societies. It is such a cheap, effective, non-toxic, low-risk solution to the rising incidence of heart disease, diabetes, chronic back pain, cancers and many other conditions that it can seem incredible that we have not been able to deliver widespread population change. This book does not present a method to effect instant population-wide uptake of health advice but it does explain why changing lifestyle behaviours is so difficult for so many people and not quite as straightforward as Professor Wiseman suggests. Furthermore this book points the reader in the direction of techniques and interventions proven to have at least some success in increasing the likelihood of successful behavioural change.

So what are the key health behaviours that the government would like us to change? The word lifestyle is used confidently by health professionals, the media and individuals but what does it mean and which health behaviours are included under its umbrella? Initially, the medical profession started to refer to 'lifestyle diseases' to reflect the role that lifestyle choices play in certain diseases. Doyle (2001) suggested that the six major lifestyle diseases are coronary heart disease, stroke, lung cancer, colon cancer, diabetes and chronic obstructive pulmonary disease. The rationale for their inclusion is that they 'trace mainly to imprudent living' (Doyle, 2001).

Interestingly, few authors would call sexually transmitted diseases 'lifestyle diseases', although they are clearly entirely a result of behavioural choices with none of the genetic component that plays a part in the six major lifestyle diseases identified by Doyle (2001). Sexually transmitted diseases are more usually defined as infectious diseases (ONS, 2007), an important distinction for clinicians but perhaps less so for primary care and community-based practitioners interested in public health.

In between an 'imprudent lifestyle' (Doyle, 2001) and the development of lifestyle diseases are a number of 'precursor' conditions. High cholesterol, high blood pressure and obesity are risk factors for the development of a number of the aforementioned lifestyle diseases. The distinction between these precursors, the diseases they predict and the behaviours that are associated with them is often blurred. They are often presented as diseases *per se* and interventions are prescribed by the medical profession. The Department of Health (2010) categorises high blood pressure as a cardiovascular disease. Obesity is frequently referred to using disease parameters. For instance, the phrase 'obesity epidemic' (Gard and Wright, 2005) is common and suggests that obesity is a disease and furthermore that it is somehow catching! Consequently, obesity is considered a lifestyle disease by some authors whereas others categorise it as lifestyle behaviour (Doyle, 2001).

The behaviours that are usually cited as being involved in the aetiology of lifestyle diseases are poor diet, lack of physical activity, cigarette smoking (Doyle, 2001; Blaxter, 1990; Egger et al., 2011) and, increasingly, excess drinking (Burke et al., 1997; Blaxter, 1990).

Sexual practices are also often described by public health professionals as health and/or lifestyle behaviours (Wardle and Steptoe, 2005). Despite not being directly linked to what clinicians refer to as lifestyle diseases, sexual practices nevertheless are still considered by most public health practitioners to be an aspect of lifestyle worthy of both concern and intervention (Egger *et al.*, 2009; Wardle and Steptoe, 2005). Furthermore, sexual practices are a clear cause of preventable and treatable diseases. Consequently, the promotion of safer sex is also included in this book.

Over the past couple of decades the unhealthy lifestyles that predominate in Western societies have been presented by the media as a new and modern crisis. Stories about drunken young women, rising levels of obesity and type 2 diabetes are no longer restricted to the health pages but frequently take the front pages of national papers and make the lead story of television news bulletins. However, it is important to recognise that people have been drinking too much and eating the wrong things for many centuries. In Victorian times there were many gin addicts and in Elizabethan times diets were poor and dangerous levels of drinking were widespread (Plant and Plant, 2006). Perhaps the main difference between then and now is the level of understanding we have. We have a better understanding of the relationship between our lifestyle and our health than previous generations. However, as long ago as Roman times, the importance of a moderate lifestyle was recognised. For example, Pythagoras suggests that 'No man, who values his health, ought to trespass on the bounds of moderation, either in labour, diet or concubinage' and Hippocrates has suggested that

> Persons of a gross relaxed habit of body, the flabby, and red-haired, ought to use a drying diet ... Such as are fat, and desire to be lean, should use exercise fasting; should drink small liquors a little warm, should eat only once a day, and no more than will just satisfy their hunger'.
>
> cited in Haslam, 2007, p. 32

The connection between obesity and angina was emphasised in 1811 by Robert Thomas who wrote:

> It is found to attack men much more frequently than women, particularly those who have short necks, who are inclinable to corpulency, and who at the same time lead an inactive or sedentary life ... he should endeavour to counteract disposition to obesity, which has been considered a predisposing cause.
>
> Thomas, 1811

It was towards the end of the eighteenth and during the nineteenth century that lifestyle approaches to health in Western societies were subsumed in the battle to control infectious diseases. Developing industrial societies and their new, crowded, urban ways of living promoted the spread of infectious diseases such as smallpox, scarlet fever, etc. (Scambler, 2008). In reality, better sanitation, nutrition and living conditions led to the decline of infectious diseases, but at the same time as these public health measures were being instigated, doctors were simultaneously starting to understand that diseases such as smallpox and measles were caused by single infectious agents. Vaccines were developed against these and people were protected from the associated diseases.

Antibiotics to treat bacterial infections were discovered and on the back of these major discoveries the biomedical principle that all disease can be traced to specific causal mechanisms emerged and dominated the practice and development of medicine over the next century (Scambler, 2008). Many would argue that the biomedical model of disease still remains the underlying principle behind the majority of medical practice in Western societies. However, in actuality, a number of models of disease and health (such as genetic, environmental and lifestyle models) influence medical practice and public health initiatives; it is just that the biomedical model usually takes prominence.

Infectious diseases have declined throughout the twentieth and twenty-first centuries and in some cases have been completely eradicated. The major health problems for modern developed societies are the chronic or so-called 'lifestyle diseases' identified by Doyle (2001). These chronic conditions are complex and cannot easily be traced to specific causal mechanisms. They are influenced at a number of levels – biologically, psychologically and sociologically. That is to say, the genes we inherit and the environment we inhabit are central to whether we go on to develop a chronic disease. Pivotal to the genetic and environmental circumstances of an individual is the way they respond to their environment and to their biological make-up. One individual may recognise that diabetes 'runs' in their family and make active choices to try to prevent it. Another with the same understanding of their family history may decide that it is inevitable that they will develop the disease and continue with damaging health choices. Similarly, one person may use smoking as a coping strategy to deal with the adverse environmental circumstances they find themselves in whereas the next may use exercise as a coping strategy. In this text we recognise that the socio-cultural circumstances in which an individual finds themselves can severely limit their lifestyle choices but we argue that usually some level of choice remains. This text explores how to encourage positive lifestyle change whilst recognising that the biological and environmental circumstances of each individual will vary enormously and have a large role to play in the degree of volitional choice each person has.

The biomedical model of disease is often characterised as curative but also has a preventative remit, albeit one that is frequently focused on vaccination or the avoidance of a specific causal organism. Chronic diseases are not generally something that you catch; rather they are a long-term response to stressors such as poor diet, lack of exercise, excess alcohol, high blood pressure, poverty or environmental hazards. Consequently, the lifestyle model of disease, first promoted by the Greeks/Romans, is once again taking precedence and influencing health policy.

A lifestyle model of disease is very focused on prevention. Lifestyle changes are clearly still pertinent once a disease is diagnosed and can slow the progress of the disease and reduce complications, but fundamentally the principle of lifestyle change is to prevent disease. This can be viewed as a threat to the medical profession and to commercial companies that make a profit from curing disease. However, lifestyle approaches have their own commercial spin-offs and the proliferation of private gyms and diet products is a visible sign of the commercial potential of a lifestyle approach to health and disease prevention.

Lifestyle approaches to health, whilst having the potential to generate profit for commercial operators, are attractive to governments because of the potential to shift the responsibility for health from the government to the individual. In this way, whilst some can see a way to profit from lifestyle approaches to health, the government can see a potential low-cost solution to healthcare. Many policy documents emphasise the role of individual choice in health-related behaviour and stress personal responsibility. There is a danger that this approach can be seen as a 'way out' for governments who can fairly cheaply provide individuals with the information they need to make informed choices about their lifestyle and leave them to get on with it. However, this is a short-sighted approach because when such tactics don't work the NHS is still 'burdened' with the job of treating people who have developed chronic diseases. Indeed, many commentators remain concerned about the lifestyle approach to disease, arguing that by emphasising individual choice the huge social factors involved in inequities in health can be ignored.

It is certainly true that early responses to the evidence that chronic diseases are influenced by behaviour did focus on knowledge-based health promotion campaigns that left the individual to resolve any behavioural flaws. However, the evidence from decades of educational health promotion is that it doesn't produce lifestyle change. Recently, public health policy makers at all levels have made position statements about expanding the medical definition of 'lifestyle' to take into account the social nature of lifestyle behaviour (Ashton and Seymour, 1988; Bruce, 1991; Hansen and Easthope, 2007). 'New public health', as it has been described, aims to discard health education initiatives in favour of enhancing people's life skills and creating supportive environments (McPearson, 1992; Ashton and Seymour, 1988). 'New public health' operates with a biopsychosocial understanding of health which requires education and lifestyle modification to be part of general public policy, the workplace and education, not restricted to health promotional campaigns (Hansen and Easthope, 2007). The lifestyle model of disease, rather than being individualistic, can at its best enable individuals to take control of their health and influence policy to enable them to do so. The importance of supportive environments in promoting behavioural change has been emphasised recently by the impressive impact of the public smoking ban on rates of heart attacks, reduced by 10 per cent in England and 14 per cent in Scotland (Nursing Times, accessed 2009).

If we are to move away from a health promotion approach to lifestyle behaviour towards developing people's 'life skills' then a sound basis in the psychology of behavioural change will be necessary. To move from providing knowledge to improving the ability to change requires a psychological approach. We need to work with people within their current socio-economic resources whilst pressurising governments to provide the resources to enable change.

As recognised by the World Health Organisation (1986), lifestyle is more than simply an individual choice. The way we live is dictated by our economic and cultural circumstances (Frieden, 2010). Indeed, the use of the term 'lifestyle change' reflects the importance of socio-demographic factors in health behaviour change rather better than the term 'health promotion'. Ethnicity, sex, age, socio-economic circumstances and cultural groups all interplay to influence the way we choose to behave (Blaxter, 1990). The evidence for socio-demographic influences on lifestyle choices is irrefutable (Craig and Mindell, 2008).

The UK government and more recently the devolved institutions of Wales, Scotland and Northern Ireland have been collecting demographic mortality and morbidity data for some time, enabling comparisons between the health of different demographic and socio-economic groups. More recently, data on physical activity, eating habits, drinking and smoking have also been included. Each of these UK institutions has commissioned surveys on a continuing basis to enable comparisons between behaviours over time and to monitor health targets. The demographic data collected in each survey includes sex, age and socio-economic class. Each of these will be explored in the coming section to detail how these demographic factors can influence health and well-being so that the healthcare professional is able to recognise and understand the influence that some of these variables exert.

Both biological sex and gender are related to health and health outcomes, but it is generally accepted that it is gender rather than biological sex that influences lifestyle choices. Indeed, the gender influence on health is primarily mediated through lifestyle choices. Many studies confuse the terms sex and gender. Sex is the biological underpinning – our genetic make-up. Gender, on the other hand, is socially constructed; it is more concerned with how we think and behave (Annandale and Hunt, 2000).

A woman born between 2008–2010 has a life expectancy of 82.3 years, a man 78.2 years (ONS, 2011a). Men and women also have different morbidity rates. For example, women are less likely to suffer from cardiovascular disease and more likely to suffer from breast cancer than men (ONS, 2007). Prostate cancer is a solely male disease as women do not have a prostate gland. Male and female differences in morbidity and mortality are influenced by biological sex (physiological and hormonal differences) but also by gender and gender role casting (Annandale and Hunt, 2000). The difference in male and female mortality rates is diminishing and this is generally held to be due to changing gender roles in Western societies rather than to biological factors, although early menarche may play a part in the rising prevalence of some female hormonally linked cancers. Unfortunately, not all gender role adaptations are positive and some of these changes in gender expectations have resulted in women adopting unhealthy, traditionally male lifestyle behaviours (Emslie *et al.*, 2002). The influence of gender over health is mediated through the lifestyle choices that men and women make. The implications of gender roles for the various lifestyle behaviours will be developed and discussed in the relevant chapters.

Age is different from every other demographic variable in that the majority of us will experience old age. There are clear differences in health and health outcomes between different age categories and, unlike sex/gender differences, a large factor will be physiological changes over the lifespan rather than cultural expectations about age-related behaviour. Nevertheless, cultural expectations of how people of different ages should behave do play a role in the way that, for example, teenage mothers approach their pregnancies and older people participate in exercise and sport. Furthermore, despite the fact that presumably we must all hope to become older, older people experience considerable discrimination, which has implications for their health and well-being and for their lifestyle choices (Scambler, 2008). Hence, it is important to explore the impact of the cultural influences of age on lifestyle and health and this will be addressed in each of the lifestyle behaviour chapters.

Socio-economic is a broad term encompassing many variables and is assessed using a range of different factors. Social class, income, work, housing, physical and social environments have all been found to influence our health directly and also indirectly through their influence on lifestyle choices (Doyle, 2001). The definition of social class adopted by this text has been provided by the seminal Black Report (Townsend and Davidson, 1989) which first clearly stated the link between health and social class in modern society:

> Segments of the population sharing broadly similar types and levels of resources, with broadly similar styles of living and (for some sociologists), some shared perception of their collective condition.

In essence, different classes have differential power to access material resources: homes, cars, white and electronic goods etc.

Explanations for behavioural choices are both contentious and politically sensitive. In 1989 Townsend and Davidson recognised that there were a number of explanations for differing levels of health in different sections of society. The key most plausible explanations are a materialist explanation and a behavioural explanation. Simply, a materialist explanation suggests that most of the class differences in health can be explained by the environmental circumstances in which individuals find themselves. A behavioural explanation suggests that most of the class differences in health can be explained by the choices that individuals make. At first sight, these explanations would seem to argue for different causes of disease but actually the distinction is more subtle. To use late-onset diabetes as an example, a behaviourist explanation would argue that a proportion of the class difference in diabetes morbidity can be explained by what individuals choose to eat. A materialist explanation does not refute the claim that diet is a major cause of late-onset diabetes but questions the degree of choice that individuals actually have about the food that they eat. Another way of framing the dichotomy is in terms of individual or collective responsibility. In the first case, the right of individuals to do as they wish with their own lives is emphasised; in the second, the inability of individuals to exert control over their environment is considered key (Blaxter, 1990). At first sight, a lifestyle model of health would appear to operate within behaviourist or individualistic explanations for lifestyle choices. However, for these authors the use of the term lifestyle behaviours rather than health behaviours is a deliberate attempt to recognise the role of socio-environmental factors in decisions individuals make about behaviours that impinge on their health. The challenge for health practitioners is to identify how to enable individuals to make positive changes to their lifestyle within the socio-economic circumstances in which they live. In other words, it is hoped that recognising that social and environmental circumstances are an integral aspect of lifestyle choice does not rule out the possibility of effective behavioural change within those parameters. Clearly, a blanket-style approach to lifestyle change is unlikely to be successful and lifestyle interventions must be tailored to the circumstances in which individuals find themselves.

One popular way of describing the role of the environment in behavioural choice is to refer to obesogenic environments. The common use of the term obesogenic environment reflects the widening acceptance of the role of factors external to the individual in the development of obesity. The complexities of what contributes to an obesogenic environment are not well understood. We know that roads and cars promote sedentary modes of travel through their ease and convenience and discourage active transport by being a danger to pedestrians and cyclists, but cars also enable people to travel to leisure activities that support health and well-being. We understand that the easy availability of high-calorie food and the increasing portion size in restaurants promote over-eating of the 'wrong' types of food but there is far greater availability of healthy food choices as well. Other factors such as shift working, alcohol and drug consumption, media output, etc. all contribute to an obesogenic environment. The key to what makes an environment obesogenic would seem to be understanding and influencing the cultural responses we make to that environment (Jones *et al.*, 2007).

Lifestyle behaviours have multiple functions; they are not simply or even primarily health focused. Lifestyle behaviours play a key role in developing and maintaining social relationships. They can be mood enhancing or a way of coping with stressful circumstances. Lifestyle behaviours are often pleasurable. Furthermore, the roles they play in our lives change during the lifespan. Lifestyle behaviours are all under some degree of volitional control, although the amount of control individuals have over their lifestyle choices is debatable and likely to vary a lot between people. The term lifestyle reflects that these are behaviours we do regularly and probably habitually. Lifestyle behaviours have the majority of their positive consequences in the present and the majority of their negative outcomes in the future. Any lifestyle behavioural change intervention consequently requires individuals to be future orientated. When you start to consider the complexity of lifestyle behaviours it becomes apparent why change is not as straightforward as it first appears.

It is true that, to some extent, the rise in chronic diseases is actually a reflection of the success of modern healthcare and social reform in that more people live long enough to experience the chronic conditions associated with old age. However, there is considerable evidence that, in addition, people take less exercise (Department of Health, 2011), drink more alcohol (HM Government, 2012), are less safe in their sexual practices (Center for Disease Control, 2007) and eat poorer diets (Fox and Hillsdon, 2007) than they did in previous recent generations. Smoking is the only lifestyle behaviour where incidence is declining, although a considerable minority of the population continue to smoke (Cancer Research UK, 2012). It is important to try to understand why unhealthy lifestyles have become so widespread, particularly since Western societies seem to be exporting these deleterious practices to developing nations (Wagner and Brath, 2011).

The lifestyles of societies are constantly evolving and will change in response to modernisation and social reform. We can see this in the different patterns of lifestyle choices in countries at different stages of modernisation and with different cultural norms (WHO, 1986). Life in modernised societies is easier and requires less physical effort than it did in previous generations (Department of Health, 2011; Fox and Hillsdon, 2007). Employment is more likely to be sedentary, housework is less demanding and far fewer people are physically active in the process of travelling. There is no evidence that people are less active in their leisure time than they were in previous generations but because the majority of physical activity is now leisure, people's total physical activity has declined (Department of Health, 2004). The increase in cheap fast-food outlets, high-calorie snacks and ready-prepared meals all contribute to the poorer diets we eat today (Myslobodsky, 2003; Blouin *et al.*, 2009). Alcohol has become considerably cheaper than it was in previous generations and is more readily available (Plant and Plant, 2006; Babor *et al.*, 2010). Cultural acceptance of heavy drinking remains a stable facet of British life but a key change here is that it used to be unacceptable for young women to drink heavily; however, changing gender expectations are making it more acceptable for young women to match young men in their excessive drinking (Plant and Plant, 2006). It is probably in terms of sexual behaviour that cultural expectations have altered most dramatically, with sex outside marriage and children out of wedlock virtually normalised in secular society (Schubotz *et al.*, 2003). There are many positives from a more liberal attitude towards sex. It has enabled better education and communication about safe sex, empowering some women to control their sexual destinies and consequently protect themselves from sexual infection and unwanted pregnancy.

Beck (1990) coined the phrase 'risk society' to acknowledge that we live in a world where perceptions of risk are heightened, and the identification and management of risk are a major concern at all levels of society. Risk assessment in the workplace is now a legal requirement. Similarly, in schools and colleges all activities must be risk assessed, which may result in a reduction of school trips if procedures to mitigate the risk cannot be simply and cheaply instigated. Alongside risk assessment has emerged the concept of informed consent. Many professionals, health practitioners included, must ensure that they have the informed consent of an individual before embarking on a treatment programme or other intervention. All these procedures combine to create the impression that we live in a high-risk environment, when in reality we are probably safer from environmental hazards and disease than at any previous point in history. The perception of a high-risk environment is further perpetuated by the media who bombard us with 'risk' stories. Stories about crime, environmental and health risks dominate the media because they meet key news agendas in that they are negative and often sensational: 'Drinking a glass of wine a day increases your risk of breast cancer by 6%'. Lifestyle risks such as the risk of breast cancer from alcohol consumption are just some of a range of risks that we need to manage daily. For many people the best way to deal with the plethora of risk messages that they receive on a daily basis is to ignore them (Thirlaway and Heggs, 2005).

Lifestyle behaviours are embedded in daily life. There are four aspects to most people's lives: sleeping, travelling, occupation and leisure (Buckworth and Dishman, 2002). However, it is impossible to describe a typical 24 hours for someone working in the UK. The complexities of modern life in terms of work patterns and outside responsibilities mean that fewer and fewer people work a nine to five day. However, if you consider an average night's sleep to be about eight hours, the average working day to be eight hours and an average journey to and from work to be an hour then there are about seven hours left a day for leisure and/or caring and household responsibilities. Obviously, many people will take longer to travel to work, sleep for longer or less, have greater or fewer responsibilities outside of work, but most people will have some time each day that is not taken up with travelling, work, caring or sleeping. Many people do not work for longer than eight hours at a time. People in the UK work some of the longest hours in Europe and also many people work fewer but longer days each week, e.g. those in the police force and nursing. Shift work is common and it is associated with unhealthy lifestyle choices (Folkard *et al.*, 2005; Lowden *et al.*, 2010). Probably one of the major changes in daily living in the UK has been the huge increase in parents with young children who work (ONS, 2011b). This means that people are busy with household responsibilities outside of work that may previously have been completed during the day. In summary, given that the physically active nature of housework and shopping has reduced (Department of Health, 2004) and that there has been a reduction in time available for physically active pursuits, it is not surprising that changes in the pattern of a 'normal' day have had consequences for both lifestyle and health.

While we are travelling we could be physically active, we could eat or smoke. However, smoking has recently been banned in all public places, including public transport vehicles, in the UK. This is the first major piece of legislation for many years that pertains to volitional lifestyle behaviour and evidence is emerging that the public ban has had a significant positive effect on heart attack rates in the UK (Nursing Times, accessed 2009). Private cars are not subject to the legislation so it is possible that the ban may encourage people to use their cars if they wish to smoke on a journey, but there is no evidence yet of this.

For the majority of people the trip to work, school or college is the most frequent journey. A minority of people take the opportunity to walk or cycle to their place of work or study but the majority will drive or use public transport. A steady decline in walking trips has been witnessed with the number of people making trips by foot 28 per cent lower in 2010 than in 1995 (Department for Transport, 2011). Factors believed to contribute to the decline of regular travel by foot or bicycle include: perceived and actual safety; the provision of facilities to segregate conflicting road users; and the proximity of local shops/workplace (Jones *et al.*, 2007). However, encouragingly evidence is starting to emerge that integrated projects to increase active transport, such as the sustainable transport towns project, can have a positive impact on walking and cycling (Sloman *et al.*, 2010).

Work and caring for relatives are the primary occupations for most people and the majority of jobs these days are predominantly sedentary (Department of Health, 2004). Similarly, most caring roles do not involve physical activity, although they can require heavy lifting. At work, most people will eat at least one meal and the quality of available food will influence the food choices. Jeffery *et al.* (2006) found no relationship between the proximity of fast-food outlets to the workplace and what people ate. There is little evidence about the influence of on-site food provision in the workplace on food choice, although the healthy workplace initiatives in Scotland (Scotland Health Improvement Agency, accessed 2009) and Wales (Welsh Assembly Government, accessed 2009) were designed to improve on-site food choice. The majority of work on on-site provision of food has been carried out with children. Previously, unhealthy food choices have dominated school food sales but the impact of new nutritional standards in schools in September 2006 is yet to be evaluated (Jones *et al.*, 2007; see Chapter 3 on eating well).

Whilst drinking alcohol at work is extremely rare, the workplace culture of drinking outside of working hours has been found to be significantly related to both drinking with work colleagues and non-work-related drinking (Delaney and Ames, 1995; Barrientos-Gutierrez *et al.*, 2007). The establishment of healthy drinking norms in the workplace could have beneficial effects for drinking both with work colleagues and more widely.

Patterns of leisure activity have changed dramatically with the development of sedentary activities such as watching television, using computers and the myriad of electronic games consoles available. The relationship between time spent in such sedentary leisure activities and reductions in time spent in physically active leisure pursuits has been, and still is, the subject of much concern, particularly in children (Department of Health, 2011). At the same time the number of health clubs and gyms has proliferated and a small increase in the proportion of people taking leisure-time physical activity has been reported (Department of Health, 2004). Television cookery programmes are popular but it would seem that watching cookery programmes rather than actually cooking is the popular leisure pursuit! Other popular leisure activities such as going to the cinema are associated with unhealthy food availability and large portion sizes. Similarly, recent studies have highlighted the increase in portion sizes of meals served in restaurants (Steenhuis and Vermeer, 2009). Hence, leisure activities themselves can lead to an increase in unhealthy lifestyles.

Conclusion

The world we live in is both the safest yet and a highly risky place, and probably the biggest risk to health, for most people, is the lifestyle choices that they make. However, most of us continue to be concerned about dramatic risks such as aeroplane crashes, but continue to ignore the far more likely risks associated with a lifetime of smoking, eating and drinking too much and remaining sedentary. Education has little impact on people's failure to respond to risk. Choices about eating, drinking, smoking or physical activity are possible, although not for everyone in every context. Enabling choice, supporting choice, empowering choice is what all health practitioners want to achieve, and understanding how best to do this is what this book is about.

Key points

- The major lifestyle diseases are coronary heart disease, stroke, lung cancer, colon cancer, diabetes and chronic obstructive pulmonary disease.
- Unhealthy lifestyles have arisen as a response to modern society.
- We understand the risks associated with unhealthy lifestyle behaviours probably better than at any other time in history but still fail to make appropriate changes to our behaviour.
- Lifestyle change is more difficult for some people than others, depending on their socio-demographic and environmental circumstances.
- Lifestyle behaviours are complex, which makes instigating change similarly complex and difficult.

Discussion points

- The success of the ban on smoking in public places has made some commentators suggest that we should ban certain types of unhealthy food. What are the complications involved in banning certain foodstuffs?

- To what extent should lifestyle change be an individual choice or imposed on people through policy and legislation?
- Practising an unhealthy lifestyle is more common in people living in deprivation. How can we make healthy lifestyles more accessible to all?

References

Annandale, E. and Hunt, K. (2000). *Gender Inequalities in Health*. Buckingham: Open University Press.

Ashton, J. and Seymour, H. (1988). *The New Public Health: The Liverpool Experience*. Milton Keynes: Open University Press.

Babor, T. F., Caetano, R., Casswell, S., Edwards, G., Giesbrecht, N., Graham, K., Rossow, I. et al. (2010). *Alcohol: No Ordinary Commodity: Research and Public Policy: Research and Public Policy*. Oxford: Oxford University Press.

Barrientos-Gutierrez, T., Gimeno, D., Mangiane, T.W., Harrist, R.B. and Amick, B.C. (2007). Drinking social norms and drinking behaviours. *Occupational and Environmental Medicine*, 64: 602–608.

BBC. (2006). Available at: http://www.worcestershirehealth.nhs.uk/whs_recruitment/recruitment_waht/_medical_dental/WD06_07.asp (accessed 7 June 2012).

Beck, U. (1990). *Risk Society: Towards a New Modernity*. London: Sage.

Blaxter, M. (1990). *Health and Lifestyles*. London: Sage.

Blouin, C., Chopra, M. and van der Hoeven, R. (2009). Trade and health 3: trade and the social determinants of health. *Lancet*, 373(9662): 502–507.

Bruce, N. (1991). Epidemiology and the new public health: implications for training. *Social Science and Medicine*, 32(1): 103–106.

Buckworth, J. and Dishman, R. (2002). *Exercise Psychology*. London: Human Kinetics.

Burke, V., Milligan, R.A., Beilin, L.J., Dunbar, D., Spencer, M., Balde, E. and Gracey, M.P. (1997). Clustering of health-related behaviours among 18 year old Australians. *Preventative Medicine*, 26, 724–733.

Cancer Research UK (2012). *Percentage of Population who Smoke*. Available at: http://www.cancerresearchuk.org/cancer-info/cancerstats/types/lung/smoking/lung-cancer-and-smoking-statistics#history (accessed 14 January 2013).

Center for Disease Control. (2007). *Healthy Youth! Sexual Risk Behaviours*. Available at: http://www.cdc.gov/HealthyYouth/sexualbehaviors/index.htm (accessed 20 December 2007).

Craig, R. and Mindell, J. (2008). *Health Survey for England 2006*. Volume 1: *Cardiovascular Disease and Risk Factors in Adults*. London: The Information Centre.

Delaney, W.P. and Ames, G. (1995). Work team attitudes, drinking norms and workplace drinking. *Journal of Drug Issues*, 25: 275.

Department of Health. (2004). *At Least Five a Week: Evidence on the Impact of Physical Activity and its Relationship to Health*. London: Department of Health.

——(2010). *Our Health and Wellbeing Today*. London: Department of Health.

——(2011). *Start Active, Stay Active: A Report on Physical Activity for Health from the Four Home Countries' Chief Medical Officers*. London: Department of Health.

Department for Transport (2011). *National Travel Survey: 2010*. Statistical Release. Newport: ONS.

Doyle, R. (2001). Lifestyle blues. *Scientific American*, 284: 30.

Egger, G.J., Binns, A.F. and Rossner, S.R. (2009). The emergence of 'lifestyle medicine' as a structured approach for management of chronic disease. *Medical Journal of Australia*, 190(3): 143.

Egger, G.J., Binns, A. and Rossner, S. (2011). *Lifestyle Medicine: Managing Diseases of Lifestyle in the 21st Century*. London: McGraw-Hill.

Emslie, C., Hunt, K. and Macintyre, S. (2002). How similar are the smoking and drinking habits of men and women in non-manual jobs? *European Journal of Public Health*, 12: 22–28.

Folkard, S., Lombardi, D.A. and Tucker, P.T. (2005). Shiftwork: safety, sleepiness and sleep. *Industrial Health*, 43: 20–23.

Fox, K.R. and Hillsdon, M. (2007). Physical activity and obesity. *Obesity Reviews*, 8(Suppl. 1): 115–121.

Frieden, T.R. (2010). A framework for public health action: the health impact pyramid. *Journal Information*, 100(4): 590–598.

Gard, M. and Wright, J. (2005). *The Obesity Epidemic*. London: Routledge.

Hansen, E. and Easthope, G. (2007). *Lifestyle in Medicine*. London: Routledge.

Haslam, D. (2007). Obesity: a medical history. *Obesity Reviews*, 8(Suppl. 1): 31–36.

HM Government (2012). *The Government Alcohol Strategy*. London: The Home Office. Available at: http//www.homeoffice.gov.uk/publications/alcohol-drugs/ (accessed 15 June 2012).

Jeffery, R.W., Baxter, J.E., McGuire, M.T. and Linde, J.A. (2006). Are fast food restaurants an environmental risk factor for obesity? *International Journal of Behaviour, Nutrition and Physical Activity*, 3, 2: 1–6.

Jones, A., Bentham, G., Foster, C., Hillsdon, M. and Panter, J. (2007). *Tackling Obesities: Future Choices – Obesogenic Environments – Evidence Review*. London: United Kingdom Government Foresight Programme, Office of Science and Innovation. Crown Copyright.

Lowden, A., Moreno, C., Holmbäck, U., Lennernäs, M. and Tucker, P. (2010). Eating and shift work – effects on habits, metabolism and performance. *Scandinavian Journal of Work, Environment and Health*, 36(2): 150–162.

McPearson, P.D. (1992). Health for all Australians. In H. Gardner (ed.) *Health Policy*. Melbourne: Churchill Livingstone.

Myslobodsky, M. (2003) Gourmand savants and environmental determinants of obesity. *Obesity Reviews*, 4: 121–128.

Nursing Times (accessed 2009). www.nursingtimes.net

Office for National Statistics (ONS) (2007). *Omnibus Survey Report No.33. Contraception and Sexual Health 2006/7*. Newport: ONS.

——(2011a). *2010-based Period and Cohort Life Expectancy Tables*. Available at: http://www.ons.gov.uk/ons/rel/lifetables/period-and-cohort-life-expectancy-tables/2010-based/p-and-c-le.html (accessed 16 September 2013).

——(2011b). *Social Trends. Mothers in the Labour Market 2011*. Newport: ONS

Plant, M. and Plant, M. (2006). *Binge Britain*. Oxford: Oxford University Press.

Scambler, G. (ed.) (2008). *Sociology as Applied to Medicine*, 6th edn. London: Elsevier.

Schubotz, D., Simpson, A. and Rolston, B. (2003). *Towards Better Sexual Health: A Survey of Sexual Attitudes and Lifestyles of Young People in Northern Ireland*. Research Report. Belfast: FPA in partnership with the University of Ulster.

Scotland Health Improvement Agency. *Health Improvement Agency*. Available at: http://www.healthscotland.com/ (accessed 23 November 2009).

Steenhuis, I.H. and Vermeer, W.M. (2009). Portion size: review and framework for interventions. *International Journal of Behavioral Nutrition and Physical Activity*, 6: 58.

Sloman, L., Cairns, S., Newson, C., Anable, J., Pridmore, A. and Goodwin, P. (2010). *The Effects of Smarter Choice Programmes in the Sustainable Travel Towns: Summary Report*. London: DfT.

Thirlaway, K.J. and Heggs, D. (2005). Interpreting risk messages: women's responses to a health story. *Health, Risk and Society,* 7: 107–121.

Thomas, R. (1811) *The Modern Practice of Physic*. New York: Collins and Co.

Townsend, P. and Davidson, N. (1989) *Inequalities in Health: The Black Report*. Harmondsworth: Penguin.

Wagner, K.H. and Brath, H. (2011). A global view on the development of non-communicable diseases. *Preventive Medicine*. 54, Suppl: S38–S41.

Wardle, J. and Steptoe, A. (2005). Public health psychology. *The Psychologist,* 18: 672–675.

Welsh Assembly Government (accessed 2009). http://new.wales.gov.uk/topics/health/improvement/healthatwork/corporate-standard/?lang=en

Wiseman, M. (2009). *Press Release: Biggest Ever Review: How Breast Cancer Can Be Prevented*. Available at: www.wcrf-uk.org (accessed 23 September 2013).

World Health Organisation (Health Education Unit). (1986). Lifestyles and health. *Social Science in Medicine,* 22: 117–124.

2 | Health promotion

Learning objectives

At the end of this chapter you will:
- understand health promotion, health improvement, health education and health literacy
- recognise the challenges of providing an equal opportunity to everyone to improve their health
- recognise who is responsible for the delivery of health promotion in the UK
- appreciate the challenges and complexities involved in delivering health improvement and health promotion interventions
- have evaluated some of the available health improvement and health promotion interventions in the UK.

Case study

Jemma is a primary school teacher working in a school in the suburbs of a large city. Over the past few years Jemma has become increasingly concerned about the health and fitness of the children in her school. Very few children walk to school, the majority are dropped off in a car. She is aware that there are a sizeable number of children who do not enjoy their P.E. lessons and do not participate in physical activity at playtime. Another concern is the diet of the children in the school. In a recent school project about food many reported disliking most fruit and vegetables and refused to try any during the project.

Jemma and her colleagues in the school would like to try to promote healthy eating and physical activity in their school. Jemma has been tasked with exploring what support there is in their area for promoting healthy eating and physical activity. She has been asked to draw up a proposal to present to the school governors. Jemma is now looking for advice from the local public health team and the local education authority about what interventions might be feasible for the school to adopt.

Introduction

The World Health Organisation (WHO) in 1986 defined health promotion as 'The process of enabling people to increase control over, and to, improve, their health' (WHO, 2009, p. 3).

So there are two elements to health promotion: the *process* of empowerment and the *aim* of improving health. In theory the process of empowerment leads to improvements in health but we need to recognise that this is based on the assumption that individuals and communities wish to improve their health. The WHO Ottawa Charter for Health Promotion in 1986 identified five health promotion action areas:

- Build health public policy
- Create supportive environments
- Develop personal skills
- Strengthen community action and
- Re-orient health services.

Health promotion is about improving the health of communities as a whole and of the individuals within those communities. Communities can be defined by their geographical or their demographic characteristics. So a particular city council may decide to promote active transport in their city and target all the inhabitants. Alternatively a charity such as Diabetes UK may decide to promote walking to the diabetic community. Often the aim may to be reach a particular community of individuals but the intervention may be at the level of the community, individualised or indeed a combination of both types of strategies.

It is important to recognise that health promotion, for the WHO, should be focused on reducing health inequalities. At the 1988 WHO International Conference on Health Promotion a target to reduce health inequalities by 25 per cent by the year 2000 was set: 'By the year 2000 the actual differences in health status between countries and between groups within countries should be reduced by at least 25% by improving the level of health of disadvantaged nations and groups' (WHO, 2009, p. 7).

This focus on reducing health inequalities through health promotion is reflected in the mission statements of all the four UK government bodies responsible for health promotion: Public Health England, Public Health Wales, Health Scotland and Public Health Agency Northern Ireland (Department of Health, 2011; Public Health Wales, accessed 2012; Health Scotland, accessed 2012; Public Health Agency, Northern Ireland, accessed 2012). For example the mission of Public Health England is:

To protect and improve the health and well-being of the population, and to reduce inequalities in health and wellbeing outcomes

DoH, 2011, p. 1

Public Health Wales states that:

Our purpose is to give people power to protect and improve health and well-being and reduce inequities by informing, advising and speaking up for them.

Public Health Wales, accessed November 2012

Scotland and Northern Ireland in their policy documents and mission statements give a similar emphasis to reducing health inequalities. It is therefore sobering to reflect that, instead of reducing health inequalities through our health promotion policies, strategies, interventions and practice over the past three decades the evidence suggests we have made no inroads on health equalities and in some areas inequalities may be widening. A recent report from the Department of Health in England (Department of Health, 2009a) suggested that the health inequalities between the most affluent and the most deprived have not improved. The Chief Medical Officer in Scotland in 2010 (Scottish Government, 2011) reported a similar picture of at best no improvement and at worst a widening of health inequalities. In the most recent report, which is from Wales in 2011, the Chief Medical Officer reported a slight widening of health inequalities as measured by life expectancy and healthy life expectancy (Welsh Government, 2012). Indeed it has been argued that rather than reducing health inequalities health promotion interventions can increase them. Those who are more affluent and have a higher level of formal education are more likely to modify their diets, give up smoking and increase levels of physical activity than are the less affluent with lower levels of formal education (Buck and Frosini, 2012). In 2012 Buck and Frosini in a report for the Kings Fund reported that whilst engagement with unhealthy lifestyle behaviours was decreasing overall, these reductions have been seen mainly among those in higher socio-economic and educational groups. They found that people with no qualifications were more than five times as likely as those with higher education to engage in all four *poor* behaviours in 2008, compared with only three times as likely in 2003.

Health promotion is not solely or even predominantly focused on lifestyle behaviours but also includes issues such as: accident prevention, road safety, immunisation against infectious disease, food safety, support for individuals with learning disabilities to live in the community and supporting patients in adhering to medical advice and treatments (WHO, 2009). Health promotion has previously been described as having two main activities (Shriven *et al.*, 2010):

1. Providing services for people who are ill or who have a disability and
2. Positive health activities which are about personal, social and environmental changes aimed at preventing ill health, developing healthier living conditions and lifestyles.

However, this distinction is increasingly redundant and creates an artificial divide between people who are disabled or have a diagnosis of an illness and those who are currently free from disability or a diagnosed condition. Having a disability doesn't necessarily lead to ill health and many people with disabilities are interested in preventing ill health and leading healthy lifestyles (Kroll *et al.*, 2006). Similarly, many people with a diagnosed chronic condition would describe themselves as healthy and be committed to preventing any deterioration of their health (Hobbis *et al.*, 2011). Individuals with type 2 diabetes are a good example of this. They have a diagnosis of an illness that in itself may not impact on their quality of life particularly during the early stages (Department of Health, 1999). Indeed, it may require no medical treatment and may be managed solely through lifestyle modification. However, they are a community who are at high risk of developing other associated diseases that arise from the damage that high levels of circulating blood glucose can cause to cells (see Chapter 10 on special conditions) and are an important group for health promotion to target as many health gains are possible through lifestyle modification (Department of Health, 1999).

Health promotion is a complex activity and clarity about its precise meaning and the role of related activities such as health education, health improvement, health protection and health prevention are not consistently defined or understood. The WHO in 2012 described health promotion as involving the combination of health education activities and the adoption of healthy public policies and their diagrammatic representation of the relationship between the major health concepts is a useful starting point for understanding what health promotion involves (WHO, 2012).

Health improvement

Later in this chapter it is argued that public health works in three areas: health improvement, service improvement and health protection and that health promotion is involved in all three areas. The focus of this book, which is lifestyle behaviours, is very clearly health improvement. However, across the UK the words promotion and improvement are used inter-changeably with the public health body in Scotland, Health Scotland, describing itself as Scotland's health improvement agency. It is clear though that lifestyle behavioural change could deliver improvements in health and longer life expectancy whereas other more protective health promotion activities such as vaccination schemes are more about maintaining health.

Health education

Health education activities are a central strategy to achieve the goals of health promotion. Health education has been defined by the WHO (2012) as 'Consciously constructed opportunities for learning involving some form of communication designed to improve health literacy, including improving knowledge and developing life skills which are conducive to individual and community health.'

Health education, at its broadest and best, involves educational, motivational, skill-building and consciousness-raising techniques (Figure 2.1). However, too often it is solely educational and too focused on communicating risks and benefits which are now

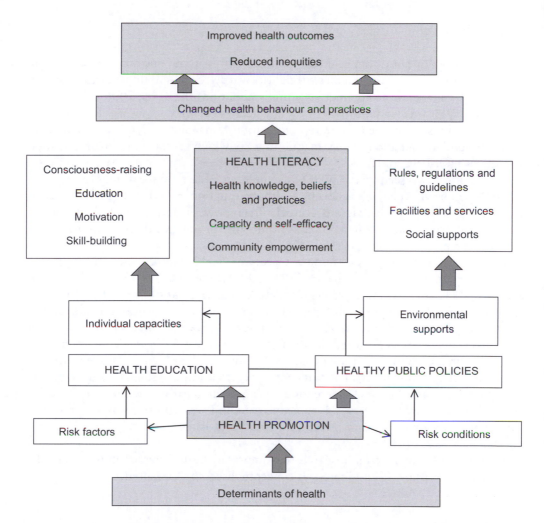

Figure 2.1 Relationship between major health concepts (adapted from WHO, 2012)

well established to have little influence on lifestyle change (Thirlaway and Upton, 2009; Whitehead, 2001). As discussed in the introductory chapter of this book, decades of health education and risk communication focused interventions have not delivered the targeted changes in lifestyle behaviours that governments required. As argued by the WHO (2012), health education should not be limited to the dissemination of health-related information. Its purpose should not only be to increase knowledge about personal health behaviour but also to develop skills that enable individuals and communities to engage in activities that address the psychological, behavioural, social, economic and environmental determinants of their health. As such the concept of health education is far broader than many lay, and indeed professional, interpretations of education.

Health literacy

Similarly to health education, health literacy is a term with no one accepted definition. Many authors view health literacy straightforwardly as the ability to read written health information and to communicate orally about health (Baker, 2006). Once again though the WHO takes a far broader view and defines Health Literacy as: 'The cognitive and social skills which determine the motivation and ability of individuals to gain access to, understand and use information in ways which promote and maintain good health' (WHO, 2012, p. 12).

Health literacy is seen by the WHO as something more than the ability to read and write. By improving people's access to health information, and their capacity to use it effectively, health literacy is viewed as crucial to empowerment (Figure 2.1). Defined in this way, improved health literacy is a key outcome for any health promotion activity but measurement of health literacy in its broadest WHO conception is a challenge. There are available measures of some aspects of health literacy such as the Rapid Estimate of Adult Literacy in Medicine (REALM) (Davis *et al.*, 1993) and the Test of Functional Health Literacy in Adults (TOFHLA) (Parker *et al.*, 1995). The REALM is a 66-item word recognition and pronunciation test that measures the domain of vocabulary. The TOFHLA measures reading fluency. Neither of these measures attempt to assess general health knowledge, which is clearly an aspect of the WHO definition of health literacy. Similarly, the key issues of motivation and empowerment are not addressed. As recently as 2011 Berkman *et al.* carried out a systematic review of the literature on health literacy interventions using a far narrower definition of health literacy: 'The ability to interpret documents, read and write prose (print literacy), use quantitative information (numeracy), and speak and listen effectively (oral literacy)' (Berkman *et al.*, 2011).

Consequently, interpreting research that improves health literacy must always be scrutinised to see how health literacy is conceptualised and measured.

Social capital

Social capital is a concept developed to formalise and acknowledge the role that the cultural norms and informal networks that exist in communities can play in the economic viability and health of communities. It was defined by the government Performance and Innovation Unit in 2002 as: 'The networks, norms, relationships, values and informal sanctions that shape the quantity and co-operative quality of a society's social interactions.'

Building social capital may be one way of empowering communities to improve their health and for the WHO it is a key aspect of health literacy (Figure 2.1). Shared values and normative beliefs can shape the way that health promotion is perceived and understood by individuals within different communities. The potential that building social capital offers for using community and civic pathways to promote and improve health has been promoted by some as a useful means of tackling inequalities in health (Morgan and Swann, 2004).

However, as Blaxter (2004) discusses, understanding what social capital is and how to measure it in communities is difficult. Communities are hard to define, they are fluid and perceived differently by the various individuals within them. Many people are members of more than one community. Furthermore, different professional groups view social capital differently, measure it differently and will try and build it within communities differently as well. So policy makers and political scientists may view social capital in terms of activism and wish to promote activism within communities, whereas social workers, community workers and sociologists may take a more structural view looking at the networks and community groups that exist within a defined community. Psychologists tend to take a more individualised view of social capital focusing on the relationships that people have been able to establish within a community. Within the discipline of psychology there are well-established valid and reliable measures of social support, social relationships and social isolation (Blaxter, 2004).

Walker and Coulthard in 2004 used the data from the 2000/01 General Household Survey to identify five key aspects of social capital that should all be measured if a comprehensive measure of social capital is to be made:

1. Civic Engagement
2. Neighbourliness
3. Social Networks
4. Social Support
5. Local Area.

These five aspects cover the breath of social capital but they are rarely all assessed in one questionnaire and interventions to improve social capital often focus on one particular aspect. The link between social relationships, social support, social isolation and health are well established across many different communities (Kumar *et al.*, 2012; Uchino, 2009) but community level interventions to improve social capital are often focused on local resource improvement or the development of community groups and the way these feed individuals' social support networks is not well understood (Morgan and Swann, 2004).

Social marketing

Social marketing was first named and introduced in the 1970s by Kotler and Zaltman (1971). In their seminal paper, Kotler and Zaltman (1971) argue that marketing concepts and techniques that are commonly used to sell commodities and goods may be effectively applied to promote health and social change in areas such as driving safely and family planning. Since its introduction, social marketing has been defined as: 'A process that applies marketing principles and techniques to create, communicate, and deliver value in order to influence target audience behaviours that benefit society as well as the target audience' (Kotler *et al.*, 2006, cited in Cheng *et al.*, 2010, p. 2).

Although similar in principle to traditional marketing methods, social marketing is different because it is used to achieve specific behaviour change for the good of society as well as the target group whose behaviour it is aiming to influence. Its focus is to enable, encourage and support behavioural change and/or maintenance and this will often involve the development or re-structuring of services to support and facilitate this change (French *et al.*, 2009). Its efficacy as a framework for behaviour change interventions has been demonstrated in a recent systematic review (Stead *et al.*, 2007). This review concludes that social marketing has the potential to achieve behavioural change across different contexts and levels of influence, including the individual, environment and wider policy levels (Stead *et al.*, 2007). Its utility as an approach to behaviour change is therefore diverse.

Fundamentally, social marketing relies on the principles derived from commercial marketing, in particular the marketing mix strategies, otherwise termed the 4Ps:

1. Product (e.g., condoms; quit smoking kits; screening tests; breastfeeding practice)
2. Price (e.g., monetary cost; time or effort; risk of embarrassment/disapproval)
3. Place (e.g., distribution of product)
4. Promotion (e.g., advertising; public relations; personal selling; public service announcements).

Kotler and Lee (2008) explain that social marketing aims to influence the target audience's behaviour in four different ways:

1. *Accepting* a new behaviour (e.g., becoming an organ donor)
2. *Rejecting* a potential undesirable behaviour (e.g., unsafe sex)
3. *Modifying* a current behaviour (e.g. increasing daily fruit and vegetable consumption)
4. *Abandoning* an established undesirable behaviour (e.g., quitting smoking).

Social marketing has been used extensively in health promotion programmes both at national and international levels. In the UK, campaigns that have applied social marketing to increase the adoption of healthy behaviours for target populations have included the Change4Life campaign, which aims to reduce childhood obesity (Department of Health, 2009); Food Dudes, which aims to increase fruit and vegetable consumption in primary school aged children (Horne *et al.*, 2009); and England's National Marketing Strategy for Tobacco Control (2007–2010).

Cheng *et al.* (2010) have clearly outlined how the principles and techniques within social marketing have been successfully applied in practice over the years. These broadly include:

1. *Health promotion-related behavioural issues*: obesity; teen pregnancy; tobacco use; breastfeeding; sensible drinking
2. *Injury prevention-related behavioural issues*: domestic violence; drink driving campaigns; seatbelt use
3. *Environmental protection-related behavioural issues*: waste recycling; water conservation; air pollution from cars
4. *Community mobilisation-related behavioural issues*: organ donation; blood donation; childhood immunisation.

Kotler and Lee, 2008 in Cheng *et al.*, 2010, p. 3

However, care must be taken when designing health promotion campaigns using social marketing techniques because it is possible to unintentionally reach a different audience and/or change behaviour in an unexpected direction. One example of this is a sensible drinking campaign aimed at young adults that, rather than encouraging heavy drinkers to drink less, encouraged light drinkers to drink more (Welscher *et al.*, 2003). More about this intervention can be found in Chapter 7 on sensible drinking.

Who delivers health promotion?

The simplest but perhaps least helpful answer to this question is everyone. The health of the public is the concern of the whole of society and all members of society have a stake in the health of the nation, community or group to which they belong. Indeed it is this philosophy of health being the responsibility of everyone within a community that has driven the interest in social capital and its relationship to health. The sharing of beliefs, knowledge and skills is crucial to the lifestyle decisions individuals make and the habits they develop. Every individual within a community or group will contribute to that shared understanding whether it is teaching boy scouts how to play hockey or introducing friends or family to a new food at a meal. However, formal health promotion activities in the UK, as they do in many other countries, come under the remit of public health. The UK Faculty of Public Health defines public health as:

> Public health is the science and art of preventing disease, prolonging life and promoting health through the organised efforts of society.
>
> UK Faculty of Public Health, accessed November 2012

Public health works in three spheres as described by Griffiths *et al.* in 2005:

> **Health Improvement** (inequalities, education, housing, employment, family/community, lifestyles, surveillance and monitoring of specific diseases and risk factors)
>
> **Improving services** (clinical effectiveness, efficiency, service planning, audit and evaluation, clinical governance, equity)
>
> **Health protection** (infectious diseases, chemical and poisons, radiation, emergency response, environmental health hazards).

It is clear that whilst health promotion may be relevant in all three spheres, lifestyle behavioural change, which is the focus of this book, falls predominantly in the sphere of health improvement.

Health promotion and health improvement both require a wide range of competencies and are multidisciplinary activities involving people from many professions and backgrounds. In essence there are four levels of involvement in health promotion/improvement (see Figure 2.2). There are a relatively small number of public health specialists at the top of the health promotion triangle who are involved in the strategic development and funding of health promotion activities within their regions. They will usually have at least a level 7 qualification in public health and are often, although not

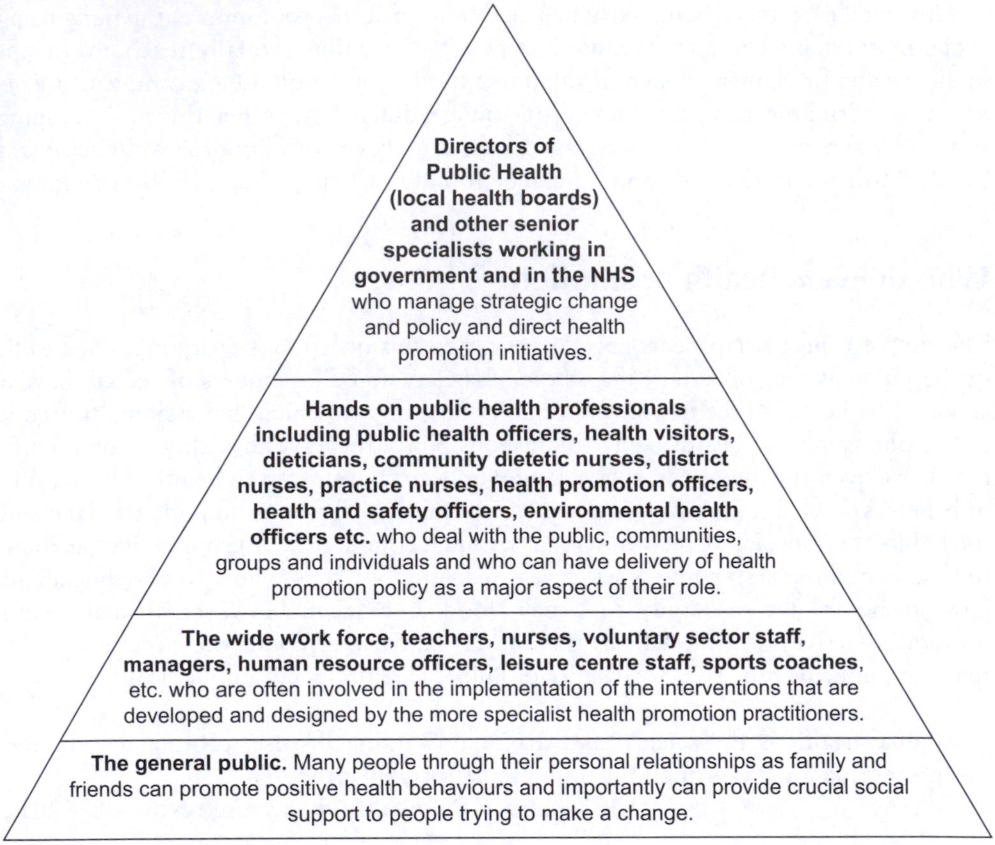

Directors of
Public Health
(local health boards)
and other senior
specialists working in
government and in the NHS
who manage strategic change
and policy and direct health
promotion initiatives.

Hands on public health professionals
including public health officers, health visitors,
dieticians, community dietetic nurses, district
nurses, practice nurses, health promotion officers,
health and safety officers, environmental health
officers etc. who deal with the public, communities,
groups and individuals and who can have delivery of health
promotion policy as a major aspect of their role.

The wide work force, teachers, nurses, voluntary sector staff,
managers, human resource officers, leisure centre staff, sports coaches,
etc. who are often involved in the implementation of the interventions that are
developed and designed by the more specialist health promotion practitioners.

The general public. Many people through their personal relationships as family and
friends can promote positive health behaviours and importantly can provide crucial social
support to people trying to make a change.

Figure 2.2 People involved in public health

exclusively, originally medical practitioners. The next level of practitioners who deliver or manage health promotion activities may include specialist public health practitioners or health promotion officers but will also include other health professionals with a significant interest in public health such as community dieticians, health visitors and district nurses. Finally, there are many other non-health professionals who have the opportunity to get involved with and deliver health promotion interventions, such as teachers like Jemma. The final level is the community members themselves whose impact, either positively or negatively, on health promotion can be considerable.

Many health professionals during the course of their career recognise that they have become focused on the health promotion aspects of their role and are interested in pursuing this aspect of their work. Until recently though there was no clear career path for health professionals interested in health promotion or health improvement. However, in 2008, Skills for Health in the UK developed a set of national standards for specialist practice in public health (see Figure 2.3). It is clear that all nine areas of competence are relevant to health promotion. This is a starting point towards developing a pathway for both medical and non-medical practitioners towards a career in health promotion.

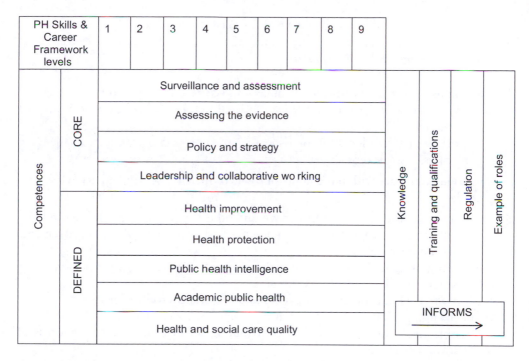

Figure 2.3 The Public Health Skills and Career Framework cube (adapted from Public Health Skills and Career Framework, 2008)

The UK Public Health Register was established in 2003 and provides a regulatory body for public health specialists and practitioners. It is currently voluntary but it provides registrants, who perhaps may not be able to register with other more specialist professional bodies, with a regulatory body who can give their professional work a 'kite' mark of approval. Using the Public Health Skills and Career framework developed by Skills for Health and drawing on other competency documents, the UK Public Health Register has developed a set of 12 standards that registrants must demonstrate to enter the register, and must maintain to stay on the register (Table 2.1). It provides a body where members of the public can take any complaints about competency of practitioners and so protects the public from incompetence by both requiring registrants to have levels of competence and by removing anyone found not to uphold their standards from the register. It aims to enable a wide range of different specialists to demonstrate their expertise in public health and perhaps move into public health strategy and management. Currently, there is a dominance of medical practitioners at the strategic level of public health which may lead to over-medicalisation of public health. The Faculty of Public Health is the professional body for public health practitioners whilst the UK Public Health Register manages the regulation of practitioners and the protection of the public from any malpractice from its registrants. This division between the regulatory body and the professional body is standard practice within many health professions. The Health and Care Professions Council (HCPC) is the statutory regulatory body for many healthcare professionals for whom registration is mandatory, such as physiotherapists, podiatrists, psychologists, dieticians

Table 2.1 Public Health Register standards

Area 1: Professional and ethical practice

1 Recognise and address ethical dilemmas and issues – demonstrating:
   a) knowledge of existing and emerging legal and ethical issues in own area of practice
   b) the proactive addressing of issues in an appropriate way (e.g. challenging others' unethical practice).

2 Recognise and act within the limits of own competence seeking advice when needed.

3 Continually develop and improve own and others' practice in public health by:
   a) reflecting on own behaviour and practice and identifying where improvements should be made
   b) recognising the need for, and making use of, opportunities for personal and others' development
   c) awareness of different approaches and preferences to learning
   d) the application of evidence in improving own area of work
   e) objectively and constructively contributing to reviewing the effectiveness of own area of work.

4 Continually develop and improve own and others' practice in public health by:
   a) reflecting on own behaviour and practice and identifying where improvements should be made
   b) recognising the need for, and making use of, opportunities for personal and others' development
   c) awareness of different approaches and preferences to learning
   d) the application of evidence in improving own area of work
   e) objectively and constructively contributing to reviewing the effectiveness of own area of work.

Area 2: Technical competencies in public health practice

5 Promote the value of health and well-being and the reduction of health inequalities – demonstrating:
   a) how individual and population health and well-being differ and the possible tensions between promoting the health and well-being of individuals and the health and well-being of groups
   b) knowledge of the determinants of health and their effect on populations, communities, groups and individuals
   c) knowledge of the main terms and concepts used in promoting health and well-being
   d) knowledge of the nature of health inequalities and how they might be monitored
   e) awareness of how culture and experience may impact on perceptions and expectations of health and well-being.

6   Obtain, verify, analyse and interpret data and/or information to improve the health and well-being outcomes of a population / community / group – demonstrating:
    a) knowledge of the importance of accurate and reliable data / information and the anomalies that might occur
    b) knowledge of the main terms and concepts used in epidemiology and the routinely used methods for analysing quantitative and qualitative data
    c) ability to make valid interpretations of the data and/or information and communicate these clearly to a variety of audiences.

7   Assess the evidence of effective interventions and services to improve health and well-being – demonstrating:
    a) knowledge of the different types, sources and levels of evidence in own area of practice and how to access and use them
    b) the appraisal of published evidence and the identification of implications for own area of work.

8   Identify risks to health and well-being, providing advice on how to prevent, ameliorate or control them – demonstrating:
    a) knowledge of the risks to health and well-being relevant to own area of work and of the varying scale of risk
    b) knowledge of the different approaches to preventing risks and how to communicate risk to different audiences.

Area 3: Application of technical competencies to public health work

9   Work collaboratively to plan and/or deliver programmes to improve health and well-being outcomes for populations/communities/groups/families/individuals – demonstrating:
    a) how the programme has been influenced by:
        i.   the health and well-being of a population
        ii. the determinants of health and well-being
        iii. inequalities in health and well-being
        iv. the availability of resources
        v.   the use of an ethical framework in decision making/priority setting.
    b) how evidence has been applied in the programme and influenced own work
    c) the priorities within, and the target population for, the programme
    d) how the public/populations/communities/groups /families/individuals have been supported to make informed decisions about improving their health and well-being
    e) awareness of the effect the media has on public perception
    f) how the health concerns and interests of individuals, groups and communities have been communicated
    g) how quality and risk management principles and policies are applied
    h) how the prevention, amelioration or control of risks has been communicated.

Area 4: Underpinning skills and knowledge

---

10 Support the implementation of policies and strategies to improve health and well-being outcomes – demonstrating:
   a) knowledge of the main public health policies and strategies relevant to own area of work and the organisations that are responsible for them
   b) how different policies, strategies or priorities affect own specific work and how to influence their development or implementation in own area of work
   c) critical reflection and constructive suggestions for how policies, strategies or priorities could be improved in terms of improving health and well-being and reducing health inequalities in own area of work
   d) the ability to prioritise and manage projects and/or services in own area of work.

11 Work collaboratively with people from teams and agencies other than one's own to improve health and well-being outcomes – demonstrating:
   a) awareness of personal impact on others
   b) constructive relationships with a range of people who contribute to population health and well-being
   c) awareness of:
      i.   principles of effective partnership working
      ii. the ways in which organisations, teams and individuals work together to improve health and well-being outcomes
      iii. the different forms that teams might take.

12 Communicate effectively with a range of different people using different methods.

---

and most recently, in England, social workers. Each profession also has a discipline specific professional body. It is possible that if registration of public health practitioners were to become mandatory that the HCPC may take over the regulatory function from the UK Public Health Register.

The development of a set of competencies for public health practice is a step towards the development of a more formal career path for public health practitioners (and also health promotion officers) who previously have had little guidance about the skills and competencies they need to develop to progress in the field. It also enables those with a very specialist area of work, for example dieticians or environmental health officers, who wish to move into public health to identify the gaps in their competence and undergo CPD activities that will support their development as public health practitioners.

Jemma has recognised that she can play a role in health promotion. She is now looking for advice and support from more specialist health promotion practitioners to inform her approach.

Delivering and evaluating health promotion/improvement interventions

As stated previously, in theory the process of empowerment leads to improvements in health. However, giving people the resources, the knowledge, skills and environment doesn't always lead to a change in behaviour and/or a measureable health gain. Sometimes empowerment can take decades to deliver an improvement. For example, promoting eating fruit at break time instead of crisps, sweets and chocolate in schools may lead to a reduction in levels of type 2 diabetes in the population but not for three or four decades after the intervention was implemented. Often health promotion is assessed by far shorter term targets of changes in health-related behaviour and/or improvements in illness and disease within targeted populations.

The term health gain emerged in policy documents in the late 1980s as governments and policy makers started to be interested in measuring the effectiveness of their policies and associated interventions. Health gain has been defined as: 'A measurable improvement in health status, in an individual or population, attributable to earlier intervention' (Nutbeam, 1998).

How you define an improvement in health status is a key element of evaluation of health promotion interventions. Increasingly, the efficacy of interventions is being questioned and if funding depends on clear demonstration of benefit the outcome measure for improvement becomes crucial. Many empowerment focused activities that enable people, but do not force or persuade individuals, are not able to demonstrate changes in primary measures of health status (such as weight loss, reduction in blood pressure, or reduction in diagnosis of disease) within the available time for evaluation. Consequently, it is important to measure aspects of health status that are more likely to change in a shorter time frame but are known to predict better health in the longer term. The process of health improvement may be lengthy and the final outcome of better physical health may be very long term so we may need to measure outcomes that we know are likely to occur during the process. Within behavioural change you can argue that there are a range of relevant 'process' measures (Table 2.2). So for example if you introduce a school policy of fruit only at break times you are unlikely to see changes in weight in the children but could demonstrate an increase in the required behaviour. Health literacy, as defined earlier, has the potential to be a useful outcome measure for health promotion activities as long as the measurement tool limitations are understood.

Table 2.2 Potential outcome measures for a health promotion activity using example of a 'bike to work scheme'

	Knowledge outcome (Time scale: immediate)	Psychological outcome (Time scale: short term)	Behavioural outcome (Time scale: short term)	Physiological change outcome (Time scale: medium to long term)	Disease outcome (Time scale: long term)
Promotional activity					
Example					
Bike to work scheme by city council: includes information leaflets, tax-free bike purchase schemes and building of more cycle lanes and parking facilities	Better understanding of value of physical activity Knowledge about local facilities Increased health literacy	Reduction in stress from physical activity Increase in self esteem Improvement in self efficacy Better mental health Increased health literacy (depending on measurement)	Increase in physical activity Reduction in sedentary time	Increase in aerobic fitness Increase in strength Reduction in weight	Lower levels of lifestyle related diseases

Applying this to Jemma

When Jemma evaluates her intervention, behaviour change will probably be the most appropriate measurement in a population of school children. Measuring fitness or weight in school-aged children is a contentious issue as it is highly personal information. Furthermore, changes in these criteria are unlikely to be evident in the short to medium term (Table 2.2).

Public health specialists such as directors of public health are responsible for the strategy direction of health promotion within their region. Guided by national strategy they will decide how resources will be allocated within their region. Ideally, their planning should be guided by strategic assessment of the needs of the particular communities within their region as well as by national targets. One particular technique promoted to help policy makers and practitioners plan their health promotion activities is a health needs assessment (HNA). It is only one of several similar approaches. Other approaches are: health impact assessment (HIA), integrated impact assessment (IIA) and health equity audit (HEA). Although there are similarities in these approaches, a key difference is their starting point. HNA starts with a population and assesses their health needs with a view to developing an intervention. In this way it is in line with the WHO aim of empowering communities to improve their health by ensuring that they are involved in the decisions about what is appropriate for their community.

Health needs assessment (HNA)

HNA can be a useful tool for tackling inequalities through targeting services and support towards the most disadvantaged groups (Department of Health, 2003). Health needs can be:

- Perceptions and expectations of the profiled population (felt and expressed needs)
- Perceptions of professionals providing the services
- Perceptions of managers of commissioner/provider organisations, based on available data about the size and severity of health issues for a population, and inequalities compared with other populations (normative needs)
- Priorities of the organisations commissioning and managing services for the profiled population, linked to national, regional or local priorities (corporate needs).

Adapted from Cavanagh and Chadwick, 2005

A good HNA will involve comparing and balancing these different needs when selecting priorities for action. The information can then be used as a basis for bringing about change through negotiation with stakeholder groups (Cavanagh and Chadwick, 2005).

Often a health challenge will be identified centrally, such as reducing the prevalence of obesity in the population, and then a health needs assessment will identify potential strategies and interventions that would be helpful within a specific population. In 2005 NICE produced guidance for effective HNA which identified five steps in the process (Table 2.3).

HNA can provide a clear protocol for planning and delivering health promotion work that can be adapted to a wide range of behaviours. By starting with the population it takes a client-centred perspective from the outset. However, a comprehensive HNA requires considerable resourcing that is often not available within health promotion budgets. However, much of the good practice identified by NICE (Table 2.3) can still

Table 2.3 Five steps for an effective health needs assessment

---

Step 1
Getting started
What population?
What are you trying to achieve?
Who needs to be involved?
What resources are required?
What are the risks?

Step 2
Identifying health priorities
Population profiling
Gathering data
Perceptions of needs
Identifying and assessing health conditions and determinant factors

Step 3
Assessing a health priority
for action
Choosing health conditions and determinant factors with the most significant size and severity impact
Determining effective and acceptable interventions and actions

Step 4
Planning for change
Clarifying aims of intervention
Action planning
Monitoring and evaluation strategy
Risk-management strategy

Step 5
Moving on/review
Learning from the project
Measuring impact
Choosing the next priority

---

be applied even if the funds for a full HNA are not available. Consulting with stakeholders, agreeing priorities and planning for action are key aspects of the HNA that can be applied to smaller scale projects with limited funding to improve the outcomes of the project. For further information on carrying out a HNA see Cavanagh and Chadwick (2005).

Applying this to Jemma

Whilst Jemma has not carried out a HNA she has identified a health priority for children in her school. She now needs to determine effective and acceptable interventions and actions and start to plan for change.

Whilst taking a HNA approach to health promotion has many advantages, often health promotion activities are more top-down activities with health promotion officers responding to policy directives and government targets. However, health promotion can also be localised and driven by the particular interests of a well-motivated individual or organisation. For example, in Wales Diabetes UK Cymru have supported screening events through local pharmacies in order to reach the 50,000 undiagnosed diabetics predicted to be currently living in Wales.

Individual level interventions

There are numerous individualised and family focused health promotion interventions to try to improve the health of people in the UK. Some of these are standardised, evaluated UK-wide interventions, others are localised and access to schemes will vary significantly depending on where you live. There are pluses and minuses to both locally derived health promotional activities and more standardised initiatives, with the latter usually being evidence-based and evaluated and the former being more tailored and specific to the local community. Some programmes have been developed within the public sector and others within the private sector. It is then down to local funding bodies which may be the NHS, a local authority or third sector organisations to decide whether to fund particular programmes. For example both standardised and local programmes are available on lifestyle for individuals with type 2 diabetes and there is more about these programmes in Chapter 10 on specific conditions.

To demonstrate the range of health promotion/improvement initiatives that can co-exist in any one area this text will use weight management interventions in Wales as an example. In Wales health promotion/improvement is co-ordinated by Public Health Wales. Listed on the Weight Management pages of their Physical Activity and Nutrition Networks Wales website, there are a number of different funded initiatives in different parts of Wales (physicalactivityandnutritionwales.org.uk, accessed

January 2013). As part of the 'BIG Way of Life' project there are 14 different local projects all trying to promote healthy eating, activity and play using one of three different models: Healthy Friends, Healthy Places and Healthy Home Tutors. The Healthy Friends model uses older children as mentors for younger children, the Healthy Home Tutors model delivers advice and support programmes to children and their families and the Healthy Places model aims to increase healthy eating and activity through engaging and interesting community activities and events. It is clear that these BIG Way of Life projects are tapping into aspects of social capital. The Healthy Friends model is focusing on social relationships as a mediator of change whilst the Healthy Places model is more focused on the local community and creating opportunities with that community. Exactly how these projects are realised is a local decision but strategically they are supported by Public Health Wales. There are also self-help community weight management groups, fat clubs as well as more established and standardised programmes such as the MEND programme running in different areas of Wales.

The Mind, Exercise, Nutrition, Do it programme (MEND) is a multi-component, community-based childhood obesity intervention that has been well evaluated and utilised widely in the UK. See Box 2.1 'Research into practice' (Sacher *et al.*, 2010). The programme is based on evidence-based principles of education, skills training and motivation and involves sessions about behavioural change, nutrition education and physical activity. It involves intensive twice weekly two-hour sessions with small groups of children who are obese and their carer/s. All MEND leaders are required to attend a four-day training programme to ensure consistency of delivery and the programme provides all the handouts, manuals and teaching aids.

The children involved in the evaluation of MEND by Sacher *et al.* (2010) were aged between 8 and 12 and attended the nine-week programme with at least one parent or carer. See research into practice Box 2.1

Moving away from weight management to consider other behaviours, one UK-wide individualised health promotion scheme is the exercise referral scheme. Whilst this is a UK-wide scheme, it is delivered locally and has been adapted in different communities to suit local requirements and facilities. Individuals can be referred by a health practitioner from primary or secondary care to the exercise referral scheme. Initially, clients were referred predominantly to gyms where they were given between a 10- and 16-week tailored gym programme and free access to the local facilities for that period. The scheme has now expanded considerably and there are a range of referral programmes that individuals can be directed towards, including a number of outdoor 'green activities'. The period of the scheme is acknowledged to be rather short and the scheme is keen to explore longer support periods or perhaps a less intense on-going support package. Further information about the exercise referral scheme can be found in Chapter 6 on being active.

So the individualised health promotion activities across the UK are a mixture of standard programmes that different government bodies may or may not choose to adopt and locally generated schemes sometimes funded by government, sometimes by

---

Box 2.1 Research into practice

Randomised controlled trial of the MEND program: a family-based community intervention for childhood obesity (Sacher *et al*., 2010)

The aim of this study was to evaluate the effectiveness of the Mind, Exercise, Nutrition, Do it (MEND) Programme.

One hundred and sixteen obese children (BMI >or= 98th percentile) were randomly assigned to the MEND intervention or waiting list control (6-month delayed intervention). Parents and children attended eighteen 2 hour group educational and physical activity sessions held twice weekly in sports centres and schools, and were then given a 12-week free family swimming pass.

Participants in the intervention group had a reduced waist circumference z-score (-0.37; $P < 0.0001$) and BMI z-score (-0.24; $P < 0.0001$) at 6 months when compared to the controls. Significant between-group differences were also observed in cardiovascular fitness, physical activity, sedentary behaviours and self-esteem. At 12 months, children in the intervention group had reduced their waist and BMI z-scores by 0.47 ($P < 0.0001$) and 0.23 ($P < 0.0001$), respectively, and benefits in cardiovascular fitness, physical activity levels and self-esteem were sustained.

High-attendance rates (86 per cent) suggest that families found this intensive community-based intervention acceptable. Further larger controlled trials are currently underway to confirm the promising findings of this initial trial.

---

lottery funding and sometimes by national and/or local charities. This is the case across all aspects of health promotion/health improvement. Alongside the individualised health promotion/improvement activities that are happening in the community will be more specialised, individualised health promotion delivered by healthcare practitioners in one-to-one settings either in primary or secondary care. Health service interventions are often only initiated once individuals have clearly identified health or behavioural problems such as morbid obesity, an alcohol dependency, type 2 diabetes or other lifestyle-related conditions. Many such interventions such as brief interventions for alcohol dependence delivered by General Practitioners are discussed within the chapters on specific behaviours. One of the challenges for health promotion is to try to direct health promotion resources away from secondary care settings and those with health problems into the community to try to prevent the currently well ever needing the services of secondary care. Regardless of health condition the considerable pressures from secondary care for resources to care for the currently ill can often limit the resources available to attempt to prevent the condition arising in the first place.

An individualised programme such as MEND is not really what Jemma is looking for. Jemma is hoping for a whole school approach to improving the eating and physical activity habits of all children in the school rather than identifying particular children with a problem, such as weight. Jemma is quite interested in the healthy friends model but initial exploration of the way other such local schemes have worked indicates it seems more appropriate in secondary schools than primary schools.

Community level interventions

Community level interventions in the UK may be delivered by the Department of Health across the UK. Alternatively, some may be Scottish, English, Welsh or Northern Ireland only initiatives or more localised still. Many interventions will sit under the umbrella of a wide-scale promotional campaign. UK wide campaigns are often media based, traditionally involving television advertising and poster campaigns. However, internet-based campaigns and initiatives are increasing with the Change4Life intervention being the most high profile example of a recent campaign where the internet is a central communication tool. Change4Life was launched in 2009 and was originally aimed at parents with school-aged children. It now also encompasses adults. Change4Life states that its aim is:

> To inspire a broad coalition of people, including the NHS, local authorities, businesses, charities, schools, families, community leaders – in fact anyone working with families or individuals – to play a part in improving the nation's health and well-being by encouraging everyone to eat well, move more and live longer.
> Change4Life, accessed January 2013

As such Change4Life is an example of a complex intervention that has a main intervention which is the website that individuals and families can join but also interacts with and introduces its users to a range of other national and local initiatives. It is based on the principles of social marketing, attempting to apply commercial marketing technologies to the development of a programme designed to influence the voluntary behaviour of target audiences (Piggin and Lee, 2011). It also provides resources to other schemes, such as posters about healthy eating and sponsorship forms. Change4Life set out from the onset to utilise and work with as many organisations as possible and it has a partnership arrangement with many health promotion/improvement organisations and other businesses. For example, it lists the British Dietetic organisation and the British Heart Foundation as its partners alongside ASDA and Kelloggs. This partnership involves sponsorship in some instances which generates considerable funds for the scheme (Lancet, 2009). The decision to include major supermarkets and food providers as partners to the initiative has caused considerable controversy. Although the Change4Life website carefully avoids any mention of obesity, choosing to focus on encouraging healthy behaviours, it was nevertheless marketed by the government as their way to become 'the first major nation to reverse the rising tide of obesity' (Lancet, 2009, p. 96). An editorial in the Lancet argued that the scheme and its aims were undermined by allowing sponsorship from the very companies (PepsiCo, Kelloggs, ASDA, etc.) that make or sell the products that contribute to obesity (Lancet, 2009). Others argue that only by involving industry and food producers will we achieve a 'long-lasting transformation into a healthy society' with businesses such as supermarkets having the potential to reach consumers that traditional health promotion fails to reach (Hancock 2009).

Change4Life uses a non-judgemental informal style to present easy exercise and diet ideas. It attempts to provide motivation to change through interactive elements. Interestingly Change4Life makes no reference to obesity on its website or in its marketing materials. The Department of Health (2009b) explain that they decided not to use the word obese for three reasons: 1) because the campaign was for everyone not just the obese, 2) that not everyone who is obese recognises that they are obese and 3) that for some families the term obese is considered insulting and they wouldn't use it or allow their children to use it (Department of Health, 2009). This decision is supported by a body of psychological evidence that demonstrates the ineffectiveness of 'risk-based communications' in changing lifestyle behaviours (Thirlaway and Upton, 2009). However, Piggin and Lee (2011) argue that removing reference to obesity from the campaign conceals the real aim of the Change4Life initiative. They argue that simply removing the word obesity fails to tackle the problems with weight stigma in society. However, it is important to recognise that eating well and being physically active is important for everyone, regardless of their weight, and that considerable health benefits can be achieved by eating well and being physically active even if you are overweight and do not lose weight as a result of making changes (Moore et al., 2012).

Many different local initiatives, such as a scheme to increase fresh fruit and vegetable provision in local convenience stores in deprived urban areas, piloted in North-East England, have been branded under the Change4Life logo (Adams et al., 2012) making the effectiveness of the whole scheme very difficult to evaluate. However, the Change4Life scheme is not alone in facing these challenges; evaluation is problematic for the majority of wide-scale complex health promotion interventions. The government has published a first review of Change4Life, one year in, which is very positive about how the initial stages of the campaign have progressed meeting targets of: reach, awareness, logo recognition, responses to questionnaires, sign up and sustained interest (Department of Health, 2010). They also report that sign up for Change4Life is reaching a wide range of different groups including a large proportion of low income families, a key target audience of the campaign. Evidence of actual behavioural change is limited and primarily based on mothers' self-report of their children's behaviour but reported changes are positive. For example, 83 per cent of mothers reported they did at least four of the eight recommended behaviours compared with 77 per cent the previous year. Twenty per cent said they did all eight recommended behaviours compared with 16 per cent the previous year (Department of Health, 2010). An evaluation of food purchasing behaviours in participating supermarkets has also been carried out and again there are some positive findings. Change4Life families changed their beverage purchase patterns, buying more low fat milks and low sugar drinks than a comparison group (Department of Health, 2010). These initial findings from Change4Life must be interpreted cautiously. They simply describe some changes and there has been no independent evaluation to date. However, Change4Life was always intended to be a long-term intervention so it is encouraging that some positive changes can be described fairly early into what is a planned three-year campaign.

Another example of a UK-wide complex intervention is the January 2013 'smoking causes genetic mutations' campaign. In January 2013 the Department of Health launched its new 2.7 million pound campaign to encourage people to stop smoking. The campaign involved television adverts that focus on the fact that smoking causes genetic mutations. According to the Department of Health (2012): 'The health harms message focuses on the fact that every 15 cigarettes smoked causes a mutation that can lead to cancer and aims to increase motivation to quit.'

This is another interesting campaign. It doesn't actually present a new risk of smoking but focuses on our better understanding of how smoking causes disease. It utilises some unpleasant images of mutations growing on cigarettes and appears to hope that informing people that smoking damages your health through genetic mutation will be a motivating risk factor. However, there is limited evidence to suggest that using genetic risk information will be any better at promoting lifestyle change than non-genetic risk information (Davies and Thirlaway, 2012). However, the informational campaign is not stand alone and is supported by clearly signposted free quit smoking kits that are available in local pharmacies. In the autumn of 2012, pharmacies were pre-warned of the new campaign and asked to order their quit smoking kits in advance. Furthermore, local public health teams and smoking cessation clinics will provide the motivational and behavioural support to any new clients that the campaign brings to their doors. For example, the NHS Stop Smoking Service is a national network of advisers who provide professional support during the first few weeks that an individual attempts to stop smoking. There are regional variations in how these advisers work (www.nhs.uk/Livewell/smoking, accessed January 2013). Stop Smoking Wales offers six weekly group support sessions to anyone trying to give up smoking in Wales. They also provide a wealth of other support and advice through their website and their telephone service (www.stopsmokingwales.com, accessed January 2013). These permanent smoking services provide the individualised support and backup to wide-scale media promotion campaigns. One criticism of a campaign of this type is that it is not targeted at the most 'at risk' communities and that its message may not reach smokers from more deprived communities who are most likely to smoke.

Both these UK-wide health improvement campaigns, Change4Life and the January 2013 Stop Smoking campaign, have the potential to reach and influence the least deprived more effectively than the most deprived and thereby improve the overall health of the nation whilst failing to address health inequalities. Conversely however, targeting interventions at the most deprived communities can also fail to be effective and universal approaches such as Change4Life at least do not stigmatise particular groups in society.

Other community level interventions can be at school or organisational level. An intervention that has been very successful at increasing the fruit and vegetable consumption of primary school aged children is the Food Dudes Healthy Eating Programme (Horne *et al.*, 2009). It is an evidence-based programme based on the known determinants of children's food preferences:

1. rewards
2. role modelling
3. repeated tasting.

Role modelling of eating fruit and vegetables is provided by a video series introducing the Food Dudes who are cartoon characters and are the 'good guys' in battle with the bad guys General Junk and his Junk Punks. Children are rewarded for trying fruit and vegetables each time they try them which encourages repeated tasting. Rewards include stickers, stationery and lunch boxes all with Food Dude characters depicted on them. The Food Dude programme provides all the materials for schools and will start the intervention off with an intensive introduction. All the studies carried out on the programme so far show increases in children's fruit and vegetable consumption which in some cases generalised to the home setting. The increases in consumption were greatest in those that ate the least initially and another good outcome reported in some studies from the programme is that unhealthy snacks reduced as fruit and vegetable intake increased (Horne *et al.*, 2009). Programmes like Food Dudes can be targeted at particular schools and so could be targeted at more deprived communities and perhaps contribute to reducing inequality. More about the Food Dude programme can be found in Chapter 5.

Applying this to Jemma

Jemma found reports of the Food Dude programme through her city council healthy living network that she joined on the recommendation of her local public health team. Jemma is keen to get involved and thinks the programme looks very good. Her only concern is whether the Food Dude team will be able to come and deliver it in her school. She is concerned that they might not get selected.

Working effectively with others

Promoting lifestyle change is usually a multidisciplinary undertaking and can be a top-down activity when public health practitioners attempt to deliver a policy through localised initiatives and need to get various different professionals involved. Alternatively health promotion can be a bottom-up activity when individuals or organisations attempt to improve the health of their particular community and look towards policy and health promotion specialists to support them in their endeavour.

Within healthcare services multidisciplinary has been defined as: 'When professionals from different disciplines (such as social work, nursing and occupational therapy) work together to address the holistic needs of their patients/clients, in order to improve delivery of care and reduce fragmentation' (Department of Health, 2009c).

Multidisciplinary working refers therefore to the approach, methods and practices required for a group of practitioners to work together (Welsh Government, 2011). Much of the extensive literature on multidisciplinary working has focused on the challenges of bringing together health and social care disciplines to provide continuous care for individuals but the same principles for good practice apply to the still more diverse area of health promotion.

In some literature the terms inter-disciplinary or inter-professional are used. Inter-disciplinary has been defined as: 'The sharing of exclusive knowledge with the professional team' (Welsh Government, 2011).

Individuals from different professions working together are often described as a multidisciplinary team (MDT). A multidisciplinary team has been defined within traditional healthcare settings as:

> A team usually from both health and social care backgrounds. It does not refer only to an existing multidisciplinary team such as an acute ward. It should include those who have an up-to-date knowledge of the individual's needs, potential and aspirations.
>
> Department of Health, 2009c

In practice the term multidisciplinary team (MDT) is used to describe very many different structures, practices and groups. The MDT can be a permanent group of staff from different professions all employed by the same organisation and based in the same physical space where the multidisciplinary working is often integrated in to the day-to-day working and where team meetings to discuss one patient or one project are frequent and regular. Alternatively, it can be a group of professionals who regularly work together from different organisations. In this instance more formal meetings are often required to bring people from different locations and organisations together. Finally, informal discussions between two or more professionals can be referred to as a multidisciplinary team meeting.

Multidisciplinary working is perhaps easiest to deliver effectively in healthcare settings such as specialist units where consultants, nurses, physiotherapists, psychologists, dieticians, social workers, etc. are all located in one physical area. Whilst successful teams are not assured through the sharing of geographical space, it is far easier to communicate and to establish a common purpose and agreed methods of delivery when everyone is located together (Heitkemper *et al.*, 2008).

Whilst multidisciplinary working may be easier in on-site settings it remains essential for community-based health promotion (Tzenalis and Sotiriadou, 2010). As we increasingly recognise how many factors interact to influence the lifestyle choices that individuals make, building a supportive physical, cultural and socio-economic environment in which the population can live and work healthily cannot be the responsibility of one group, or indeed solely the province of government health departments. What is essential for effective health promotion is collaboration across different healthcare professionals, government agencies and public or private sectors (Tzenalis and Sotiriadou, 2010). Slowly, we can see governments in the UK responding to the challenge of multidisciplinary, multi-sector health promotion. Change4Life attempts to draw together a range of public sector, third sector and private organisations to promote behavioural change. Active transport policies are joint Department of Health and Department of Transport initiatives. The full impact of environmental and cultural change initiatives may not be seen for many years but they are an encouraging step towards supporting change in the population.

It is acknowledged within the literature on multidisciplinary working that certain factors are key if a group of different professionals are going to come together and create a high performing MDT (Tzenalis and Sotiriadou, 2010; Welsh Government, 2011). The key factors consistently reported across the literature are:

1. Good communication, which can be facilitated by the use of a common language and an avoidance of discipline specific jargon
2. Good leadership
3. Effective administration
4. An identified key worker.

These four factors enable the three core capabilities for multidisciplinary working to be achieved:

1. Successful multidisciplinary meetings
2. Co-ordinated assessment and planning
3. Integrated systems and practices.

Frequently reported barriers to successful multidisciplinary working include: a lack of commitment at senior level, professional rivalry, competing budgets and sharing of data (Tzenalis and Sotiriadou, 2010; Welsh Government, 2011).

Health promotion activities are sometimes delivered by MDTs that do indeed have meetings, an identified leader and administrative support. Frequently, these teams may come together to deliver a particular initiative, such as a new advice booklet for newly diagnosed diabetics, and then disband. Task specific groups are sometimes referred to as 'Task and Finish Groups'. However, health promotion is often delivered by a diverse group of professionals who seldom get the opportunity to meet and so cannot function as a traditional MDT. For example, an individual with type 2 diabetes could receive advice about their lifestyle from their GP, their practice nurse, the community dietician, the community diabetic nurse, the exercise professional in the leisure centre or the community pharmacist depending on the resources available in their community. These professionals are unlikely to get together to discuss a co-ordinated prevention strategy for that individual so the likelihood of the individual receiving conflicting advice is high. The key factors that apply to more traditional multidisciplinary working can still apply:

1. Effective communication between professionals (even if it is virtual rather than face-to-face and around general principals of advice rather than individual patient prevention plans)
2. A clear leader for diabetes prevention in each area
3. A key worker who facilitates the referral of the patient to all the other potential lifestyle support practitioners
4. Effective administration that supports the sharing of data between practitioners.

Applying this to Jemma

Jemma is mostly likely to achieve her aim of improving the health of the children in her school if she has the support of the whole school and the wider community. So if her local public health team are running healthy school initiatives or funding the Food Dudes initiatives she will be able to apply to get involved in the schemes they are supporting. She could also investigate any continuing professional development opportunities to increase her understanding of how to promote health in her school.

As for any project her aim is most likely to be realised if she takes a strategic and planned approach and follows as far as is possible the guidelines for a Health Needs Assessment. If she involves the relevant stakeholders – children, parents and staff – from the outset and plans her intervention including their perceptions of needs then she stands a greater chance of success. Careful planning and on-going evaluation using realistic outcome measures give any intervention the best chance of success.

Conclusion

Health promotion is a wide-reaching umbrella that encompasses a large range of different behaviours and a large range of diverse initiatives from very large-scale media driven campaigns to very localised small-scale schemes. The role of the various public health agencies is to support the diversity of initiatives that all undoubtedly have a role to play in the health of the nation and to try to ensure that its wide and diverse workforce is as well trained and up to date as possible. The four public health bodies play an important role in trying to take public health and health improvement outside of traditional health settings, to move the activity further 'up stream' and encourage non-health practitioners to get involved in promoting health behaviours. Schools, workplaces and all organisations that interact with the public have a role to play in supporting behavioural change and public health bodies can provide valuable expertise and resources to support them.

Key points

- Health promotion has the reduction of health inequalities as a central ambition but often health promotion activities, whilst improving the health of the nation as a whole, are least effective in the most deprived. Consequently, they have the potential to increase, rather than decrease, health inequality.
- Health education and health literacy can be interpreted as being about knowledge and ability to comprehend and communicate about health. However, the WHO and most public health organisations conceptualise them more broadly to include aspects of motivation and empowerment.
- Health promotion activities are frequently complex interventions that are hard to evaluate as their benefits may be realised decades after the intervention. Consequently, it can be challenging to demonstrate the effectiveness of an intervention and to justify its funding. More innovative and process orientated evaluations are required.
- Health promotion is a multidisciplinary activity often requiring the co-operation and collaboration of non-health professionals and organisations. Working effectively across disciplines and with non-health organisations has the potential to deliver health benefits but can be controversial if it involves organisations that produce or promote unhealthy products.
- Health promotion activities do not often deliver short-term tangible benefits to physical health but the beneficial impact that they may have over the course of the lifespan may be considerable.

Discussion points

- Should health promotion be targeted at specific groups such as overweight children or people at high risk of developing diabetes or are more community-wide interventions to encourage general healthy behaviours more appropriate?
- What sort of evidence would you require about the effectiveness of a health promotion intervention in order to utilise it in your practice?
- How important is it to include significant others in any intervention to change an individual's behaviour?

Further resources

http://www.healthscotland.com/
http://www.fph.org.uk/what_is_public_health
http://www.wales.nhs.uk/sitesplus/888/home
http://www.nhs.uk/change4life/pages/change-for-life.aspx

References

Adams, J., Halligan, J., Watson, D.B., Ryan, V., Penn, L., Adamson, A.J. and White, M. (2012). The Change4Life convenience store programme to increase retail access to fresh fruit and vegetables: a mixed methods process evaluation. *PLOS* One 7(6): e 39431.

Baker, D.W. (2006). The meaning and the measure of health literacy. *Journal of General Internal Medicine*, 21(8): 878–883.

Berkman, N.D., Sheridan, S.L., Donahue, K.E. *et al.* (2011). *Health Literacy Interventions and Outcomes: An Updated Systematic Review*. Executive Summary, Evidence Report/ Technology Assessment. Rockville, MD: Agency for Healthcare Research and Quality. Available at: http://www.ahrq.gov/clinic/epcsums/litupsum.htm

Buck, D. and Frosini, F. (2012). *Clustering of Unhealthy Behaviours Over Time: Implications for Policy And Practice*. London: The Kings Fund.

Blaxter, M. (2004). Questions and their meanings in social capital surveys. In A. Morgan and C. Swann (eds), *Social Capital for Health: Issues of Definition, Measurement and Links to Health*. London: Health Development Agency.

Cavanagh, S. and Chadwick, K. (2005). *Health Needs Assessment at a Glance*. London: NICE.

Cheng, H., Kotler, P. and Lee, N. (2010). *Social Marketing for Public Health: Global Trends and Success Stories: Global Trends and Success Stories*. London: Jones and Bartlett Publishers.

Davies, L. and Thirlaway, K. (2012). Effect of genetic explanations of type 2 diabetes on patients' attitudes to treatment efficacy. *Journal of Diabetes Nursing*, 16(4): 132–139.

Davis, T.C., Long, S.W., Jackson, R.H. *et al.* (1993). Rapid estimate of adult literacy in medicine: a shortened screening instrument. *Family Medicine*, 25: 391–395.

Department of Health (1999). *National Service Framework for Diabetes Standards*. London: Department of Health.

——(2003). *Tackling Health Inequalities: A Programme for Action*. London: Department of Health.

——(2009a). *Tackling Health Inequalities: 10 Years On – A Review of Developments in Tackling Health Inequalities in England over the Last 10 Years*. London: Health Inequality Unit, Department of Health.

——(2009b). *Change4Life Principles and Guidelines for Promotion*. London: Department of Health.

——(2009c). *The National Framework for NHS Continuing Healthcare and NHS-funded Nursing Care*. London: Department of Health.

——(2010) *Change4Life One Year On*. London: Department of Health. Electronic version only: www.dh.gov.uk/publications (accessed 23 January 2012).

——(2011). Public Health England's Operating Model. London: Department of Health. Available at: www.dh.gov.uk/publications_(accessed 23 January 2012).

——(2012). *Smoking Health Harm Campaign Launched*. Available at: http://www.dh.gov. uk/health/2012/12/smoking-health-harm/ (accessed 23 January 2013).

French, J., Blair-Stevens, C., McVey, D. and Merritt, R. (2009). *Social Marketing and Public Health: Theory and Practice*. New York: Oxford University Press.

Griffiths, S., Jewell, T. and Donnelly, P. (2005). Public health in practice: the three domains of public health. *Public Health*, 119: 907–913.

Hancock, C. (2009). Change4Life – correspondence. *Lancet*, 373(9665): 721.

Health Scotland (accessed November 2012). http://www.healthscotland.com/

Heitkemper, M., McGrath, B., Killien, M., Jarret, M., Landis, C., Lentz, M., Woods, N. and Hayward,K. (2008). The role of centers in fostering interdisciplinary research. *Nursing Outlook*, 56(3): 115–122.

Hobbis, S., Hendry, L., Sanders, L. and Thirlaway, K. (2011). Retirement and lifestyle behaviours: a thematic analysis. *Health Psychology Update*, 20(2): 2–8.

Horne, P.J., Hardman, C.A., Lowe, C.F., Tapper, K., Le Noury, J., Madden, P., Patel, P. and Doody, M. (2009). Increasing parental provision and children's consumption of lunchbox fruit and vegetables in Ireland: the Food Dudes intervention. *European Journal of Clinical Nutrition*, 63: 613–618.

Kotler, P. and Lee, N.R. (2008) *Social Marketing: Influencing Behaviours for Good* (3rd edn). Thousand Oaks, CA: Sage Publications.

Kotler, P. and Zaltman, G. (1971). Social marketing: an approach to planned social change. *The Journal of Marketing*: 3–12.

Kotler, P., Lee, N.R. and Rothschild, M. (2006). Cited in H. Cheng, P. Kotler and N.R. Lee (2010), *Social Marketing for Public Health: Global Trends and Success Stories*. London: Jones and Bartlett Learning, p. 2.

Kroll, P., Jones, G.C., Kehn, M. and Neri, M.T. (2006). Barriers and strategies affecting the utilisation of primary preventative services for people with physical disabilities: a qualitative inquiry. *Health and Social Care in the Community*, 14(4): 284–293.

Kumar, S., Calvo, R., Avendano, M., Sivaramakrishnan, K. and Berkman, L.F. (2012). Social support, volunteering and health around the world: cross-national evidence from 139 countries. *Social Science and Medicine*, 74(5): 696–706.

Lancet (2009). Change4Life brought to you by PepsiCo (and others). *Lancet*, 373 (9658): 96.

Moore, S.C., Patel, A.V., Matthews, C.E. *et al.* (2012). Leisure time physical activity of moderate to vigorous intensity and mortality: a large pooled cohort analysis. *PLOS 9*, 11: e1001335.

Morgan, A. and Swann, C. (2004). Introduction: issues of definition, measurement and links to health. In A. Morgan and C. Swann (eds), *Social Capital for Health: Issues of Definition, Measurement and Links to Health*. UK: Health Development Agency.

Nutbeam, D. (1998). Evaluating health promotion – progress, problems and solutions. *Health Promotion International*, 13: 27–43.

Parker, R.M., Baker, D.W., Williams, M.V. and Nurss, J.R. (1995). The Test of Functional Health Literacy in Adults (TOFHLA): a new instrument for measuring patients' literacy skills. *Journal of General Internal Medicine*, 10: 537.

Performance and Innovation Unit (2002) *Social Capital: A Discussion Paper*. London: Performance and Innovation Unit.

Piggin, J. and Lee, J. (2011). 'Don't mention obesity': contradictions and tensions in the UK Change4Life health promotion campaign. *Journal of Health Psychology*, 16(8): 1151–1164.

Public Health Wales (accessed November 2012). http://www.wales.nhs.uk/sitesplus/888/home

Sacher, P., Kolotourou, M., Chadwick, P.M., Cole, T.J., Lawson, M., Lucas, A. and Singhal, A. (2010). Randomised controlled trial of the MEND program: a family-based community intervention for childhood obesity. *Obesity*, 18(S1): S62–S68.

Scottish Government (2011). *Chief Medical Officer Annual Report 2010. Health in Scotland 2010 Assets for Health*. Edinburgh: The Scottish Government.

Shriven, A., Ewles, L., Simnett, I. and Parish, R. (2010). *Promoting Health: A Practical Guide*. London: Bailliere Tindall.

Stead, M., Gordon, R., Angus, K. and McDermott, L. (2007). A systematic review of social marketing effectiveness. *Health Education*, 107(2): 126–191.

Thirlaway, K.T. and Upton, D. (2009). *The Psychology of Lifestyle: Promoting Healthy Behaviour*. London: Routledge.

Tzenalis, A., and Sotiriadou, C. (2010). Health promotion as multi-professional and multi-disciplinary work. *International Journal of Caring Sciences*, 3(2): 49.

Uchino, B.N. (2009). Understanding the links between social support and physical health: a lifespan perspective with emphasis on the separability of perceived and received support. *Perspectives on Psychological Science*, 4(3): 236–255.

UK Faculty of Public Health (accessed November 2012) http://www.fph.org.uk/what_is_public_health

Walker, A. and Coulthard, M. (2004). Developing and understanding indicators of social capital. In A. Morgan and C. Swann (eds), *Social Capital for Health: Issues of Definition, Measurement and Links to Health*. London: Health Development Agency.

Welsh Government (2011). *Multi Disciplinary Working: A Framework for Practice in Wales*. Cardiff: Welsh Government.

——(2012) *Our Healthy Future: Chief Medical Officer for Wales Annual Report 2011*. Cardiff: Welsh Government.

Whitehead D (2001). Health education, behavioural change and social psychology: Nursing's contribtion to health promotion? *Journal of Advanced Nursing* 34(6), 822–832.

WHO (1986) *Ottawa Charter for Health Promotion*. Geneva: World Health Organisation.

——(2009) *Milestones in Health Promotion: Statements from Global Conferences*. Geneva: World Health Organisation.

——(2012) *Health education: theoretical concepts, effective strategies and core competencies*. Geneva: World Health Organisation.

3

Health and health inequalities

Learning objectives

At the end of this chapter you will:
- be able to define health inequality
- understand the nature of health inequalities and the factors that contribute towards them
- understand the measurements of health
- be able to demonstrate an understanding of the measurement of socio-economic status and how it relates to health status
- appreciate the complexity of tackling health inequalities
- understand the psychological, social and policy basis of tackling health inequalities.

Case study

Dave is a 43-year-old manual labourer who was born, grew up and now lives in one of the most deprived areas of Wales. Dave did not have a high attendance at secondary school and did not manage to pass any of his GCSE exams. Once he had finished school at 16 he had no inspiration to gain a career and was spending most of his time with his friends watching TV and playing computer games. At the age of 23 Dave began working as a manual labourer and has stayed in the trade on and off ever since.

Dave is currently living at home with his elderly mother (his father died of lung cancer when he was 26 years old, he was a heavy smoker) and has a 2-year-old daughter called Kelly. Dave does not maintain much contact with the mother of his child and therefore rarely visits his daughter. He spends a lot of his spare time in his local pub (he drinks heavily, particularly at the weekends) with his friends and in this time he regularly goes for a cigarette with a group of friends.

Since the age of 14 Dave has been a heavy smoker and occasionally takes drugs. Dave has always been in a smoking environment as both his father and mother have smoked throughout his childhood. His mother still continues to be a heavy smoker. Alongside this he hasn't visited the dentist since he was 25. Dave recently visited his GP due to experiencing tightness in his chest mainly when undertaking physical activity through his role as a manual labourer. He has since been diagnosed with angina. Dave is concerned about the pains he is experiencing in his chest and wants to understand how he can help relieve the pain and improve his health.

Applying this to Dave

Think about Dave's situation – how does his behaviour, his environment and his overall situation impact on his health?

Introduction

The first definition to be made is – what is meant by health inequalities? Health inequality is the variation in health outcomes and mortality rates between individuals usually dependent on some demographic variable (e.g. socio-economic class, gender and ethnicity). Although there are health inequalities according to a range of factors, this chapter will mainly focus on socio-economic differences – one of the major barriers to a long and healthy life expectancy. The discrepancy in life expectancy or in health status outcomes may be a result of many factors such as level of income, environment, health behaviours, lifestyle choices and a complex inter-relationship between all of them. A House of Commons report identified the extent of health inequalities within society while attempting to understand the causes:

> Health inequalities are not only apparent between people of different socio-economic groups – they exist between different genders, different ethnic groups, and the elderly and people suffering from mental health problems or learning disabilities also have worse health than the rest of the population. The causes of health inequalities are complex, and include lifestyle factors – smoking, nutrition, exercise to name only a few – and also wider determinants such as poverty, housing and education. Access to healthcare may play a role, but this appears to be less significant than other determinants.
>
> Barron, 2009, p.122

A recent Strategic Review of Health Inequalities post-2010 (Marmot, 2010) concluded that there is a vital need to reduce preventable health inequalities. It suggested that health inequalities should be tackled in every social class and not just the most disadvantaged communities. In making such changes and reducing the gap in health inequalities it is predicted that society as a whole would benefit. Furthermore, the reduction of this gap is a matter of social justice and is a necessity to make society fairer for all: 'Health inequalities that are preventable by reasonable measures are unfair. Putting them right is a matter of social justice' (Marmot, 2010).

Inequalities exist throughout the world and are apparent within all developed countries. Indeed, within Europe there are differences between countries – with the greatest inequalities appearing in Hungary and Poland and the least in certain areas of Spain (Euriothine report, 2007).

Exploring life expectancy in the UK, it can be seen that overall, life expectancy has improved (Table 3.1) year on year, although there is still some inequity between males and females. Although life expectancy is improving overall, health inequalities are very much still apparent between different groups in society. For example, it is still evident that the lower social group you are in, the lower your life expectancy and healthy life expectancy will be (see Table 3.2).

Table 3.1 Life expectancy at birth: by sex and country (2005–2010)

Country	2005–2007 Males	2005–2007 Females	2006–2008 Males	2006–2008 Females	2007–2009 Males	2007–2009 Females	2008–2010 Males	2008–2010 Females
U.K	77.3	81.5	77.5	81.7	77.9	82.0	78.2	82.3
England	77.6	81.8	77.9	82.0	78.3	82.3	78.6	82.6
Wales	76.8	81.2	77.0	81.4	77.2	81.6	77.6	81.8
Scotland	74.8	79.7	75.0	79.9	75.4	80.1	75.8	80.4
Northern Ireland	76.2	81.3	76.4	81.3	76.8	81.4	77.1	81.5

Source: Office for National Statistics, 2011a

Table 3.2 Life expectancy and healthy life expectancy in years at birth by social class, 2001–2003 (England)

Social class	Males LE	Males HLE	Females LE	Females HLE
Professional (I)	80.2	76.7	85.5	80.0
Managerial & technical/intermediate (II)	78.9	73.9	82.8	76.6
Skilled non-manual (IIINM)	78.4	73.0	82.2	75.5
Skilled manual (IIIM)	76.4	69.3	80.6	71.9
Partly skilled (IV)	75.9	68.1	79.9	70.8

Social class	Males		Females	
	LE	HLE	LE	HLE
Unskilled (V)	73.5	64.2	78.7	68.6
England	77.1	70.7	81.3	73.7

Source: White and Edgar, 2010

Defining and measuring social class

Research into society seldom considers it as a whole and more usually considers the position of a group (or groups of people) within society. In this way individual members of society can be categorised into different groups.

Some types of stratification are easy to apply (e.g. age bands) whereas others are more difficult and contentious when defining (e.g. social class). Although there are a number of ways in which society can be stratified in this chapter we will explore social status in most detail.

The definition of social class has been provided by the seminal Black Report (Townsend and Davidson, 1982), which first clearly stated the link between health and social class in modern society. This definition is the one used whenever social class is referred to in this chapter:

> Segments of the population sharing broadly similar types and levels of resources, with broadly similar styles of living and (for some sociologists), some shared perception of their collective condition.

In essence, different classes have differential power to access material resources – homes, cars, white goods, electronic goods and so on (Giddens, 2006). There are a number of different methods for measuring social class.

First, in the subjective method, you simply ask what social class people think they are in. Although this has been used in the past, there are a number of problems with this approach since it relies too much on self-perception rather than any objective measure of social class. The objective method, in contrast, uses a range of measures such as occupation, car ownership, unemployment, income, post code, education and so on. These are all indicators that can be objectively measured. It is these measures that have been the ones most frequently used in the research. The two most widely used measures are both based on occupation: the Registrar General's Standard Occupation Classification and the Socio-Economic Groups (SEG). Although both of these methods have been supplanted by another method (which will be discussed later) it is worth outlining these older methods in the first instance since much of the previous research has relied on these methods (in particular the Registrar General Classification system) and many healthcare workers still use it as a short-hand for classifying people.

The Registrar General's Standard Occupation Classification measurement was employed in the census from 1901 until relatively recently. It is based on the occupation of the individual head of the household (usually defined as the man – it was defined in less enlightened times!) who is classified into one of six groups (see Table 3.3).

In order to overcome some of the difficulties associated with the Registrar General's classification, the socio-economic groups listed below were developed by attempting to increase the number of categories into which individuals could be assigned. It was not based on status; rather it was based upon similar occupations:

1. Employers and managers in central and local government, industry, commerce – large establishments
2. Employers and managers in central and local government, industry, commerce – small establishments
3. Professional workers – self employed
4. Professional workers – employees
5. Intermediate non-manual workers
6. Junior non-manual workers
7. Personal service workers
8. Foreman and supervisors – non-manual
9. Skilled manual workers
10. Semi-skilled manual workers
11. Unskilled manual workers
12. Own account workers (other than professional workers)
13. Farmers – employers and managers
14. Farmers – own account
15. Agricultural workers
16. Members of the armed forces
17. Occupation inadequately described.

However, again it was rather subjective and offered little more than an extension of the RG's system. In order to overcome these difficulties a new government social classification system was developed: the National Statistics Socio-Economic Classification (NS-SEC). This new method of classification was used in the 2001 census. The NS-SEC is an occupationally based classification but has rules to provide coverage of the whole adult population (see Table 3.4).

Table 3.3 The Registrar General's Standard Occupation Classification measurement

Class	Title	Examples
I	Professional	Lawyer, doctor, University professor
II	Intermediate	Farmer, nurse, office manager, health care professionals
III(NM)	Skilled non-manual	Cashier, secretary
III M	Skilled manual	Machine fitter, miner, bus driver
IV	Partly skilled	Postman (sic), traffic warden
V	Unskilled	Labourer, messenger, window cleaner

Table 3.4 The National Statistics Socio-economic Classification (NS-SEC)

The National Statistics Socio-economic Classification analytic classes

1	Higher managerial and professional occupations
	1.1 Large employers and higher managerial occupations
	1.2 Higher professional occupations
2	Lower managerial and professional occupations
3	Intermediate occupations
4	Small employers and own account workers
5	Lower supervisory and technical occupations
6	Semi-routine occupations
7	Routine occupations
8	Never worked and long-term unemployed

Indices of multiple deprivation (IMD)

More recently, focus has moved away from socio-economic status to measures of deprivation. Deprivation is a broad concept that has many dimensions. It refers to a range of problems that arise due to a lack of resources or opportunities that we might expect to have access to in our society (Welsh Government, 2011). It encompasses a wide range of domains which cover health, education, employment, housing, income, access to services and community safety. Multiple deprivation, as the term suggests, collectively refers to these different types or domains of deprivation. Each country in the UK has its own index of multiple deprivation which is used to measure relative deprivation for small geographical areas within that country (Table 3.5). This index is able to identify and understand how deprivation is distributed across a country so that polices, funding and resources can be targeted to the most deprived or disadvantaged areas (Scottish Government, 2012).

As Table 3.5 demonstrates, each country's index of multiple deprivation (IMD) is made up of domains or categories. These domains are used to calculate an overall relative measure of deprivation for small geographical areas within each respective country in the UK. A percentage score is given to each domain within the index and this is calculated in order to establish the relative importance of that domain as an aspect of deprivation (Welsh Government, 2011). For example, higher percentage scores, or weightings as they are termed, have greater importance than domains that have lower weightings. Table 3.5 clearly shows that domains with the greatest weighting across all indices are income and employment. This indicates that, relative to the other domains, income and employment are the two most important aspects of deprivation across all four IMD.

The indices detailed in Table 3.5 are not homogenous; consequently it is difficult to accurately compare deprivation across England, Wales, Scotland and Northern Ireland. First, the weightings and indicators that are used to construct each deprivation domain are not the same across indices. For example, the living environment/housing domain is weighted differently across the four home countries (Table 3.5). A weight of 9.3 per cent is attributed to this domain in the English 2010 Indices of Deprivation. This score is calculated from indicators that specifically measure poor housing quality, lack of central heating, air quality and road traffic accidents. By comparison, the 2010 Northern Ireland Multiple Deprivation Measure (NIMDM) applies a weight of 5 per cent to the living environment domain, and to further complicate comparisons the indicators that are used to construct this measure differ from the English version of the index. Indicators that are used to construct the living environment domain in the NIMDM include: decent home standard, housing health, safety rating system, homelessness acceptances and a local area problem score (Payne and Abel, 2012).

Other factors also limit direct comparability of the indices in Table 3.5. The differing timescales and the fact that the data does not refer to the same year affects any direct comparison of data. Furthermore, the 2011 Welsh IMD has eight separate domains of deprivation, with the inclusion of physical environment, which is in contrast to the other three indices which just have seven. Finally, each index is developed according to national policy and these policies can differ across each constituent country. These differences are perhaps even more pronounced since devolution has evolved.

Many people are familiar with the term socio-economic status and it would be an oversight not to briefly explain how this compares to IMD. Standard economic and social measures of SES tend to include income, household expenditure, occupation and income, although other factors may also apply (Vyas and Kumaranayake, 2006). Perhaps the most striking difference between IMD and SES is that IMD measures relative deprivation at the small area level. This contrasts to SES which measures social/economic status at the individual or household level. The IMD also includes much wider environmental measures of deprivation such as crime, housing and access to services. These domains extend beyond the standard measures of income, education and employment which are used to calculate SES.

Table 3.5 Deprivation domains and their relative weightings for each constituent country in the UK

Domains	England 2010 Weight	Scotland 2012 Weight	Wales 2011 Weight	Northern Ireland 2010 Weight
Income	22.5%	28%	23.5%	25%
Employment	22.5%	28%	23.5%	25%
Education	13.5%	14%	14%	15%
Health	13.5%	14%	14%	15%
Access/barriers to services	9.3%	9%	10%	10%
Living environment/housing	9.3%	2%	5%	5%
Crime/community safety	9.3%	5%	5%	5%
Physical environment	Not measured	Not measured	5%	Not measured

Source: adapted from Payne and Abel, 2012

Health inequalities related to sex and ethnicity

The relationship between sex and health has been explored in a number of different ways depending on how health is defined and measured. In terms of mortality, the life expectancy of men and women in various countries is presented in Table 3.6. There is a difference between men and women with women consistently living longer than their male counterparts. This is true from the poorer countries with low life expectancies (e.g. Nigeria) to those richer countries (e.g. France) with higher life expectancies (WHO, 2012).

At a UK level, the data also support this view with women living longer than men. Table 3.1 demonstrates the differences in life expectancy between men and women since the start of the century (National Statistics, 2012a). It is possible to note that the life expectancy of both men and women has increased by some three years over the previous years – an impressive rate of improvement and this looks as if it is continuing.

Also presented on the graph is 'healthy life' expectancy – an important fact which takes into account the quality of life and health of the individuals concerned. Again this figure has improved considerably over the 20-year period. Gender differences between the health of males and females have been widely acknowledged. Data from the Office for National Statistics highlight this trend in reporting that a larger proportion of females live in to their 80s in comparison to males. In 2010, 62 per cent of females in the UK died after the age of 80, compared to 43 per cent of males (Office for National Statistics, 2012a).

Applying this to Dave

Dave is male – his 'macho behaviour' such as drinking excessively, smoking and drug taking can all impact on his health.

Table 3.6 Life expectancies by country

Country	Male life expectancy	Female life expectancy
France	75.9	83.5
Albania	67.3	74.1
Denmark	74.8	79.5
USA	74.6	79.8
Canada	77.2	82.3
Nigeria	48.0	49.6
China	69.6	72.7

There are also differences in health between ethnic groups. In April 2011 Pakistani and Bangladeshi men and women in England and Wales reported the highest rates of both poor health and limiting long-term illness, while Chinese men and women reported the lowest rates. Figure 3.1 shows the percentages of people in different ethnic groups suffering from poor health and limiting illness in 2001. Some specific conditions are also noted to be higher in certain ethnic groups (ONS, 2012a):

- South Asian people are reported to have high rates of heart disease and of hypertension.
- Black Caribbean people are reported to have high rates of hypertension, but not of heart disease.
- All ethnic minority groups are reported to have high rates of diabetes, but low rates of respiratory illness.
- Black Caribbean people, particularly young men, have high rates of admission to hospital with severe mental disorders (psychosis).

Health inequalities – determinants of health

There are many models and frameworks used to explain the determinants of health in relation to inequalities within society (Evans and Stoddart, Field Model of Health and Wellbeing, 1990; Dahlgren and Whitehead, Social Determinants of Health Rainbow, 1991). Dahlgren and Whitehead (1991) consider a social ecological theory and emphasise the relationship between the individual, who has fixed factors such as age and sex, and their environment, which is changeable. The model comprises of several layers which orientate around the individual (see Figure 3.2):

1. Individual lifestyle factors – e.g. the decision to smoke and drink alcohol
2. Social and community networks – e.g. social relations and support
3. Living and working conditions – e.g. unemployment and housing
4. General socio-economic, cultural and environmental factors.

If health inequalities are to be successfully tackled, it is important that all avenues that contribute – from the individual to the societal – are explored and addressed.

Lifestyle behaviours are known to influence health and health inequalities. Such lifestyle behaviours include:

- Smoking
- Drinking alcohol
- Drug use
- Lack of exercise.

Specific chapters on smoking cessation, alcohol reduction and promotion of exercise exist in this book so they will be considered in passing rather than any great detail here. However, it is worth noting that there tends to be a relationship between individual poor lifestyle factors and socio-economic status (although this generalisation covers a

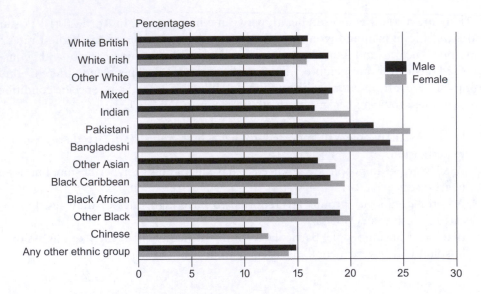

Figure 3.1 Age-standardised limiting long-term illness: by ethnic group and sex, April 2001, England and Wales

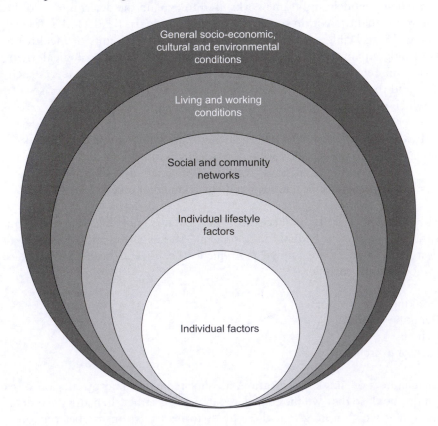

Figure 3.2 Social determinants of health rainbow

complex relationship in some areas). For example Wardle and Steptoe (2003) showed that boys and girls from more deprived neighbourhoods were more likely to have tried smoking, to eat a high fat diet, and to be overweight. Girls living in more deprived areas were also less likely to eat five servings of fruit and vegetables or to exercise at the weekend. Most differences persisted after controlling for ethnicity. A clear deprivation gradient emerged for each risk factor.

Taking smoking as an example, its relation to socio-economic class is well known. For instance it can be seen from the data in Table 3.7 that those individuals in a manual job role are more than twice as likely to smoke compared to those in a non-manual job role.

This not only emphasises the social gradient in smoking but also the population who are more likely to suffer health consequences of the behaviour. Cancer is one of the conditions linked to smoking as well as one of the main conditions linked to health inequalities (Marmot, 2010). Evidently, targeting smoking behaviour in those in the most deprived areas would improve health status. However, this may not just be about targeting individuals but about addressing systematic inequalities in society and providing support for those in the most deprived areas of the UK – the argument being that people smoke because of their environment. Improving their environment, therefore, will help reduce unhealthy behaviours.

One particular issue which requires fundamental consideration is the normative culture of differing socio-economic groups. Our social and community networks consist of a variety of individuals including friends, peers and family members. We learn the behaviours that others close to us exhibit through observation, imitation and modelling. Hence, it is possible that risky health behaviours and behaviours which have adverse health consequences are learned from significant others, consequently unhealthy behaviour begets unhealthy behaviours. For example, research suggests that peer influence and peer norms are considered an important factor in adolescents' sexual behaviour (Bauermeister et al., 2009) and perceived behaviour of peers, rather than peer approval, has been linked to adolescents' risky sexual online behaviour, particularly among males (Baumgartner et al., 2011).Once such behaviours have been taken up, they are socially reinforced by those around us who also carry out the same behaviours such as smoking, drinking and drug use (see specific chapters for details).

Our living and working conditions can also significantly affect our health. From the obvious – working as a miner or in a steel foundry can potentially be more damaging

Table 3.7 Percentage of individuals smoking cigarettes in 2010

Socio-economic classification	Men	Women	Total
Managerial and professional	14	12	13
Intermediate	20	20	20
Routine and manual	29	28	28
Total	21	20	20

Source: General Lifestyle Survey, Office for National Statistics, 2010

to health than working in an office due to the inherent risks of the work place – to the less obvious psychological factors. For example, a review of over 200 reports of research exploring the stress hormone, cortisol, found that the key factors are the unavoidable 'threats to the social self' – those threats to self-esteem and social status (Dickerson and Kemeny, 2004). Those that are 'lower on the social hierarchy' and receive 'signals of rejection' from the rest of society are more likely to be stressed and ill.

Unemployment is a key concern following the recent economic troubles which can also impact on health. From January to March 2012 there were an estimated 2.63 million unemployed people (Office for National Statistics, 2012b). It is well documented that individuals who are unemployed have higher rates of poor health. This may be related to lower income or a lack of social support gained through working (Backhans and Hemmingsson, 2012) or the clear signals of rejection from the rest of society (Dickerson and Kemeny, 2004).

All these factors have to be taken into account when attempting to address health concerns and, of course, if there are health inequalities then the task is magnified. To take one such example, in their report on reducing infant mortality a number of key recommendations (DoH, 2010c) were made which crossed a number of boundaries:

- Improving access to services amongst different ethnicities
- Improving poor housing conditions and overcrowding, which may play a role in sudden infant death syndrome
- Optimising infant and maternal nutrition, including reducing maternal obesity and promoting breastfeeding
- Reducing maternal smoking: smoking in pregnancy increases infant mortality by about 40 per cent
- Reducing teenage pregnancy: infant mortality rates are 60% higher within this age group than 20–39-year-olds.

From the individual behaviours (e.g. reducing smoking and teenage pregnancies) to the community and environmental (e.g. reducing poor housing conditions) the importance of a co-ordinated approach is evident.

Box 3.1 Applying research in practice

Social class differences in secular trends in established coronary risk factors over 20 years: A cohort study of British men from 1978–1980 to 1998–2000 (Ramsay et al., 2011)

This study investigated the risk factors of developing coronary heart disease in different socio-economic groups. This was completed over a 20-year period in an attempt to see if variations appeared over time and between different socio-economic groups. A total of 7735 British men aged between 40–59 years were followed up between 1978 and 2000. Participants' socio-economic position, anthropometric and physiological measures were taken at baseline and at the 20-year assessment period.

Results showed a narrowing of systolic blood pressure between socio-economic groups in the 20-year study period. However, other risk factors such as BMI and cholesterol levels indicated differences between socio-economic status, with individuals from manual occupations showing a greater increase in BMI, a smaller reduction in non-HDL cholesterol and a smaller increase in HDL cholesterol. In addition, smoking rates did not differ between social classes.

It is concluded that men in the lower three socio-economic positions, over a 20-year period, did not show as much change in relation to risk factors for coronary heart disease as men in the higher three socio-economic positions. This infers that there are still social inequalities related to risk factors of coronary heart disease within the male population.

Applying this to Dave

It might be suggested that Dave's social and community networks are influencing his smoking behaviour. He is and has been surrounded by people who smoke all his life including his parents and friends. Therefore his living conditions, environmental factors and social networks all contribute to the maintenance of this behaviour. Dave will need more support in any attempt to quit smoking as he is regularly surrounded by that environment.

Assessment of health

The ability to assess health in a reliable and robust fashion is of key importance when investigating and considering health inequalities. The most cited definition of health is that provided by the WHO (World Health Organization, 1946): 'Health is a state of complete physical, mental and social well-being and not merely the absence of disease or infirmity.'

It was first conceptualised just after the Second World War and emphasises that peace and health are inseparable and made something clear from the outset: disease and infirmity cannot be isolated from subjective experience and any definition of health must include a social and psychological dimension.

The definition sets a high standard: does anybody actually achieve this high status? However, the definition does provide something that countries and local communities should aspire to and so it can be extremely useful as a guide and prompter for development. However, others have argued that the definition provided is merely definition of happiness rather than health (Saracci, 1997) and that this has important consequences in the allocation of resources for 'proper' health care. However, the WHO definition has remained as it was first conceptualised in 1946 and, as mentioned, has become the byword for health in health care practice in the twenty-first century (Blaxter, 1995). Notwithstanding this, the measurement of health is just as problematic. Given the central role these play in resource allocation, target setting and achievement they are worthy of further note.

Mortality statistics

One way of measuring health is to simply count the number of people that die in a particular area, or in a particular month or are from a particular group. In this way it is possible to compare these rates from group to group (e.g. between men and women) or from area to area (e.g. between Edinburgh and Cardiff) or from period to period (e.g. from the nineteenth century to the present day). That area, group or time period with the highest death rate is, obviously, the unhealthiest. Since death rates have been collected from the mid-nineteenth century to the present day it is possible to investigate a number of important factors.

To start with, the figure was just totalled up – the *crude death rate*. It is then possible to use this to provide an overview of the death rate over the years (since we also know the population of the country at the time), then we can provide a simple overview of say XX per 1000 (the death rate in 2013). Data can then be collected and analysed at the simple level and we can compare area, group or historically (see Table 3.8).

This information can provide some useful, comparable, information. For example, within the UK there is some variation in mortality rates between the constituent countries. In 2010, Scotland had the highest mortality rates for both males and females, 785 and 552 deaths per 100,000 population respectively whereas England had the lowest rates for males and females, 638 and 456 deaths per 100,000 population

Table 3.8 Death rates by year

Year	Males: deaths (thousands)	Males: death rate (per 1000 population)	Females: deaths (thousands)	Females: death rate (per 1000 population)
1976	300.1	12.5	298.5	11.8
1981	289.0	12.0	288.9	11.3
1986	287.9	11.8	293.3	11.4
1991	277.6	11.2	292.5	11.2
1996	268.7	10.4	291.5	11.0
2001	252.4	9.9	277.9	10.4
2004	245.2	9.4	269.0	9.9
2011	234.6	6.5	249.7	4.7

respectively. Northern Ireland has experienced the largest declines in mortality for both males (51 per cent) and females (43 per cent) since 1980. In contrast males and females in Scotland have shown the smallest declines in mortality rates over the last 30 years at 44 per cent and 35 per cent respectively.

However, there are problems with this approach – the death rate in Bournemouth may be quite high whereas in Amersham it may be lower. This is not because Bournemouth is a particularly unhealthy place to live but that it is the place where people go to retire and hence it is bound to have a higher death rate. Crude death rates ignore the fact that many different factors impact upon the death rate (for example, an individual's sex, age or their previous health) and because of these problems they are not often used any more when sensitive statistics are required.

Standardised Mortality Ratios

The Standardised Mortality Rate (SMR) compares the mortality rate for the whole population with that of a particular region or group (the so-called *index population*) and expresses this as a ratio. Thus, the observed death rate is divided by the expected rate (derived from the index population) and then multiplied by 100.

SMRs are calculated in order to be able to make comparisons of death rates from a single cause (e.g. heart attacks, breast cancer) between geographical areas or different groups (according to sex, class, ethnicity and so on). The SMR for deaths from a particular disease is calculated by expressing the actual number of deaths in the group of interest in the index area as a ratio of the expected number of deaths from the standard population data. In most analyses a value of 100 equals the average mortality. Any value greater than 100 indicates above average mortality and less than 100 equates to a mortality better than average. For example, if we look at Table 3.9 we can see the SMR for the Coronary Heart Disease in selected areas of England.

Table 3.9 SMR rates due to coronary heart disease in England, 2012

Area	SMR
Buckinghamshire CC	83.5
Cambridgeshire CC	87.3
Cumbria CC	112.5
Derbyshire CC	110.1
Devon CC	88.9
Dorset CC	80.1
East Sussex CC	81.1
Essex CC	91.8
Gloucestershire CC	95.8
Hampshire CC	84.2
Hertfordshire CC	90.0

Area	SMR
Kent CC	96.5
Lancashire CC	113.0
Leicestershire CC	93.2
Lincolnshire CC	99.1
Norfolk CC	94.1
Northamptonshire CC	91.6
North Yorkshire CC	107.6
Nottinghamshire CC	100.1
Oxfordshire CC	78.3
Somerset CC	85.3
Staffordshire CC	101.3
Suffolk CC	95.5
Surrey CC	79.7
Warwickshire CC	84.1
West Sussex CC	86.1
Worcestershire CC	86.3

Source: http://www.apho.org.uk/resource/item.aspx?RID=97087

The data can be used to determine where in the country death rates are at their highest. From Table 3.9, it is evident that the higher SMR rates are in Lancashire compared to the lower rates in Oxfordshire. Similarly, the SMR can be used to compare countries (see Table 3.10) which indicates the crude death rate, the death rate per 1000 population and the overall SMR. As is obvious, in comparing mortality rates, England does better than the other home countries, particularly Scotland (General Registrar Office for Scotland, 2012).

Table 3.10 Death rates in the home countries, 1981–2001

	Number of deaths			Death rate per 1,000 population			SMR		
	1981	1991	2000	1981	1991	2000	Persons	Males	Females
Scotland	63.8	61.0	57.8	12.3	12.0	11.3	118	117	117
England	541.0	534.0	501.0	11.6	11.1	10.0	98	98	98
Wales	35.0	34.1	33.3	12.4	11.8	11.3	102	102	102
Northern Ireland	16.3	15.1	14.9	10.6	9.4	8.8	105	105	105
United Kingdom	658.0	646.2	608.4	11.7	11.2	10.2	100	100	100

Morbidity statistics

Morbidity statistics are often used to determine the prevalence of illness and disease. Again such databases are used to make comparisons across years and population groups. The databases provide a wide range of statistics from information on the prevalence of specific cancers to individuals who have drug dependency and mental health disorders. In the UK this information can be found on websites such as that of the Office for National Statistics, the Department of Health and Health Protection Agency. Such statistics are only concerned with the population as a whole and not at an individual level.

Individual health measurement tools

Measuring health at an individual level can be undertaken from several perspectives, by looking at either physical or psychological health, or potentially a combination of the two – Health Related Quality of Life (HRQoL). There are a number of measures for assessing the latter, for example the short-form 36-item questionnaire (SF-36; Brazier *et al.*, 1992). This is a generic health survey consisting of eight constructs, which combined, assesses the physical and mental health of an individual by considering the areas shown in Figure 3.3.

When interpreting the results of such questionnaires it is always suggested that slight caution should be used due to the nature of the measures. As the measures rely on self-reports, potential biases or socially desirable answers may be used.

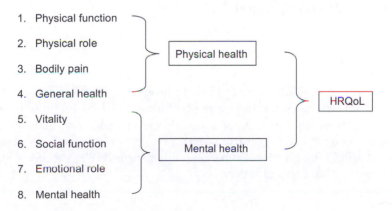

Figure 3.3 The short-form questionnaire

Applying this to Dave

Dave could undertake an assessment of quality of life in relation to his angina. This will enable his health care professionals to understand the impact of his illness on him from a social and psychological perspective.

Health promotion

Health promotion is the process of enabling people to increase control over their health and its determinants, and thereby improve their health. It is a core function of public health and contributes to the work of tackling communicable and non-communicable diseases and other threats to health (World Health Organisation, 2005).

In a broad sense, health promotion combines disease prevention and health education in an attempt to inspire individuals to maintain a healthy lifestyle (see Chapter 2 for more detail).

Approaches to health promotion

Approaches to health promotion vary and will be considered in more detail in the next chapter. However, it is worth giving a brief outline of five main approaches and how these can be linked to health inequalities.

Medical model

In order to ensure individuals remain in good health, the medical model encourages individuals to undertake efforts to ensure good health such as immunisation. This is done through persuasion. For example, the NHS launched a national immunisation programme in 2008 to protect girls from developing cervical cancer. Girls aged between the ages of 14 and 17 are given the human papilloma virus (HPV) vaccine in an attempt to reduce rates of adult cervical cancer.

Behavioural model

The behavioural model considers the individual's behaviours and attitudes and aims to change these in an attempt to improve health. The government has considered this angle of health promotion in schemes such as the school fruit and vegetable scheme (SFVS). This programme runs as part of the 5 A Day programme and has been shown to increase children's consumption of fruit and vegetables (Teeman et al., 2010). In using this approach, health promoters take an expert-led, top-down role in an attempt to impact upon the individuals' behaviour. Strategies are used in an attempt to persuade the individual to undertake beneficial health behaviours.

Educational model

This model aims to give the individual the required information on healthy lifestyles, such as the benefits of smoking cessation, in order for them to make an educated decision concerning their health behaviours. Within this model, the method of persuasion is not considered and it focuses on providing knowledge in order to empower the individual to adopt healthy behaviours. Therefore, in this sense, health promotion is purely seen as an information provider aimed at empowering the individual to consider their attitudes towards health behaviours.

Client-led model

This model is predominantly concerned with empowering the individual to understand the health impact of their behaviour. In doing so the client takes control of their health behaviours in a bottom-up process. The health professional is simply there to guide and advise the client in the behaviour they wish to change. For example an individual may decide, with the support of their GP, that they want to lose weight. The health professional is simply there to guide the client and support them in accomplishing their goal. This can be through providing information, support and recourses.

Societal-led model

The societal-led model does not intend to change the individual's behaviour but that of society as a whole. In making health behaviours more accessible to all individuals no matter what socio-economic background they are from, health promotion can tackle health and health inequalities. In doing so poor health-related behaviours can be made less accessible. For example, there have been recommendations to increase tax by 20 per cent on unhealthy foods which are considered high in fat and sugar (Mytton *et al.*, 2012), therefore attempting to install a top-down process when tackling issues such as obesity and cardiovascular disease.

Applying this to Dave

Dave could make use of health promotion materials that can be found in local chemists and GP surgeries. He could take a bottom-up approach and start to take control of his health-related behaviours by considering promotional materials on angina and smoking. This may not only help to educate him but to also motivate him to change. Alternatively, other models could be applied – but these are much more difficult and long-term in nature.

Interventions to reduce health inequalities

Interventions aimed to improve the overall health of individuals and reduce health inequalities have been considered an essential part in the government's agenda for many years (Department of Health, 2003, 2004, 2010a). It is clear that the health service cannot tackle this alone and a multi-disciplinary approach involving a combination of local services will prove the most beneficial (Department of Health, 2010b).

The Department of Health (2012) outlined a move to integrate public health into local government, allowing services to be planned in the context of broader social determinants of health such as poverty, education, housing and employment. The Public Health Outcomes Framework will be refocused around positive health outcomes and reducing inequalities in health rather than focused on performance targets. The intended outcomes of the change are to increase healthy life expectancy and reduce differences in healthy life expectancy between communities.

By instigating this change, the DoH hopes that by taking central control away, health promotion messages can be tailored to a more local target audience. The government proposed to 'reach across and reach out' by being:

- Responsive – Owned by communities and shaped by their needs
- Resourced – With ring-fenced funding and incentives to improve
- Rigorous – Professionally-led, focused on evidence, efficient and effective
- Resilient – Strengthening protection against current and future threats to health.

Department of Health, 2010b, p. 6

Specific interventions aimed at a community level have been rolled out throughout the country, such as the Coventry South Cancer Project, under this directive. This scheme aims to tackle health inequalities in the Coventry South area which was known to have a high rate of cancer and mortality. In an attempt to reduce these, health promotional material was generated. Posters and advertisements displaying cancer related symptoms were displayed in local pubs, free health assessments were offered and a stop smoking clinic and healthy walk group were devised. By taking this multi-angled approach, health messages are able to reach a wider audience and therefore impact on health and reduce health inequalities.

As part of this intervention, men from deprived areas were specifically targeted. Taking a community stance on the intervention enabled individuals to be approached who don't voluntarily go to seek medical advice. In conducting ad hoc drop-in sessions in community venues of hard-to-reach individuals, the health professionals were able to motivate individuals to be more aware of the signs of cancer. In order to tackle health inequalities it could mean that programmes such as this are needed to deliver health messages to hard to reach populations.

In using this multi-angled approach to reduce health inequalities several psychological principles can be used, such as motivational interviewing, which will enable the individual to understand what behaviour they want to change; it enables the client to make the decision and does not tell the client what they need to change. For example it could be used as part of the Coventry South Cancer project and motivate men to be more aware of the signs of cancer. It is thought that when an individual is self-motivated in changing behaviour, behaviour change is more successful.

England's approach to tackling health inequalities focused on developing a cross-governmental plan with a number of inequalities targets to be achieved by 2010. Based on the most recent data, these targets look unlikely to be met. England finds itself in a similar position to Northern Ireland in that it has seen considerable gains in the absolute levels of health in its whole population, however there has also been an underlying widening of the gap between social groups.

The Public Health Strategy in the other countries of the UK is similarly comprehensive. In Wales, a five-year Public Health Strategy for Wales (2010–2015) has been developed to address the public health challenges of the country. Although the general health of the Welsh population appears to be improving as measured by life expectancy, closer inspection of the data reveals that a widening gap between the health of the wealthiest and the health of the poorest is evident. These findings indicate that deprivation remains a significant determining factor in people's health status. Objectives within the strategy clearly outline the need to improve health and reduce health inequalities by addressing the wider socio-economic and environmental determinants of health.

A review of the 10-year public health strategy for Northern Ireland 'Investing for Health' concluded that similar to the other countries in the UK, Northern Ireland has also witnessed an overall improvement of population health since its publication in 2002. This finding however disguises the persistent inequalities in health that exist between the wealthiest and the poorest in the country, a trend that is evident across all the countries in the UK. The health of people in Northern Ireland was also identified as being poorer than those in England on specific measures of health. The review identifies that the 2002 public health strategy requires updating in order to take account of the changing social and economic landscape and policy developments. A new strategic public health policy for Northern Ireland is currently being developed to address these issues.

'Partnership for Care' (Scottish Executive, 2003), the Scottish Health White Paper, clearly states in its introduction that an 'unacceptable' health gap between the wealthiest and poorest groups exists in Scotland. Although a general improvement in population health is again observed, there is acknowledgement within the document that health outcomes are strongly linked to deprivation and inequality. 'Better Health Better Care' (2007) is an action plan that has subsequently been developed by the Scottish Government in order to improve and sustain the health of the Scottish population. An emphasis has been placed specifically on providing disadvantaged communities with access to fast, local quality healthcare in order to improve health and reduce inequalities. This action plan reflects the work undertaken by the Ministerial Task Force for Health Inequalities (Equally Well, 2008). Their report provides a detailed analysis of Scotland's health inequalities and their determinants.

Interventions

Interventions designed to tackle health inequalities can be described as 'upstream' or 'downstream' though, in reality, there is a continuum between the two. Upstream interventions act on the social determinants of health, or act to create a healthier environment or culture (e.g. legislation on smoking in public places). Downstream interventions seek to address an existing health problem or risk factor (e.g. smoking cessation services). Another key distinction is whether an intervention is applied at a whole population level (e.g. alcohol minimum unit pricing) or at the individual level (e.g. alcohol brief interventions). Further information on such interventions is available in the individual chapters on these topics.

Tackling health inequalities at an individual level is important due to the variations within society and individual differences. In attempting to change health inequalities, the government recognises the need to provide individuals with more support when attempting to change lifestyle behaviours such as smoking. Therefore putting various interventions into place, such as health trainers, was considered essential. Health trainers work in disadvantaged communities with individuals who are engaging in risky behaviours and tailor their support to the needs of the individuals in that specific community. The 2008 handbook *Improving Health, Changing Behaviour* (Department of Health, 2008) further outlined the job of accredited health trainers. The role would require motivating individuals to change their behaviour while also stressing the importance and benefits of a healthy lifestyle. In turn this would enable individuals to understand consequences of risky health behaviours. In attempting to motivate individuals the health trainers use psychological principles and evidence-based behaviour change techniques such as goal setting, confidence building and coping strategies. Results have indicated that the intervention was effective in reaching deprived areas and individuals who engage in risky behaviours. Individuals who were participating in the intervention were seen to have a good level of intention to change their behaviour but lower levels in self-efficacy, coping planning and action planning (Wilkinson *et al.*, 2011). Therefore, it is suggested that with the help of intervention, the participants' self-efficacy can be increased which can therefore result in behaviour change. The importance of self-efficacy in relation to health behaviour change has been highlighted in Chapter 4. It is recognised that self-efficacy is one of the best predictors of behaviour change. For example, Cleland *et al.* (2010) reviewed factors associated with resilience to physical inactivity in women from socio-economically disadvantaged backgrounds. It was found that the strongest related factors to achieving the recommended levels of physical activity were factors such as self-efficacy.

Policy level developments addressing health inequalities

It is clear from Chapter 2 that in order to reduce health inequalities, health promotion must be a central focus. As previously outlined, public health strategies for England, Wales, Northern Ireland and Scotland recognise that health inequalities must be tackled so that socially disadvantaged groups are able to enjoy good health at a level that is comparable to those who are wealthier. A recent report by the Health Committee for the House of Commons (House of Commons Health Committee, 2009) has comprehensively examined the extent of health inequalities in the UK. This document focuses on policy developments tackling health inequalities and their evaluation and identifies initiatives which have been designed specifically to deal with these inequalities.

Traditional health promotion strategies such as large public health campaigns that aim to raise awareness of health issues are effective, but only it seems for the more advantaged groups in society who have greater access to time, resources and finances (House of Commons Health Committee, 2009). As a result we have witnessed a widening of health inequalities because the health of those in higher socio-economic groups is improving at a faster rate. Herein the complexity lies. The report explains that the health of disadvantaged groups is not necessarily worsening, it is just not improving at the same rate as their wealthier counterparts. These socially disadvantaged groups are unable, it seems, to access the same opportunities for good health as the more advantaged groups in society and this has led to the observed inequalities in health that are apparent in the UK today. Knowing that good health is not equally distributed in society, it is important that scarce resources are targeted to those in greatest need.

Sure Start

Specific health inequality initiatives have been developed by the UK government in an attempt to close the widening gap between the wealthiest and the poorest in society. The Sure Start initiative, which was launched in the UK in 1998, is a good example of how the government has developed and targeted services to families living in deprived areas in an attempt to tackle inequalities. This government-led initiative identifies that early years are a crucial stage in the lifespan to address health inequalities through policy development (House of Commons Health Committee, 2009). Promoting a healthy start in life is the emphasis of the Sure Start initiative and this is particularly important because lifestyle factors can have a huge impact on a young child's development and future health. A mother's lifestyle during pregnancy can affect the health of her unborn child, and once born lifestyle factors such as breastfeeding, diet and parental smoking can impact significantly on a child's health and development (House of Commons Health Committee, 2009). The importance of the early years in governmental policies addressing health inequalities cannot be overstated.

Sure Start programmes are typically designed around a set of objectives that relate to children's social and emotional development, health, ability to learn and strengthening of communities (Roberts 2000). The breadth of these objectives acknowledges that health is indeed a multidimensional concept and supports the WHO's definition of health which is described at the beginning of this chapter. These objectives are:

- To improve social and emotional development
- To improve health

- To improve the ability to learn
- To strengthen families and communities
- To increase productivity of operations.

Roberts, 2000

Preventive work and family support are central components of the programme. The importance of social support in relation to behaviour change is discussed more fully in Chapter 4; however, one way social support is believed to improve health is by enhancing healthy lifestyles. In terms of Sure Start, social integration and specific social support for parenting skills and health promotion are ways that social support may operate to enhance behaviour change in harder to reach, disadvantaged families.

National evaluation of the programme has reported modest success. A recent evaluation showed that children in Sure Start areas showed better social development at three years, exhibiting more positive social behaviour and greater independence and self-regulation than their counterparts in non-Sure Start areas (Melhuish *et al.*, 2008). Parents were also described as exhibiting more positive parenting skills and providing a better home learning environment for their preschool children in these Sure Start locations (Melhuish *et al.*, 2010). Despite these positive outcomes, it has yet to be demonstrated that improvements in child behaviour and parenting skills will translate into future health gain and a narrowing of health inequalities for either children or parents (House of Commons Health Committee, 2009).

Inequalities and lifestyle

The causes of health inequalities are clearly complex, and include lifestyle factors such as smoking, exercise and nutrition, to name a few. As outlined earlier in this chapter, smoking in particular is considered to be a significant cause of health inequalities in the UK. Policy level developments that have had a positive impact in reducing these inequalities include the introduction of legislation to ban smoking in public places and banning point of sale tobacco advertising (House of Commons Health Committee, 2009).

Social marketing

Social marketing has also been heralded as a promising new approach to achieve specific behaviour change particularly in harder to reach or disadvantaged groups (House of Commons Health Committee, 2009). As discussed in Chapter 2, social marketing aims to influence a target audience's behaviour in order to promote positive behaviour/s for health or social change. Change4life is one such example of a national social marketing initiative that aims to tackle childhood obesity in the UK. In an attempt to address health inequalities in socially disadvantaged groups, a social marketing approach to health promotion is potentially able to communicate health messages in a more tailored and evidence-based way in an attempt to influence positive behaviour change (House of Commons Health Committee, 2009).

Financial incentives

A recently debated topic and potential intervention that aims to improve medical adherence and participation in vaccination and screening programmes is the use of financial incentives. It is thought that using these schemes could be a useful method in tackling health inequalities. Incentives can be in a variety of forms such as vouchers for money off at local retailers to gifts for adherence and attendance. The idea of incentives related to specific behaviours has been previously shown to be effective (Burr *et al.*, 2007). Although research has supported the use of incentives for one-off behaviours such as screening and testing for diseases (Zenner *et al.*, 2012) these are behaviours which do not require long-term maintenance. It is recognised that more research is needed on the use of incentives in producing long-term health behaviour changes which aim to change habits as results of studies using incentives have not always been shown to be positive (Oliver and Brown, 2012).

Applying this to Dave

Individual level interventions such as those above could help Dave improve his health. For instance, if his local area had health trainers they could help keep Dave motivated to reduce smoking habits. In doing so conjointly Dave's level of self-efficacy could be assessed and further developed.

Conclusion

Health inequalities are of key concern to all governments across the UK and it is considered that the ill health that results from them is mainly preventable. Changing the health behaviour of individuals is acknowledged as challenging but the systematic changes required to society even more so. In order to change behaviour and tackle health inequalities and the social gradient in health it is necessary to target individuals, cultures and social policy.

Key points

- Health inequalities are the variation in health outcomes and mortality rates between individuals.
- Various factors impact upon health and health inequalities such as age, gender, level of education, socio-economic status and ethnicity.
- A relationship exists between income and health which has produced a social gradient.
- Emphasis to reduce the gap in health inequalities has been enforced by the government.

- Multi-layered approaches such as Dahlgren and Whitehead's (1991) social determinants of health rainbow are useful as they acknowledge the complexity involved when trying to tackle health inequalities.
- It is important to consider the individual's beliefs and reasons behind health related and risky behaviours.
- Measures based on psychological principles can be used to unravel beliefs regarding health related behaviours.
- Self-efficacy is important when aiming to change health related behaviour.
- It is important to ensure health promotion and health interventions reach all individuals in the population if health inequalities are to be successfully tackled.

Points for discussion

- Critically discuss the statement – socio-economic status determines health.
- Consider and discuss the evidence for the various measures of health.
- Describe and evaluate how social factors impact upon health inequalities.

Further resources

Marmot, M. (2010). *Fair Society, Healthy Lives*. UCL: Marmot Review. Available at: www.instituteofhealthequity.org/projects/fair-society-healthy-lives-the-marmot-review (accessed 23 September 2013).

Department of Health (2010). *Healthy Lives, Healthy people: Our Strategy for Public Health in England*. London: Department of Health.

World Health Organization (1998). *Health Promotion Glossary*. Geneva: WHO.

Naidoo, J. and Wills, J. (2010). *Developing Practice for Public Health and Health Promotion*, 3rd edn. Edinburgh: Bailière Tindall.

References

Barron, K. (2009). *Health Committee Health Inequalities: Third Report of Session 2008–09*. Vol. 1: report, together with formal minutes. London: Stationery Office.

Backhans, M.C. and Hemmingsson, H. (2012). Unemployment and mental health – who is (not) affected? *European Journal Public Health*, 22(3): 429–433.

Bauermeister, J., Elkington, K., Brackis-Cott, E., Dolezal, C. and Mellins, C. (2009). Sexual behavior and perceived peer norms: comparing perinatally HIV-infected and HIV-affected youth. *Journal of Youth and Adolescence*, 38(8): 1110–1122.

Baumgartner, S.E., Valkenburg, P.M. and Peter, J. (2011). The influence of descriptive and injunctive peer norms on adolescents' risky sexual online behavior. *Cyberpsychology, Behavior and Social Networking*, 14(12): 753–758.

Better Health Better Care Action Plan (2007). Edinburgh: The Scottish Government. Available at: http://www.scotland.gov.uk/Publications/2007/12/11103453/0 (accessed 4 April 2012).

Blaxter, M. (1995). *Health and Lifestyles*. London: Routledge.

Brazier, J.E., Harper, R.R., Jones, N.B., O'Catham, A.A., Thomas, K.J., Usherwood, T.T. and Westlake, L.L. (1992). Validating the SF-36 health survey questionnaire: new outcome measure for primary care. *BMJ: British Medical Journal (International Edition)*, 305(6846): 160.

Burr, M.L., Trembeth, J., Jones, K.B., Green, J., Lynch, L.A. and Roberts, Z.E.S. (2007). The effects of dietary advice and vouchers on the intake of fruit and fruit juice by pregnant women in a deprived area: a controlled trial. *Public Health Nutrition*, 10(6): 559–565.

Cleland, V., Ball, K., Salmon, J., Timperio, A. and Crawford, D. (2010). Personal, social and environmental correlates of resilience to physical inactivity among women from socio-economically disadvantaged backgrounds. *Health Education Research*, 25(2): 268–281.

Dahlgren, G. and Whitehead, M. (1991). *Policies and Strategies to Promote Social Equity in Health*. Stockholm: Institute for Future Studies.

Department of Health (2003). *Tackling Health Inequalities, A Programme for Action*. London: Department of Health.

——(2004). *Choosing Health: Making Healthier Choices Easier*. London: Department of Health.

——(2008). *Improving Health: Changing Behaviours. NHS Health Trainer Handbook*. London. Department of Health.

——(2010a). *Equity and Excellence: Liberating the NHS*. London: Department of Health.

——(2010b). *Healthy Lives, Healthy People: Our Strategy for Public Health in England*. London: Department of Health.

——(2010c). *Tackling Health Inequalities in Infant and Maternal Health Outcomes: Report of the Infant Mortality National Support Team*. London: Department of Health.

——(2012). *Healthy Lives, Healthy People: Improving Outcomes and Supporting Transparency*. London: Department of Health.

Dickerson, S.S. and Kemeny, M.E. (2004). Acute stressors and cortisol responses: a theoretical integration and synthesis of laboratory research. *Psychological Bulletin*, 130(3): 355.

English Indices of Deprivation (2010). Available at: https://www.gov.uk/government/uploads/system/uploads/attachment_data/file/6871/1871208.pdf (accessed 10 October 2012).

Equally Well: Report of the Ministerial Task Force on Health Inequalities – Volume 2 (2008). Edinburgh: The Scottish Government. Available at: http://www.scotland.gov.uk/Resource/Doc/226607/0061266.pdf (accessed 23 September 2013).

House of Commons Health Committee. (2009). *Health Inequalities*. Third Report of Session 2008–9. Volume 1. London: The Stationery Office Ltd.

Marmot, M. (2010). *Fair Society, Healthy Lives*. UCL: Marmot Review. Available at: www.instituteofhealthequity.org/projects/fair-society-healthy-lives-the-marmot-review (accessed 23 September 2013).

Melhuish, E., Belsky, J. and Barnes, J. (2010). Evaluation and value of Sure Start. *Archives of Disease in Childhood*, 95(3): 159–161.

Melhuish, E., Belsky, J., Leyland, A.H. and Barnes, J. (2008). The National Evaluation of Sure Start Research Team. Effects of fully-established Sure Start Local Programmes on 3 year old children and their families living in England: a quasi-experimental observational study. *The Lancet*, 372: 1641–1647

Mytton, O., Clarke, D. and Rayner, M. (2012). Taxing unhealthy food and drinks to improve health. *BMJ (Clinical Research Ed.)*, 344: e2931.

Northern Ireland Multiple Deprivation Measure (2010). National Statistics Publication. Available at: http://www.nisra.gov.uk/deprivation/archive/Updateof2005Mcasures/NIMDM_2010_Report.pdf (accessed 12 October 2012).

Office for National Statistics. (2010). *General Lifestyle Survey, A Report on the 2010 General Lifestyle Survey*. London: Office for National Statistics.

——(2011). *Life Expectancy at Birth and at Age 65 by Local Areas in the United Kingdom, 2004–06 to 2008–10*. London: Office for National Statistics.

——(2012a). *Mortality in the United Kingdom, 2010*. London: Office for National Statistics.

——(2012b). *Labour Market Statistics, May 2012*. London: Office for National Statistics.

Oliver, A. and Brown, L.D. (2012). A consideration of user financial incentives to address health inequalities. *Journal of Health Politics, Policy & Law*, 37(2): 201–226.

Partnership for Care: Scotland's Health White Paper (2003). Edinburgh: The Scottish Government. Available at: http://www.scotland.gov.uk/Resource/Doc/47032/0013897.pdf (accessed 15 January 2013).

Payne, R. and Abel, G. (2012). UK indices of multiple deprivation – a way to make comparisons across constituent countries easier. *Health Statistics quarterly/Office for National Statistics*, (53): 22

Public Health Wales Strategy 2010–2015 (2010). Public Health Wales. Available at: http://www.wales.nhs.uk/sitesplus/888/news/17240 (accessed 15 January 2013).

Ramsay, S.E., Whincup, P.H., Hardoon, S.L., Lennon, L.T., Morris, R.W. and Wannamethee, S.G. (2011). Social class differences in secular trends in established coronary risk factors over 20 years: a cohort study of British men from 1978–80 to 1998–2000. *PLOS ONE*, 6(5): 1–5.

Roberts, H. (2000). What is Sure Start? *Archives of Disease in Childhood*, 82: 435–437.

Saracci, R. (1997). The World Health Organization needs to reconsider its definition of health. *BMJ* 314: 1409.

Scottish Government (2012).*Scottish Index of Multiple Deprivation 2012.A National Statistics Publication for Scotland*. Edinburgh: The Scottish Government. Available at: http://simd.scotland.gov.uk/publication-2012/ (accessed 22 January 2013).

Teeman, D., Lynch, S., White, K., Scott, E., Waldman, J., Benton, T., Shamsan. Y., Stoddart, S., Ransley, J., Cade, J. and Thomas, J. (2010). *The Third Evaluation of the School Fruit and Vegetable Scheme*. London: Department of Health.

Townsend, P. and Davidson, N. (1982). *Inequalities in Health: Black Report*. London: Pelican Series, Penguin Books.

Vyas, S. and Kumaranayake, L. (2006). Constructing socio-economic status indices: how to use principal components analysis. *Health Policy and Planning*, 21(6): 459–468.

Wardle, J. and Steptoe, A. (2003). Socioeconomic differences in attitudes and beliefs about healthy lifestyles. *Journal of Epidemiology & Community Health*, 57(6): 440–443.

Welsh Government (2011).*Welsh Index of Multiple Deprivation 2011*. Available at: http://wales.gov.uk/topics/statistics/headlines/compendia2009/110831/?lang=en (accessed 23 September 2013).

White, C. and Edgar, G. (2010). Inequalities in healthy life expectancy by social class and area type: England, 2001–03. *Health Statistics Quarterly*, 45.

Wilkinson, D., Sniehotta, F.F. and Michie, S. (2011). Targeting those in need: baseline data from the first English National Health Service (NHS) Health Trainer Service. *Psychology, Health & Medicine*, 16(6): 736–748.

World Health Organization (WHO). (1946). *Records of the World Health Organization*. New York: Constitution of the World Health Organization.

——(2005). *The Bangkok Charter for Health Promotion in a Globalized World*. Available at http://www.who.int/healthpromotion/conferences/6gchp/hpr_050829_%20BCHP.pdf (accessed 17 December 2012).

Zenner, D., Molinar, D., Nichols, T., Riha, J., Macintosh, M. and Nardone, A. (2012). Should young people be paid for getting tested? A national comparative study to evaluate patient financial incentives for chlamydia screening. *BMC Public Health*, 12(1): 261–267.

<table>
<tr><td>

4

</td><td>

Psychology in practice

</td></tr>
</table>

Case study

Caroline is a practice nurse in a semi-urban GP practice. Her role at the clinic includes health promotion. When Caroline first joined the practice she was very enthusiastic about the health promotion aspect of her role. She was convinced of the importance of a healthy lifestyle in preventing chronic disease. Caroline set up a high blood pressure clinic and a weight control clinic to support patients who had been advised by the doctor to reduce their blood pressure and/or lose weight. Caroline sees patients shortly after the doctor has told them that they are putting their health at risk; many are worried and anxious about their future health. Patients at these clinics are provided with high-quality information and advice about how to change their diet, reduce their drinking and increase their physical activity. They are directed towards local leisure-centre classes and given suggested meal plans. However, over the five years that Caroline has worked at the practice she has become disillusioned with her health promotion role. Very few people make permanent changes to their eating, drinking or exercise habits and the number of patients diagnosed with type 2 diabetes and other chronic diseases continues to increase.

At first, Caroline wondered whether her patients didn't understand the health information that she was giving them. However, a questionnaire survey amongst the clinic attendees demonstrated that the majority understood the importance of a healthy lifestyle, were aware of the government recommendations for diet and exercise and knew about the local community leisure facilities. Caroline has come to the conclusion that education is not going to result in lots of patients changing their ways and is looking for new approaches to use in her clinic. She has enrolled on a continuing professional development (CPD) module looking at psychological approaches to behavioural change in the hope that it will give her new ideas to improve her practice.

Introduction

A central strategy of health promotion has always been education. Health education involves a combination of risk communication and behavioural advice (knowledge) as well as developing life skills. As such, it assumes that people practise unhealthy lifestyle behaviours because they do not understand what is bad or good for their health and that if they had correct information and appropriate skills they would make healthy choices (WHO, 2012).

In line with an educational approach to health promotion, until recently psychology has focused on investigating how people understand and respond to the information they receive about health and behaviour. This is often described as a social cognitive approach to behavioural change. Social cognitive approaches assume that behavioural choices are a reflection of the way people see and think about the world. Consequently, if we can understand how people think then we will be able to influence the way they decide to behave. A key aspect of this approach is the recognition that different people may perceive the same thing differently. So what is unpleasant for one person may be enjoyable for another. In terms of lifestyle choices, one person may find cycling from work a pleasant way to unwind after work, whilst another cannot face cycling home at the end of a long day.

Decisions about how to behave are thought to involve some sort of cost-benefit analysis. In its simplest version, any model of behavioural change is a straightforward weighing up of these two factors. Research has then gone on to investigate what other factors are also influential. A number of different theoretical models of health behaviour have been developed to predict people's behavioural choices, all expansions of the basic cost-benefit model. It is beyond the remit of this text to provide a description and explanation of the numerous social cognitive models of behaviour.

There are a number of texts where the reader can find a comprehensive review of these models, such as Conner and Norman (2005) or Thirlaway and Upton (2009). In this chapter we will evaluate the key factors (Table 4.1) that emerge from research on the various social cognitive models of behaviour as particularly influential on behavioural change.

Promoting lifestyle change has traditionally focused on educating people to realise that they need to change and more recently on motivating people so that they wish to change. However, the focus on getting people to adopt healthier habits has been at the expense of considering how people maintain newly adopted habits (Nigg *et al.*, 2008). Lifestyle change needs to be long term to improve health outcomes but unfortunately many people who take up a healthy behaviour soon stop. For example, research has shown that about 50 per cent of people who start a formal physical activity programme drop out within six months (Nigg *et al.*, 2008). Psychological concepts such as self-regulation, habituation and stages of change do recognise the long-term issues around behavioural change and the interventions associated with these concepts go some way towards addressing the issue of sustained change (Table 4.1).

Applying this to Caroline

Caroline needs a range of skills to deal with the range of factors that could be influencing the lifestyle behaviours in her clients.

Table 4.1 Factors that may influence lifestyle behavioural change

Psychological concept	Associated intervention
Perception of risk	Education
Perception of benefits	Education
Barriers	Structural change, cognitive behavioural therapy
Social norms	Policy; education; cultural adaptation
Social support	Motivational interviewing; counselling
Self-efficacy	Motivational interviewing; goal setting
Self-regulation	Goal setting; implementation intentions
Fear	Risk communication
Habituation	Motivational interviewing; implementation intentions; cognitive behavioural therapy
Pleasure	Little known, classical conditioning
Stages of change	Various, depending on stage

Psychological concepts

Perception of risk and benefits

A perception of risk is a central factor in the majority of psychological models of behavioural change; it delivers the costs side of the basic behavioural change evaluation. It is assumed that unless people realise that behaviour is risky they will not attempt to alter that behaviour.

In 2002 the Cabinet Office Strategy Unit defined risk as 'Uncertainty of outcome, whether positive opportunity or negative threat' (Cabinet Office Strategy Unit, 2002, p. 7). However, for most people risk is negative and indicates something to worry about (Thirlaway and Heggs, 2005). Indeed, a lot of risk communication is intended to generate fear and anxiety in order to get people to change their behaviour; whether this works will be considered later in the chapter.

A more useful definition of risk for health promotion is the one provided by Connolly *et al.* (2000): 'A situation of risk presents some chance of injury, damage or loss, a hazard or dangerous chance.'

So the starting point for any health promotion activity has always been to communicate a risk because it is assumed that unless people realise that drinking is dangerous they are unlikely to stop. Similarly, people are unlikely to adopt healthy behaviours that they don't enjoy, such as eating fruit, unless they understand that not eating fruit puts their health at risk.

Health professionals collectively make a decision about what is risky and what is safe. They provide a plethora of information about the 'right' way to behave. In the UK people are advised about the number of units of alcohol they can safely consume. They are advised to eat five portions of fruit and vegetables each day and to do 30 minutes of moderate to vigorous physical activity each week. There is expert advice available on the correct way to brush your teeth, the amount of water to drink, the speed at which to drive your car. Through risk communication the government informs us both of the *cost* of practising unhealthy behaviours, such as drinking too much, and of the *cost* of avoiding healthy behaviours, such as being physically active. There is an agreed 'correct' risk perception and on the basis of that, an agreed 'correct' decision. However, health promotion has been communicating lifestyle risks for more than two decades with little impact on lifestyle choices. In general the public fail to adhere to the recommendations made by the government (Department of Health, 2010). It is often assumed that this is because they don't understand the risk correctly (Thirlaway and Upton, 2009). Indeed, in 1999 the Department of Health stated that lay risk perceptions must be challenged by more effective risk communications. However, a large body of research suggests that people understand the risks associated with an unhealthy lifestyle perfectly well but still do not change their behaviour (Blaxter, 2004; Lawton and Conner, 2007).

Applying this to Caroline

Caroline needs to recognise that providing risk information is only a small aspect of the behavioural change intervention process.

The other main communication that health promotion delivers is behavioural advice and this behavioural advice often informs about the *benefits* of change as well as giving advice about what the change should be. Similarly to risk communications, behavioural advice is generally well understood but it is not generally adhered to (Thirlaway and Upton, 2009).

Applying this to Caroline

Once Caroline has recognised that educating people about the risks (costs) of unhealthy behaviour and the benefits of healthy behaviour will not, on its own, result in behavioural change, she will need to explore what other strategies she can use to improve the uptake of and adherence to the advice she provides.

Why don't people respond to risk communications and behavioural advice about their lifestyle by changing their behaviour? Certainly, when asked to evaluate a risky communication people report feeling anxious or worried (Thirlaway and Heggs, 2005). It has been argued by Thirlaway and Upton (2009) that there are three main reasons why risk communications do not result in lifestyle behavioural change.

First, lifestyle behaviours are not practised solely for health reasons. Lifestyle behaviours have other social outcomes that are often more important for people than a future risk to health, so any cost-benefit analysis carried out by individuals may include non-health outcomes that are often not considered by health-focused health professionals.

Second, health messages are predominantly focused on long-term health outcomes. This requires people to be 'future-orientated' and most people are focused in the present (Thirlaway and Upton, 2009). Health promotion is asking people to make unpalatable changes to their life now in order to reduce a risk that is a long way in the future. Consequently, people tend to look for other, less difficult ways to reduce the anxiety that a risk communication generates. It is easier to use strategies such as deciding the source of the message is untrustworthy, or to be unrealistically optimistic about your current behaviour, than it is to actually set about changing.

Third, many established health behaviours have become habitual and are controlled not by cognitive decisions but by automatic responses to the routine situations of our daily lives (Verplanken and Melkeviko, 2008). How many of us have decided to give up biscuits with our cup of coffee only to find that we are halfway through one before we remember our decision not to eat them?

Barriers

Barriers refer to those things that are part of our wider social and physical environment that prevent us carrying out behaviours we might otherwise choose to do. Individuals tend to list a set of barriers, such as lack of time, lack of resources or poor facilities, as the reason for their failure to make positive lifestyle choices. However, what is a barrier for one person, e.g. a three-mile trip to a leisure centre, may not be seen as a barrier at all for another.

The term obesogenic environment is now widely used to refer to the physical, economic, social and cultural barriers in the environment that impede the maintenance of a healthy body weight (Lee *et al.*, 2011). Barriers to successful weight maintenance are things like the easy availability of high-fat food and the environmental obstacles to active commuting. However, recently the government-commissioned Foresight Report on obesity in the UK (Jones *et al.*, 2007) concluded that the influence of the environment on obesity was not straightforward. It is not the environment *per se* that matters but the way individuals perceive it. Jones *et al.* (2007) have raised concerns that building more cycle paths may only encourage people who already cycle rather than creating more cyclists. Non-cyclists will need support to encourage them to believe that they could use the cycle paths provided in their environment.

Applying this to Caroline

Caroline needs to work at changing her clients' perceptions of the local resources available to them to increase their physical activity. She may be supported in this as active transport policies start to change the cultural norms for cycling and walking.

Social norms

As part of their detailed analysis of obesity in the UK, the Foresight authors (Jones *et al.*, 2007) argue that normative social behaviour, that is, what is acceptable behaviour to the majority of an individual's peer group, is key to understanding and promoting positive lifestyle choices. For a number of decades psychologists have found very little evidence that social norms are influential over lifestyle choices but it appears that they may have been asking the wrong questions (Thirlaway and Upton, 2009). Psychologists have carried out a lot of research looking at what is socially acceptable or unacceptable, and how motivated people are to comply with what is expected of them. Looked at in this way, there is very little evidence that social norms influence behaviour (White *et al.*, 2009). However, more recently, the field of drinking research has focused on looking at how much individuals think their peers are drinking (McAlaney and McMahon, 2007). This is a much more promising line of research and there is a clear relationship between what people think their peers are drinking and what they themselves choose to drink. This relationship has been demonstrated both in adults at work and in students at college (McAlaney and McMahon, 2007; Barrientos-Gutierrez *et al.*, 2007). The fact that people are influenced in their drinking by what they think other people are drinking is particularly interesting because of the wealth of evidence that indicates people are generally very optimistic about their own behaviour in comparison to other people (McAlaney and McMahon, 2007).

Applying this to Caroline

Caroline could use data from individuals similar to her clients to demonstrate that their behaviour is actually more risky than that of other similar people.

Social support

There is considerable evidence that social isolation or lack of social support increases the risk of developing a range of chronic diseases (Uchino, 2006; Cohen and Janicki-Deverts, 2009). Social support clearly matters for health but what is difficult is defining and measuring something so complex. As social support is fundamentally about relationships, a simple way to investigate social support is to count how many relationships an individual has. Other studies have tried to evaluate the quality of social support using questionnaires that ask questions such as: 'Do you have someone that you can share your innermost thoughts with and confide in?' (Wang *et al.*, 2005, p. 600).

Another way to think about social support is in terms of emotional support (availability of close emotional support) and social integration (availability of peripheral contacts). Social support is a complex thing; we know that it has health benefits but it is hard to identify how it is beneficial and therefore develop any strategies to build in what is lacking for the socially isolated.

One way that social support is believed to improve health is by enhancing healthy lifestyles. For example, smokers with good social support are more likely to succeed in giving up smoking (Pirie *et al.*, 1997). Jeffery and French (1996) found that social class was related to obesity in women. One difference between women from different socio-economic groups is the perceived social support from friends for healthy diet and exercise behaviours, with women from higher social classes perceiving friends as more supportive.

What is not clear is whether general social support (good emotional support and/or strong social integration) is enough to support individuals attempting to change their behaviour or whether specific support for the attempted activity is necessary. So is it enough to get general emotional support from a partner whilst dieting, or does the partner need to be supportive of the specific dieting behaviour? Similarly, it is not clear whether specific support for changing behaviour, such as that available from personal trainers or support groups, is sufficient to support long-term behavioural change and could provide the social support necessary to facilitate change for the socially isolated. It has been argued that general social support improves health outcomes by acting as a stress buffer (Uchino, 2006). Individuals who have people with whom they can talk through stressful situations and from whom they can receive emotional support may receive direct physiological benefits in terms of lower levels of stress hormones (Uchino, 2006). Equally, they may be less likely to use alcohol, high-fat food or drugs as a stress alleviator (Gruber, 2008). Specific social support such as that provided by weight reduction groups, exercise programme classes or by personal trainers or other health professionals can work at the individual level by providing positive feedback about successful behavioural change and improving self-efficacy (Gruber, 2008) but it can also, over time, provide some of the general emotional support if the relationships persist over time.

Applying this to Caroline

Caroline needs to tailor her advice to ensure it does not threaten valuable social networks and increase stress for her clients.

Self-efficacy

Self-efficacy is the belief that you can carry out a specific behaviour in a specific situation (Bandura, 1997). Self-efficacy has been found to be the best predictor of whether people will change their behaviour across all lifestyle behaviours. University students who reported higher levels of exercise self-efficacy were more likely to be physically active (Williams and French, 2011). Gilles et al. (2006) found that those with low self-efficacy for avoiding heavy drinking in social situations drank more. Higher self-efficacy has been found to predict greater ability to resist peer pressure to have sex (Dilorio et al., 2001) and a better ability to avoid risky sexual behaviour (O'Leary et al., 2008).

Self-efficacy is behaviour specific and is not transferable. So you may have high self-efficacy for taking physical activity but low self-efficacy for practising safe sex. Increasing self-efficacy in one behaviour will not translate into increased self-efficacy in other behaviours. Given the importance of self-efficacy in behavioural change, it is crucial to understand how self-efficacy can be improved or damaged.

The dieting industry is often detrimental to the self-efficacy of individuals trying to lose weight. There are many diets on the market offering rapid weight loss that is either very difficult to achieve or very difficult to maintain. A series of failed dieting attempts can seriously damage self-efficacy for weight loss. Professionals working with individuals trying to lose weight need to be aware that if they have made multiple failed attempts to lose weight and/or maintain weight loss they are likely to have very little confidence in their ability to succeed. Repeated failure is very damaging to self-efficacy.

Self-efficacy has been argued to be enhanced by personal accomplishment, mastery, vicarious experience or verbal persuasion (Williams and French, 2011). It is important to note that some of the most common behavioural techniques such as persuasion and barrier identification are associated with lower levels of self-efficacy. The strong evidence that increasing self-efficacy can promote behavioural change has generated a number of psychological strategies to support self-efficacy, including motivational interviewing, goal setting and implementation intentions, all of which will be discussed later in the chapter.

Applying this to Caroline

Caroline may want to consider how confident her clinic participants are about making the changes she is suggesting and investigate ways of increasing their self-efficacy for the proposed change.

Self-regulation

Self-regulation in the context of behavioural change refers to efforts by people to alter their responses to situational cues such as being in a pub and not ordering an alcoholic drink. It is people trying to control the number of calories they consume, the number of units of alcohol they drink, the drugs they take, the cigarettes they consume, the time they spend in sedentary activities or the amount of physical activity they take. It is likely that at any one time a majority of people will be attempting to regulate one or more of their lifestyle behaviours. The chronic diseases that are the major health issues for people in the twenty-first century can all be argued to be influenced by people's failure to control their appetites for pleasure-giving substances or behaviours. Self-regulation is closely linked to self-efficacy because if people try and succeed in regulating a behaviour, their self-efficacy will increase. However, if they try and fail to regulate a behaviour, they risk damaging their self-efficacy and are less likely to succeed if they attempt regulation again.

Successful self-regulation involves setting goals for a particular behaviour and sticking to them. So, for instance, many people try to lose weight by going on a calorie-controlled diet where they attempt to limit the amount of calories they consume each day. Interestingly, people who are dieting are more prone to bouts of disinhibited eating than people who are not attempting to diet (Herman and Polivy, 2004). At first sight this is counterintuitive, in that people who are trying to restrict their calorie intake should be less likely to overeat. However, research consistently shows that if people on a diet are asked to consume food perceived as 'high calorie', such as a rich milkshake, they are more likely than people not dieting to over-consume afterwards when provided with palatable food (Herman and Polivy, 2004). It would seem that once dieters perceive that they have 'failed' to stick to their daily calorie quota, they feel they might as well eat whatever they like. Herman and Polivy (2004, p. 498) describe this as the 'what-the-hell' effect. This then creates a real problem for health professionals attempting to encourage weight loss because the setting of goals for calorie intake may actually put individuals at greater risk of overeating. In the field of alcohol and drug addiction many treatment programmes aim for total abstinence, which is one response to the problem of disinhibition; however, total abstinence is not an option for sustained weight loss.

Fear

When the relationship between behaviour and health was first recognised and health professionals wanted to stop unhealthy behaviours they used risk communication to try to generate fear.

Fear appeals are based on the fear-drive model which argues that fear is unpleasant and people want to avoid it. If a communication makes people feel fearful or anxious then the fear-drive model suggests that the recipient will want to reduce this unpleasant state of mind. If the communication also contains advice then individuals may try to follow this advice in order to escape from the unpleasant feelings of anxiety and fear for their future health. If following the behavioural advice leads to a reduction in fear then people are likely to continue with their changed behaviour.

Fear is intuitively appealing as a means of promoting behavioural change but the role it plays in initiating behavioural change is not clear-cut or consistent (Thirlaway and Upton, 2009). Often the response to failed fear appeals is to increase the level of fear either by increasing the graphicness of the imagery or by focusing on the worst possible outcome. Gallopel-Morvan et al. (2009) found that graphic images were more effective than text messages alone in changing behavioural intentions but it is not clear whether this translates into behaviour change. Other research suggests that increasing the level of fear generated by a message does not increase the uptake of behavioural prevention strategies. One reason may be that highly fearful messages are likely to induce denial and therefore fail to have any impact on behavioural choices (Sutton, 1982). Fear appeals may be more effective when combined with self-efficacy messages which can help individuals believe there is an effective action to minimise the risk.

Habituation

Past behaviour is a powerful predictor of future behaviour (Hagger *et al.*, 2002; Conner and Norman, 2005). Consistent patterns of past behaviours are often referred to as habits. Habits are behaviours that may once have been initiated by rational choice but are now under the control of specific situational cues that trigger the behaviour without thinking (Verplanken and Melkevik, 2008; Aarts *et al.*, 1997). So, many of the choices we make about what to eat for breakfast, the amount of coffee we consume, whether we walk or drive to work on a day-to-day basis are not conscious choices at all but things we do without thinking. Health promotion and social cognition, when looking at lifestyle behavioural change, assume that lifestyle choices are always a conscious choice, which may explain why their educational strategies are less effective than they would like.

All lifestyle behaviours have the potential to become habits or even addictions. There is a tendency to assume that behaviours such as smoking and drinking that include a physiological response to the alcohol or the nicotine are harder habits to break because of the combined physiological and psychological reinforcement. However, people struggle to give up smoking long after the physiological addiction is overcome (Thirlaway and Upton, 2009), which implies that psychological addiction can be powerful alone.

Health professionals are faced with a dual problem: they need to help people break unhealthy habits and they need to support the development of healthy habits. Many of the unhealthy habits that older adults struggle with, as the negative consequences of decades of unhealthy living start to materialise, are established in adolescence and early adulthood when health is optimal, and the costs of smoking, drinking, eating badly or not exercising are in the distant future. Important outcomes for young people are identity formation and the establishment of social relationships (Kuther and Timoshin, 2003). Drinking and eating are an integral component of many social events in the UK and alcohol in particular enhances social integration and facilitates the development of relationships. Interventions that attempt to enable young people to set up healthy drinking habits need to focus on the role of alcohol for young people in the present, rather than on the cost of alcohol consumption in the future. On a positive front, sport is often central to socialisation, particularly for young men, and supports the establishment of positive physical activity habits (Thirlaway and Upton, 2009).

Health starts to become pertinent for individuals as they start to experience ill health and the costs of unhealthy lifestyles are in the present or the near future rather than in the distant future (Lawton, 2002). Unfortunately, by the time individuals wish to change their unhealthy habits they are likely to be well established and difficult to break. Research now needs to focus on understanding how we can help people change ingrained habits, and implementation intentions are one promising avenue.

Caroline needs to recognise that her clients are not disregarding her advice and probably leave her clinic with every intention to change but find it impossible to overcome ingrained habits.

Pleasure

People usually choose to do things that they enjoy. Pleasure can be argued to be the main motivation for lifestyle choices, particularly among the young (Kuntsche and Cooper, 2010). Pleasure can be experienced as a physiological sensation, for instance the response to chocolate in the mouth. Pleasure can also be experienced as a positive emotion, for instance winning a game of sport. Frequently, a pleasurable response includes both physiological and emotive sensations. Some things are innately pleasurable, such as sweet food. Other things we learn to enjoy, such as drinking alcohol. Few young people enjoy their first taste of an alcoholic drink, which is why beverage manufacturers have developed sweetened alcoholic drinks for the teenage market to make the alcohol more palatable and support the initiation of learnt enjoyment of alcohol (Plant and Plant, 2006).

Regardless of whether the pleasure is physiological or psychological, innate or learnt, if an experience is pleasurable people are more likely to repeat it. Consequently, pleasure is fundamental in the establishment of habitual behaviours. One approach to encouraging healthy lifestyle habits would be to try to elicit pleasurable responses to healthy behaviours. However, we don't understand very well how people learn to enjoy certain behaviours and not others.

Applying this to Caroline

Presumably most health professionals understand that people do things that they enjoy but they seldom take that into account when offering advice about lifestyle change.

Stages of change

As well as looking at what external factors influence behavioural change, psychologists have also looked at the motivation state of the individual who is trying to change. This approach views change not as a one-off event but as a process, and argues that health professionals need to tailor their support for individuals to their stage of change.

According to all stage theories, a person can move through a series of stages in the process of behavioural change. Different models argue for different numbers of stages that last for differing lengths of time. The most well-known Stages of Change model comes from the transtheoretical model of change which conceptualises the process of change as having five stages as described in Table 4.2.

The model argues that it is important to understand where people are in the process of change before attempting to support them to change, because depending on the stage of change you would use different techniques to encourage a change in behaviour. For example, if people are in the pre-contemplation stage you may use education to move them into contemplation. Once people are contemplating a change then motivational interviewing may be key to encouraging people to start preparing to change. During the stages of preparation and action, strategies to increase self-efficacy may be important. Which interventions are best at different stages is not well established (Thirlaway and Upton, 2009).

Applying this to Caroline

Caroline could consider tailoring her approach so that she focused on providing behavioural advice to those clients who are contemplating or preparing to change.

Table 4.2 The stages of change, conceptualised using alcohol as the health behaviour

Stages of change	Behavioural and motivational characteristics
Pre-contemplation	Individuals are drinking and have no intention of stopping in the next six months
Contemplation	Individuals are drinking but they intend to stop in the next six months
Preparation	Individuals are drinking less and intend to stop in the next six months
Action	Individuals have stopped drinking to excess within the past six months. The perceived benefits are greater than the perceived costs. This is the least stable stage
Maintenance	Individuals have been non-drinkers for over six months and risk of relapse is small

Psychological interventions

Motivational interviewing

Miller and Rollnick (2002) suggested that motivation is fundamental to change and they suggest that motivational interviewing is the appropriate approach. Motivational interviewing can be defined as 'a client-centred, directive method for enhancing intrinsic motivation to change by exploring and resolving ambivalence' (Miller and Rollnick, 2002).

Motivational interviewing aims to increase an individual's motivation to consider change rather than showing them how to change. If a person doesn't want to change then it is irrelevant if they know how to do it or not. However, if a person is motivated to change then the interventions aimed at changing behaviour can begin.

Motivational interviewing (MI) is a technique based on cognitive-behavioural therapy which aims to enhance an individual's motivation to change health behaviour. The whole process aims to help the patient understand their thought processes, to identify how their thought processes are helping to produce the inappropriate behaviour and how their thought processes can be changed to develop alternative, health-promoting, behaviours. Motivational interviewing differs from counselling because it is directive; the healthcare professional elicits and selectively reinforces change talk that resolves ambivalence and moves the client towards change.

Motivational strategies include eight components that are designed to increase the level of motivation the person has towards changing a specific behaviour. It is important to note that the motivation is specific to one behaviour and so being motivated to quit smoking does not simply transfer to being motivated to reduce alcohol consumption. The eight components are:

- Giving advice (about specific behaviours to be changed)
- Removing barriers (often about access to particular help)
- Providing choice (making it clear that if they choose not to change that is their right and it is their choice; the therapist is there to encourage change but not to insist on change)
- Decreasing desirability (of the ambivalence towards change or the status quo)
- Practising empathy
- Providing feedback (from a variety of perspectives – family, friends, health professionals – in order to give the patient a full picture of their current situation)
- Clarifying goals (feedback should be compared with a standard (an ideal), and clarification of the ideal can provide the pathway to the goal)
- Active helping (such as expressing caring or facilitating a referral, both of which convey a real interest in helping the person to change).

Although this seems relatively simple and straightforward and, to a certain extent, it is, there are a number of key skills that you need to employ in order to be successful in motivating people to change and some of these are presented in Table 4.3.

Table 4.3 Key skills for motivational interviewing

Skill	Comment
Express empathy	There should be no criticism or blame as acceptance facilitates change
Develop discrepancy	Change is motivated by a perceived discrepancy between present behaviour and personal goal
Roll with resistance	Avoid arguing for change or providing change – see the smoker as the source of information
Support self-efficacy	The smoker's belief in the possibility of change is an important motivator for change
Use open-ended questions	Encourage the client to do most of the talking: 'What are your concerns about smoking?'
Use reflective listening	Reflect back change talk in a statement: 'I had real cravings this morning' to 'You are a little concerned about the cravings in the morning'
Use affirmation	Use to build rapport: 'You are right to be concerned about smoking in front of the children'
Summarise	Link together and reinforce what has been discussed: 'You are concerned that your smoking may cause lung cancer'
Reframe or agree with a twist	Address resistance by reinterpreting: 'My kids nag me about giving up smoking' to 'It sounds like they really care about your health'
Emphasise personal choice	Reinforce that it is the client's choice to change their behaviour
Evocative questions	
Increasing confidence	Use open questions to evoke confidence talk: 'How might you go about making this change?'
Confidence ruler	Use the ruler to ask 'What would it take to score higher?'
Strengths and successes	Review obstacles and how the client has overcome them
Reframing	'I've tried three times to quit and failed' to 'You have had three good attempts already and are learning new skills'
Prompt coping strategies	Ask for potential obstacles and putative coping strategies

Source: adapted from Miller and Rollnick, 2002

Goal setting

We all set ourselves goals in all areas of life. Some psychologists would argue that goals give meaning to people's lives (Rasmussen *et al.*, 2006). The challenge for health professionals interested in behavioural change is how to utilise goal setting to support change. Goals can vary both in terms of their difficulty (running a marathon is more difficult than running a 10 km race) and in terms of their specificity (Strecher *et al.*, 1995). Someone may have a vague goal 'to eat well' or a more specific goal 'to eat a high-fibre breakfast cereal at least five times a week'.

Evidence suggests that non-specific, vague goals such as wanting to lose weight are less likely to be achieved than more specific goals such as 'I am going to stop eating chocolate biscuits for the next fortnight' (Strecher *et al.*, 1995). Health professionals therefore can support people in their overarching goals to lose weight, get fitter, control their blood sugar etc. by helping them break down their complex and long-term goals into a set of simpler, short-term sub-goals.

A major benefit of goal-directed behaviour is the possibility of positive feedback. Feedback about goal success can significantly improve subsequent performance, probably by improving self-efficacy. However, for behavioural change, difficult, complex, long-term goals (such as weight loss or fitness) are unlikely to generate immediate positive feedback. This can lead to a reduction in self-efficacy as individuals feel they are not achieving their goal and can lead to individuals giving up and reverting to their original 'bad habits'. Indeed, research suggests that failing to achieve self-regulatory goals can promote a worsening of original bad habits (Herman and Polivy, 2004). Short-term goals are much easier to link to positive feedback and can improve self-efficacy and help people stick to their change. The majority of health behaviours that people wish to change are highly complex and will require careful planning to develop an appropriate goal-setting strategy. It is generally better to set behavioural goals such as increasing exercise rather than physiological status goals such as increasing VO2 max. Behaviours are more directly under a person's control than are physiological responses. The key strategies for successful goal setting are presented in Table 4.4.

It is emerging that having an action plan about how to achieve goals that involve particularly ingrained habitual behaviours can be further supported by 'if-then' plans that provide strategies for people to achieve their goals in difficult contexts (see following section on implementation intentions).

Successful goal setting will promote self-efficacy for changing the specified behaviour, giving the client the confidence to believe that having met previous goals, they can meet the next sub-goal and that the overarching goal is possible. Ineffective goal setting, when clients fail to meet their short-term targets, can have the opposite effect and damage self-efficacy, reducing the likelihood that clients will meet their overarching goal.

Effective goal setting needs to be tailored to the individual and supported by regular feedback and encouragement. For long-term goals, such as major weight loss, this will involve considerable and sustained input from a health professional. It is not usual for health professionals to have the resources available to provide this level of individualised support. One avenue that might be worthy of exploration is whether clients can be taught effective goal-setting techniques and could then set and reward their own goals.

Table 4.4 Key recommendations for goal-setting behavioural change strategies using weight loss as the example

Strategy	Example
Explore client motivation. This might be done using the stages of change paradigm. Pre-contemplation clients are not ready for goal setting	A client has been referred to you by her GP for weight loss support. The client has been advised to lose 3 stone. Initially, you need to establish the client's personal motivation for weight loss of this magnitude
Break down a complex goal into a series of short-term sub-goals and create an action plan	You might set the client a series of short-term goals such as stop eating biscuits at coffee time for the next fortnight
Attempt where possible to set behavioural goals rather than physiological goals	You may wish to focus on the food an individual chooses to eat or on an activity such as walking rather than pounds lost over a time frame
Evaluate client self-efficacy for the various behaviours involved in goal achievement	Your client may be more confident about restricting food intake than taking exercise and your action plan needs to be tailored to client self-efficacy
Tailor sub-goals to the client to ensure they are challenging but realistic and perceived as such by the client	Your client may wish to set goals that are unrealistic, as rapid weight loss is attractive to most individuals wishing to lose weight. You need to negotiate a goal for which you are likely to be able to deliver positive feedback
Provide regular feedback to the client	Feedback needs to be regular, supportive and reflect behavioural achievements and physiological achievements if appropriate
Goal adaptation	For long-term complex change the short-term sub-goals may need to be reviewed and renegotiated as the client's physiological status and self-efficacy change in response to behavioural adaptation

Implementation intentions

One of the problems with goal setting and with behavioural change generally is that people may have decided to change, they may want to change very strongly, but because their behaviour is habitual and ingrained they may not be able to overcome the impulse to give in, in situations where they habitually practise an unhealthy behaviour. So people who are trying to give up smoking will have key situational prompts when they find it very hard to overcome the impulse to smoke; perhaps during a coffee break, or in the pub. Gollwitzer and Sheeran (2006) have suggested that people need to develop a set of 'if-then' plans to help them deal with situations where they usually do something they are trying to stop doing. For example, if your goal is to lose weight then you need to identify when you are likely to eat high-fat food and how you will respond differently in that situation. So if you usually have a cup of tea and a biscuit mid-morning you need to formulate an alternative response to replace eating a biscuit, such as eating a low-fat cracker instead.

Building 'if-then' plans into goal-setting action plans increases the involvement and commitment of the health professional. As mentioned under goal setting, it is unlikely that many health professionals currently have the resources to provide this level of support. Encouragingly Hagger *et al.* (2012) found that using motivational and implementation interventions delivered using an online format did reduce drinking in participants with high baseline alcohol consumption. Other researchers similarly report that online interventions can be effective (Kypri *et al.*, 2009). Online behavioural change interventions have the potential to provide an efficient way of providing the personalised support that is required.

Cognitive behavioural therapy

Cognitive behavioural therapy (CBT) is more traditionally associated with mental health disorders (such as anxiety, depression, panic or agoraphobia) than with lifestyle choices (Westbrook *et al.*, 2007). However, CBT may well be useful for some individuals attempting to change their lifestyle. Indeed, motivational interviewing (described earlier in the chapter) is based on aspects of CBT. However, in some instances, perhaps when the behaviour people are attempting to change is clearly addictive, there may be a place for a more complete cognitive behavioural approach than motivational interviewing. Motivational interviewing is usually a brief therapy (1–4 sessions) for enhancing motivation to change problematic health behaviours (Ismail *et al.*, 2008). Cognitive behavioural therapy is longer (a minimum of six sessions) and aims to help the client identify, challenge and substitute unhelpful thoughts (cognitions) and behaviours with more constructive ones (Ismail *et al.*, 2008). It is beyond the remit of this book to provide a comprehensive review of CBT and the reader is advised to access one of the many available texts if they wish to explore the subject further (for instance: Westbrook *et al.*, 2007). Ismail *et al.* (2008) found that CBT improved blood glucose control in patients with diabetes 12 months after the intervention whereas motivational interviewing did not. However, given that motivational interviewing is a brief intervention and CBT is a longer-term intervention, it is possible that it is the length of the intervention that results in the better outcome rather than the type of therapy itself. Longer-term interventions have the potential to provide social support for individuals attempting to change a behaviour, and it may be the social support rather than the therapeutic approach that is important.

Working effectively with others

Lifestyle change is a complex challenge which individuals must address outside of healthcare settings in their daily lives. It is if you like an upstream activity before the descent into primary, secondary or tertiary care and consequently outside of the experience of many traditional health professionals. Few health professionals, even specialists such as dieticians, have time in their workloads to work with individuals to build self-efficacy and or provide the social support that can make lifestyle change more likely. Traditionally, health practitioners in primary care have focused on ensuring that they work effectively with secondary care to identify individuals who have clinical problems that need referral to specialist services such as addiction centres or dieticians. Increasingly, as the complexities of lifestyle change are beginning to be recognised, primary care practitioners need to build relationships with a wider range of health and non-health practitioners that are community-based and can provide additional support to those embarking on lifestyle change. Understanding how health advice is translated into the normal daily lives of individuals is a different knowledge base to understanding the relationship between health behaviours and disease. If we are to reach individuals who are living in high levels of deprivation and so attempt to tackle the widening health inequalities in society, health practitioners will probably need to work with community workers, social workers, probation officers and others who have the experience and expertise in working with individuals most at need of health interventions. Links with non-health practitioners and primary care are beginning to be established. The exercise referral scheme is one newly established pathway to link primary care to community exercise schemes (See Chapter 6, Being Active). Community pharmacies are increasingly recognised as a local resource where support for lifestyle change could be provided (Thirlaway, 2011). There are also private companies such as Weight Watchers, gyms, personal trainers that can provide valuable support for individuals embarking on change. Any primary care practitioner interested in promoting lifestyle change will need to access resources that can support change on a more regular basis than is possible as an individual practitioner.

Conclusion

The various behaviours implicated in contributing to ill health – eating, drinking, smoking, illicit drug taking and sexual behaviours – are all complex behaviours that have many different roles in individuals' lives. People need to eat to stay alive and hunger is the physiological response that ensures that people do eat and don't starve to death. Viewed in this simplistic way, understanding eating behaviour should be straightforward. People should eat enough to prevent hunger. However, people eat for pleasure, they eat for comfort, they eat because they are bored, they eat because the social situation demands it, and they eat because they have got into the habit of doing so in particular situations or at particular times. Psychological theories of behavioural change have developed to try to understand how these non-biological factors influence the choices people make. Psychological theory to date gives us some clues about the key factors that influence behaviour.

Key Points

- Education about the risks and benefits of behaviour is not an effective behavioural change strategy.
- Getting people to change their lifestyle requires them to prioritise their health and change often long-established habits.
- Getting people to change their lifestyle requires them to make unpalatable changes in the 'here and now' for an uncertain benefit in the future.
- Perceptions of barriers to healthy lifestyles are more important than actual barriers; what is insurmountable for one individual will not be a problem for another.
- Self-efficacy is key to successful behavioural change; if you believe you can change you are far more likely to succeed.
- Self-regulation involves the setting of goals, but failing to achieve goals can put people at greater risk of excessive consumption. Goal setting requires a delicate balance to arrive at a sufficiently challenging but realistic goal.
- Implementation intentions can help people achieve their goals by providing strategies to deal with settings where the undesired behaviour is an ingrained habitual response to the situation.
- Social support is complex but indisputably related to health. It is possible, but not yet established, that health professionals and/or support groups could provide useful social support for behavioural change.
- The stage of change that an individual is in may influence their response to an intervention.
- The aim of motivational interviewing is to increase an individual's motivation to change.

Discussion points

- Motivational interviewing requires a client-centred perspective and requires the professional to let the client set their own objectives for change. How can we balance that against a requirement to give professional advice?
- Many people seeking help with weight loss will have tried and failed to lose weight many times before finally seeking professional help. They are likely to have low self-efficacy. How would you go about re-building self-efficacy in such clients?
- Breaking bad habits and establishing new good habits can be a long process. How can health professionals manage to provide sustained support for individuals attempting to change their behaviour?

Further resources

Thirlaway, K.J. and Upton, D. (2009). *The Psychology of Lifestyle: Promoting Healthy Behaviour*. London: Routledge.

Conner, M. and Norman, P. (2005) *Predicting Health Behaviour*. Berkshire: Open University Press.

Change4Life 0300 123 4567 http://www.nhs.uk/Change4Life

References

Aarts, H., Paulussen, T. and Schaalma, H. (1997). Physical exercise habit: on the conceptualization and formation of habitual health behaviours. *Health Education Research*, 21: 363–374.

Bandura, A. (1997). *Self-efficacy: The Exercise of Control*. New York: W.H. Freeman.

Barrientos-Gutierrez, T., Gimeno, D., Mangiane, T.W., Harrist, R.B. and Amick, B.C. (2007). Drinking social norms and drinking behaviours. *Occupational and Environmental Medicine*, 64: 602–608.

Blaxter, M. (2004). *Health and Lifestyles*. London: Routledge.

Cabinet Office Strategy Unit. (2002). *Risk: Improving Government Capability to Handle Risk and Uncertainty*. London: Cabinet Office.

Cohen, S. and Janicki-Deverts, D. (2009). Can we improve our physical health by altering our social networks? *Perspectives on Psychological Science* 4(4): 375–378.

Conner, M. and Norman, P. (2005). *Predicting Health Behaviour*, 2nd edn. Berkshire: Open University Press.

Connolly, T., Arkes, H.R. and Hammond, K.R. (2000). *Judgement and Decision Making: An Interdisciplinary Reader*. Cambridge: Cambridge University Press.

Department of Health. (1999). *Saving Lives: Our Healthier Nation*. London: The Stationery Office.

——(2010). *Healthy Lives, Healthy People: Our Strategy for Public Health in England*. London: The Stationery Office Ltd.

Dilorio, C., Dudley, W.N., Kelly, M., Soet, J., Mbwara, J. and Sharpe Potter, J. (2001). Social cognitive correlates of sexual experience and condom use among 13 though 15 year old adolescents. *Journal of Adolescent Health*, 29: 208–216.

Gallopel-Morvan, K., Gabriel, P., Le Gall-Ely, M., Rieunier, S. and Urien, B. (2009). The use of visual warnings in social marketing: the case of tobacco. *Journal of Business Research*, 64(1): 7–11.

Gilles, D.M., Turk, C.L. and Fresco, D.M. (2006). Social anxiety, alcohol expectancies, and self-efficacy as predictors of heavy drinking in college students. *Addictive Behaviors*, 31: 388–398.

Gollwitzer, P.M. and Sheeran, P. (2006). Implementation intentions and goal achievement: a meta-analysis of effects and processes. *Advances in Experimental Social Psychology*, 38: 69–119.

Gruber, K.J. (2008). Social support for exercise and dietary habits among college students. *Adolescence*, 43(171): 557–575.

Hagger, M.S., Chatzisarantis, N.L.D. and Biddle, S.J.H. (2002). A meta-analytic review of the theories of reasoned action and planned behaviour in physical activity: predictive validity and the contribution of additional variables. *Journal of Sport and Exercise Psychology*, 24: 3–32.

Hagger, M.S., Lonsdale, A.J. and Chatzisarantis, N.L.D. (2012). A theory-based intervention to reduce alcohol drinking in excess of guideline limits among undergraduate students. *British Journal of Health Psychology*, 17: 18–43.

Herman, C.P. and Polivy, J. (2004). The self-regulation of eating: theoretical and practical problems. In R.F. Baumeister and K.D. Vohs (eds), *Handbook of Self Regulation: Research, Theory and Applications*. London: The Guilford Press.

Ismail, K., Thomas, S.M., Maissi, E., Chalder, T., Schmidt, U., Barlett, J., Patel, A., Dickens, C.M., Creed, F. and Treasure, J. (2008). Motivational enhancement therapy with and without cognitive behaviour therapy to treat type 1 diabetes. *Annals of Internal Medicine*, 149: 708–719.

Jeffery, R.W. and French, S.A. (1996). Socioeconomic status and weight control practices among 20 to 45 year old women. *American Journal of Public Health*, 86(7): 1005–1010.

Jones, A., Bentham, G., Foster, C., Hillsdon, M. and Panter, J. (2007). *Tackling Obesities: Future Choices – Obesogenic Environments – Evidence Review*. London: United Kingdom Government Foreign Programmes Office of Science and Innovation. Crown Copyright.

Kuntsche, E. and Cooper, M. L. (2010). Drinking to have fun and to get drunk: motives as predictors of weekend drinking over and above usual drinking habits. *Drug and Alcohol Dependence*, 110(3): 259–262.

Kuther, T.L. and Timoshin, A. (2003). A comparison of social cognitive and psychosocial predictors of alcohol use by college students. *Journal of College Student Development*, 44: 143–154.

Kypri, K., Hallett, J., Howat, P., McManus, A., Maycock, B., Bowe, S.J. and Horton, N.J. (2009). Randomized controlled trial of proactive web-based alcohol screening and brief intervention for university students. *Archives of Internal Medicine*, 169: 1508–1514.

Lawton, J. (2002). Colonising the future: temporal perceptions and health-relevant behaviors across the adult lifecourse. *Sociology of Health and Illness*, 24: 714–733.

Lawton, R. and Conner, M. (2007). Beyond cognition: predicting health risk behaviours from instrumental and affective beliefs. *Health Psychology*, 26: 259–267.

Lee, R.E., McAlexander, K.M. and Banda, J.A. (2011) *Reversing the Obesogenic Environment*. USA: Human Kinetics.

McAlaney, J. and McMahon, J. (2007). Normative beliefs, misperceptions and heavy episodic drinking in a British student sample. *Journal of Studies on Alcohol and Drugs*, 68(3): 385–392.

Miller, W.R. and Rollnick, S. (2002). *Motivational Interviewing: Preparing People for Change*, 2nd edn. New York: Guilford Press.

Nigg, C.R., Borrelli, B., Maddock, J. and Dishman, R.K. (2008). A theory of physical activity maintenance. *Applied Psychology: An International Review*, 57(4): 544–560.

O'Leary A., Jemmott, L.T. and Jemmott III, J.B. (2008). Mediation analysis of an effective sexual risk-reduction intervention for women: the importance of self-efficacy. *Health Psychology*, 27(2): 180–184.

Pirie, P., Rooney, B., Pechacek, T., Lando, H. and Schmid, L. (1997). Incorporating social support into a community-wide smoking cessation contest. *Addictive Behaviour*, 22(1): 131–137.

Plant, M. and Plant, M. (2006). *Binge Britain*. Oxford: Oxford University Press.

Rasmussen, H.N., Wrosch, C., Scheier, M.F. and Carver, C.S. (2006). Self-regulation processes and health: the importance of optimism and goal adjustment. *Journal of Personality*, 74(6): 1721–1747.

Strecher, V.J., Seijts, G.H., Kok, G.J., Latham, G.P., Glasgow, R., DeVellis, B., Meertens, R.M. and Bulger, D.W. (1995). Goal setting as a strategy for health behaviour change. *Health Education Quarterly*, 22(2): 190–200.

Sutton, S. (1982). Fear-arousing communications: a critical examination of theory and research. In J.R. Eiser (ed.) *Social Psychology and Behavioural Medicine*. London: Wiley, pp. 303–337.

Thirlaway, K. (2011). Lifestyle change. *Welsh Chemist Review*. Winter: 18–19.

Thirlaway, K.J. and Heggs, D. (2005). Interpreting risk messages: women's responses to a health story. *Health, Risk and Society*, 7: 107–121.

Thirlaway, K.J. and Upton, D. (2009). *The Psychology of Lifestyle: Promoting Healthy Behaviour*. London: Routledge.

Uchino B.N. (2006). Social support and health: a review of physiological processes potentially underlying links to disease outcomes. *Journal of Behavioral Medicine*, 29(4): 377–387.

Verplanken, B. and Melkeviko, O. (2008). Predicting habit: the case of physical activity. *Psychology of Sport and Exercise*, 9(1): 15–26.

Wang, H.X., Mittleman, M.A. and Orth-Gomer, K. (2005). Influence of social support on progression of coronary heart disease in women. *Social Science and Medicine*, 60: 599–607.

Westbrook, D., Kennedy, H. and Krik, J. (2007). *An Introduction to Cognitive Behavioural Therapy*. London: Sage.

White, K.M., Smith, J.R., Terry, D.J., Greenslade, J.H. and McKimmie, B.M. (2009). Social influence in the theory of planned behavior: the role of descriptive, injunctive and in-group norms. *British Journal of Social Psychology*, 48(1): 135–158.

WHO (2012). *Health Education: Theoretical Concepts, Effective Strategies and Core Competencies: A Foundation Document to Guide Capacity Development of Health Educators*. Regional Office for the Eastern Mediterranean: World Health Organization.

Williams, S.L. and French, D.P. (2011). What are the most effective intervention techniques for changing physical activity self-efficacy and physical activity behavior – and are they the same? *Health Education Research*, 26(2): 308–322.

Eating well

Case study

Robert is a 28-year-old man who works in the finance office of a large supermarket chain. Bob, as he likes to be called, has been working in an office since completing his accountancy degree a few years ago. Bob always had a problem with his weight, but since his son was born some five years ago his weight has ballooned and he now tips the scales at 23 stone (or 146 kilos). He has found that access to a regular wage packet, limited exercise, regular nights out and access to a plentiful supply of food (he has a staff discount) mean that he has put on considerable weight.

Bob is married and currently has a five-year-old son, Dave, although he and his wife are trying for another child. His wife is also obese and they fear that their weight is getting in the way of them having another child. Dave is rather chubby and takes a great delight in eating fish fingers and chips to the exclusion of most other food!

Bob now finds that his regular diet of takeaways and pre-packaged meals with limited fruit and vegetables is leading him on a downward spiral. He used to play five-a-side football with 'the lads', but given his weight and because he becomes out of breath easily he has stopped playing, merely turning up for the post-match drinking session.

Bob has recently had a health scare; he had a pain in the centre of his chest and was rushed to hospital where he was admitted overnight for observation. This caused great family concern and started to get them all to worry about their lifestyle. Although the hospital tests revealed no significant problems, his blood pressure was high (160/100 mmHg) and his BMI (44) placed him in the morbidly obese category. He was referred to you to try to reduce his weight and improve his overall weight control.

Applying this to Bob

In order to help Bob and work with him and his family to reduce his weight and improve his lifestyle it is important to consider three main things; improving his diet, reducing his weight and installing an exercise regime.

Introduction

Unlike many of the other behaviours (e.g. smoking or drinking alcohol) discussed in this text, we all eat and we all have to eat. Eating can have a protective benefit; for example, eating a healthy diet protects from a third of all cancers, diabetes, osteoporosis, heart disease, strokes and tooth decay. In contrast, having an unhealthy diet can lead to considerable health damage, such as osteoporosis, heart disease and cancer. It is estimated that obesity, on average, is associated with a 30 per cent increased mortality rate, thus indicating that BMI can be a predictor of mortality (Whitlock *et al.*, 2009). Forecast estimates suggest that moving towards the recommended diet could result in significant benefits in terms of both mortality and morbidity (see Table 5.1).

Table 5.1 Premature mortality and morbidity improvements
resulting from move towards recommended diets

	Premature mortality avoided	Quality adjusted life years (QALYs) gained
Increase fruit and vegetable intake by 136 g/day	42,000	411,000
Reduce daily salt intake from average 9 g to 6 g	20,000	170,000
Cut saturated fat intake by 2.5% of energy	3,500	33,000
Cut added sugar intake by 1.75% of energy	3,500	49,000

Source: Ofcom, 2006

Government recommendations

The national guidelines suggest that a healthy diet is a balanced diet based on five major food groups: breads, other cereals and potatoes; fruit and vegetables; milk and dairy foods; meat, fish and alternatives; and foods containing fats and sugars (see Photograph 5.1). The Department of Health (DOH) (1999) defines good nutrition in the 'Saving Lives: Our Healthier Nation' document as 'plenty of fruit and vegetables, cereals, and not too much fatty and salty food'. The NHS advice has developed over time, although the advice is still non-specific: 'Starchy foods such as rice and pasta; with plenty of fruit and vegetables; some protein-rich foods such as meat, fish and lentils; some milk and dairy foods; and not too much fat, salt or sugar' (NHS Live Well website, 2012).

In addition to this general 'eat well' guidance, there are two specific government recommendations: eat at least five portions of fruit and vegetables per day, and reduce consumption of salt to a maximum of 6g per day. The government launched Change4Life in 2009. This initiative encompasses six behaviour changes for adults, including 'fibre swap'; encouraging wholegrain, fruit and vegetable intake, '150 active minutes' to promote physical activity and 'cutting down on alcohol' (DOH, 2011a). One of the major recommendations, and the one that has been the focus of much marketing and advertising, is that at least five portions of fruit and vegetables are consumed each day (NHS, 2011; World Health Organization (WHO), 2004), with a portion being approximately 80g (e.g. one medium apple, or three heaped tablespoons of peas). In addition, there was specific guidance on salt intake with the aim being the reduction in consumption to a maximum of 6g per day.

The eatwell plate

Use the eatwell plate to help you get the balance right. It shows how much of what you eat should come from each food group.

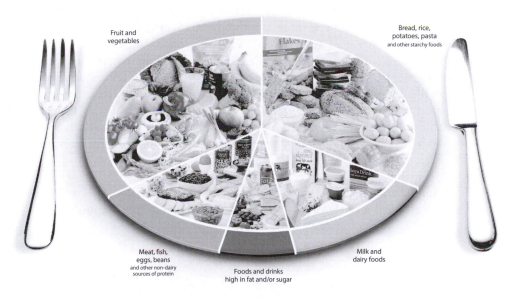

Public Health England in association with the Welsh Government, the Scottish Government and the Food Standards Agency in Northern Ireland

Photograph 5.1 Balance of a good diet

Source: From Food Standards Agency, http://www.eatwell.gov.uk/healthydiet/eatwellplate/?lang=en, © Crown copyright 2007. Crown copyright material is reproduced with permission under the terms of the Click-Use Licence

Applying this to Bob

Bob eats a limited amount of fruit and vegetables, in addition to consuming a lot of processed and takeaway convenience foods that can contain high levels of salt. Therefore Bob should cut down the amount of convenience foods he eats alongside increasing the amounts of fruit and vegetables consumed to ensure he stays within recommended government guidelines. Abiding by this will have a positive impact on his health.

Evidence from the National Diet and Nutritional Survey (2011) found consumption of fruit and vegetables was three portions or less for children per day. Boys were eating 3.1 portions a day compared to girls eating 2.7 portions (aged 11–18). In addition only

10 per cent of children and 30 per cent of adults (19–64 years) were eating the recommended '5 A Day' (Bates *et al.*, 2011).

The overall rates of daily fruit and vegetable consumption as per government guidelines for adults aged 16 years and above varied considerably by country. Wales observed the highest overall rate of adults meeting the recommended daily intake of at least five portions of fruit and vegetable as compared to Scotland which had the lowest (35 per cent and 22 per cent respectively). The percentage of adults meeting these guidelines has increased since 2003 with the exception of Wales where there has been a decline in the rate of adults consuming the recommended 5 A Day. Gender differences exist within the data. Across all four home countries, proportionately more women than men meet government guidelines to consume at least five portions of fruit and vegetables daily. At the other extreme, only Scotland and Wales explicitly report data for adults who did not consume any fruit and vegetable at all during the previous day (see Table 5.2).

Table 5.2 The percentage of men and women living in the UK achieving the government guidelines for daily fruit and vegetable consumption (based on guidelines set out in '5 A Day', DoH)

Source of data	*% of adults achieving 5 or more portions of fruit and vegetables daily*	*% of men achieving 5 or more portions of fruit and vegetables daily*	*% of women achieving 5 or more portions of fruit and vegetables daily*	*% of adults not consuming any fruit and vegetables daily*
Health Survey for England (2008)	27%	25%	29%	Not reported
Health Survey for Scotland 2010 (Bromley and Given, 2011)	22%	20%	23%	10%
Welsh Health Survey 2010 (Welsh Government, 2011)	35%	33%	36%	8%
Health Survey Northern Ireland 2010/2011 (Department of Health, Social Services and Public Safety, 2011)	33%	27%	36%	Not reported

Social class differences are also apparent, with those in the working class consuming 50 per cent less than those in professional groups. A particular area of concern is children's diet – research suggests that nearly 20 per cent of those aged between 4 and 18 years eat no fruit at all during a typical week (Scientific Advisory Committee on Nutrition (SACN), 2008). Despite considerable effort, increased marketing commitment and expenditure towards increasing the consumption of fruit and vegetables, there has been little success (SACN, 2008).

Health consequences of a poor diet

A poor diet can contribute to a range of illnesses, including both coronary heart disease (CHD) and cancer (see Table 5.3). A poor diet can also result in increased falls and fractures in older people, low birth weight, increased childhood morbidity and mortality, and increased dental cavities in children (see Table 5.4 for links between specific nutrient deficits and poor health). There is also evidence to support the link between poor diet and anti-social behaviour, not to mention growing concern over the economic implications of the population's weight gain.

The benefits of an improved diet have been highlighted in a number of public health documents and government policies. For example:

- High cholesterol levels are one of eight risk factors that account for 61 per cent of cardiovascular deaths a year worldwide. Reducing the intake of saturated fat could reduce these numbers (World Health Organization [WHO], 2009).
- The incidence of strokes could be decreased by increasing the consumption of fruit and vegetables.
- Hypertension could be reduced by reducing the salt intake and therefore have a positive impact on the incidence of cardiovascular diseases such as CHD/stroke (Bibbins-Domingo et al., 2010).
- Approximately 40 per cent of endometrial cancer and 10 per cent of breast and colon cancers would be avoided by maintaining a healthy weight (i.e. BMI of 25 or less).
- Increased dietary fibre is associated with a decreased risk of colorectal and pancreatic cancer.

Table 5.3 Diseases associated with obesity

Cardiovascular disease
Cancer
Diabetes
Stroke
Hypertension
Angina
Dental decay

Table 5.4 Health risks associated with lack of dietary elements

	Found in	Health risk
Vitamin A	Liver, cheese, eggs and oily fish	Weakening of immune system
Vitamin B6	Poultry, whole cereals and peanuts	Depression and irritability
Vitamin B12	Meat, salmon, cheese and eggs	Anaemia
Vitamin C	Oranges, peppers, broccoli, cabbage	Bleeding gums, aching joints
Vitamin D	Oily fish, eggs	Muscle weakness and aching bones
Calcium	Milk, cheese, broccoli and cabbage	Bone and tooth decay
Folic acid	Broccoli, Brussel sprouts, peas, brown rice	Anaemia
Iron	Meat, bones, whole grains and watercress	Anaemia
Magnesium	Spinach, nuts, bread	Tiredness and bone and tooth decay
Vitamin B3	Beef, pork, eggs and milk	Skin problems, dizziness, swelling of tongue
Potassium	Bananas, vegetables, nuts	Irregular heartbeat, irritability and nausea
Vitamin B2	Mushrooms, rice, eggs and milk	Skin problems, difficulty sleeping
Vitamin B1	Peas and other vegetables, pork, milk and cheese	Headaches and tiredness
Zinc	Meat, shellfish, milk and cheese	Hair loss, skin problems, diarrhoea

Obesity may be a risk factor in a number of chronic diseases such as heart disease, stroke, some cancers and type 2 diabetes (Wang *et al.*, 2011). Figures from The Health and Social Care Information Centre (2011) suggest that in 2008, 94 per cent of adults who were classified as obese suffered from high blood pressure compared to 49 per cent of adults who were not classified as obese. Greater awareness of the disease burden associated with obesity has led to concern over the economic implications of the population's weight gain. The Department of Health (2011b) estimates that overweight and obesity currently cost the NHS £5.1bn per year, around 5–6 per cent of their total budget spend. Coupled with indirect costs such as loss of earnings, it is predicted that the figure could rise to just under £50bn in 2050, if obesity rates continue unchecked.

The consequences of a poor diet are more than just obesity. For example, it has been suggested that around 38.6 per cent of lung cancer is caused by smoking cigarettes – but around 20.5 per cent can be attributable, in some part, to poor diet and obesity (Parkin, 2011) and in the United States it has been estimated that overweight and obesity contribute to 14–20 per cent of all cancer-related deaths (Kushi *et al.*, 2012). A diet involving significant intake of high-fat foods, high levels of salt and low levels of fibre appears to be particularly implicated (World Cancer Research Fund, 2007).

In addition to cancer, excessive fat intake has been implicated in disease and death from several serious illnesses, including CHD. According to recent research, cardiovascular and cancer deaths are related to the type and quality of the food we consume. It is suggested that replacing a portion of red meat per day with food such as fish and poultry can help to reduce mortality rates by up to 19 per cent (Pan *et al.*, 2012). Losing even as little weight as 5 per cent has been proven to significantly reduce health risks (Powell *et al.*, 2007). Obesity is an important issue in the poverty–poor diet–poor health cycle. A report by the Cabinet Office (2008) estimated that food-related ill health is responsible for about 70,000 premature deaths every year in the UK. Research has also concluded that the cost to the health service of dealing with poor dietary habits was significantly higher than the estimate for the annual cost of smoking, which is around £3.3 billion. They estimated that food accounts for costs of £5.8 billion a year (Scarborough *et al.*, 2011). It should be emphasised that this chapter will explore the obesity 'epidemic' and this side of the diet equation rather than the malnutrition side of a poor diet (although the latter has been suggested as costing the NHS some £13 billion a year, i.e. higher than the cost of obesity; Elia and Russell, 2009).

Applying this to Bob

Bob is at an increased risk of developing cancer, heart disease, diabetes and other chronic diseases as a result of his poor diet. Also his poor intake of fruit and vegetables could leave him with low levels of potassium, folic acid and vitamin C.

Obviously, eating the right foods can prevent illness and promote health. For example, eating fruit and vegetables may offer protection against some forms of cancer. (e.g. Aune *et al.*, 2011). Block *et al.* (1992) suggested that on the basis of 132 of 170 studies there is evidence to suggest that fruit and vegetables offer significant protection against cancer. However, recent reports (e.g. Key, 2011) suggest that this study was less convincing than initially considered given that, along with many others, it failed to take account of confounding variables such as smoking (World Cancer Research Fund, 2007) and consequently the relationship between fruit and vegetable intake and cancer may be somewhat dubious. However, specific phytonutrients (certain plant chemicals) may protect against certain cancers; cruciferous vegetables, for example, such as broccoli, cabbage and cauliflower and carotenoids such as lycopene, found in tomatoes and β-Carotene, in orange and yellow fruits and vegetables have demonstrated unique anti-carcinogenic properties (Pilátová *et al.*, 2011; Tanaka *et al.*, 2012). Key (2011) disputes the fact that fruit and vegetables offer specific 'broad spectrum' cancer protection amongst otherwise well-nourished individuals, but does draw a link between their role in decreasing nutrient deficiencies and consequentially reducing cancer risk in those with a poor diet. Other studies have indicated that fruit and vegetable intake is also of benefit for stroke and heart disease (Scarborough *et al.*, 2011).

Assessment of diet

There are many ways of assessing diet, but the most easily employed within a clinical setting would be the recording of a food diary (see Table 5.5). In this case, the individual patient or client would be asked to record their daily intake of a range of foodstuffs (based on the five categories in the eatwell plate).

The other method of assessing the consequence of diet is to infer it from body measurements. The most common form of body measurement is the Body Mass Index (BMI). BMI is calculated using the equation weight (kg)/height (m^2) or can be read from a graph (see Figure 5.1). Although BMI is a good way of assessing body fat levels for the average person, there are problems when using this method to assess muscular people (overestimates possible) and the elderly (possible underestimate of true BMI). For example, athletes and well-trained body builders have a very low percentage of body fat, but their BMI may be in the overweight range. This is because BMI does not distinguish between fat mass and lean mass. Similarly, others have argued that it is overestimated in tall people and underestimated in shorter people with the need for a new, revised formula (see: http://people.maths.ox.ac.uk/trefethen/bmi.html). However, this suggestion has not been widely accepted and certainly the simple formula for BMI calculation is easy to calculate and understand.

For adults, BMI provides a simple guide to whether weight matches height appropriately. For children, however, BMI is more complex because weight varies with height as children grow. It is calculated the same way as for adults but then compared to typical values for other children of the same age and biological sex.

Table 5.5 Your food diary

Think back over the last week. On how many days did you eat fruit, vegetables, fried food and high-fat dairy food? Fill in the table below.

Food type	How many days in a week do you eat this type of food?
Fruit (e.g. bananas, apples, mangoes, pears and plums)	
Vegetables (carrots, peas, broccoli)	
Fried food (e.g. burgers, fried chips, chicken)	
High-fat dairy food (e.g. ice cream, full fat milk, cheese, butter)	

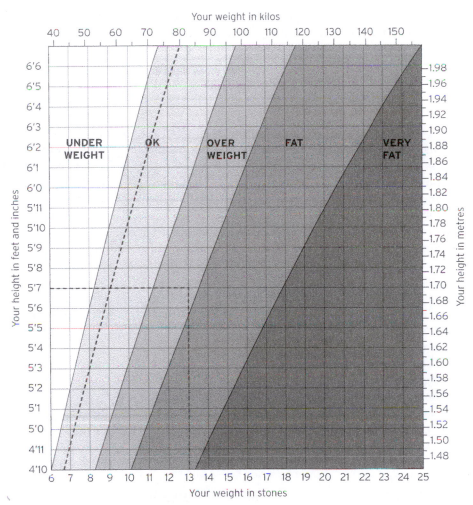

Figure 5.1 BMI measurements

For adults, BMI provides a simple guide to whether weight matches height appropriately. For children, however, BMI is more complex because weight varies with height as children grow. It is calculated the same way as for adults but then compared to typical values for other children of the same age and biological sex.

Applying this to Bob

Bob weighs 23 stone (146 kilos), and his BMI is 44, this places him in the very fat category on the BMI measurement graph. This puts Bob at high risk of developing weight related health problems.

Using the UK National BMI percentile classification system for children aged 2–15 years, overweight and obesity are categorised as shown in Table 5.6.

Although it is rather crude and imprecise, BMI is a useful measure of adiposity and correlates well with the risk of obesity-related diseases (Brown *et al.*, 2010). In many studies, BMI is calculated using self-report height and weight. However, a recent systematic review has demonstrated that this self-report BMI may be lower than a measured BMI, i.e. some obese individuals are being misclassified as being non-obese based on self-reported BMI (Connor Gorber *et al.*, 2007). Importantly, this self-report misclassification is not random: moderately obese individuals are more likely to side with non-obese than severely obese, the latter having a BMI which is further away from the obese/non-obese cut-off value. Consequently, you should always take recordings of height and weight rather than rely on self-report, as this may be an underestimate. Another issue may be the time of day measurements are taken. There are certain diurnal variations in weight which may result in over or underestimation of BMI (Routen *et al.*, 2011). Again, care should be taken to ensure consistency of recordings.

An alternative method for assessing body size is to measure waist circumference. Although most people can measure their own waist size, they usually do it at the smallest point rather than the appropriate place (see Table 5.7). The final method for assessing body shape is the waist-to-hip ratio (see Table 5.7). The waist-to-hip ratio is a simple measure of where fat is stored on the body. Most people store their body fat in two places: around their waist and around their hips. Storing extra weight around your waist (apple shaped) puts a person at a higher health risk than someone carrying extra weight around their hips and thighs (pear shaped). Waist-to-hip ratio is calculated by dividing the waist measurement by hip measurement.

Table 5.6 UK National BMI percentile classification for children aged 2–15 years

Description	BMI *centile for child's exact age*
Not overweight	85th centile or below
Overweight	Over 85th to 95th centile
Obese	95th centile or over

Table 5.7 How to get waist and hip measurements

Use a measuring tape to take the waist and hip measurement:
Waist: This measurement should be taken at the smaller section of the natural waist, usually located just above the belly button.
Hips: Hip measurement should be taken at the hips on the widest part of your buttocks.
Healthy waist-to-hip ratios
A healthy waist-to-hip ratio for women is **0.8** or lower.
A healthy ratio for men is **1.0** or lower.
Ratios above **0.8** for women and **1.0** for men are associated with obesity and are linked to greater risk of health complications and diseases.

Both BMI and waist sizes come with cut-offs that suggest whether the individual has a problem with their size or not (see Table 5.8).

Why do people eat unhealthily?

There have been a number of explanations for why people eat what they do, and these have ranged from the genetic through to the social-environmental, taking in media and cognitive factors along the way. Although it is impossible in this brief review to cover all these different proposals, it is worth exploring some of them to examine how they translate into interventions.

The media

The media is often cited as one of the major reasons for the increase in diet problems in the developed world (Boyce, 2007). There have been a number of studies that have linked TV viewing and childhood obesity, with the conclusion that television viewing is associated with obesity (Sodhi, 2010). There are a number of potential explanations for this link, but two predominate. On the one hand, it may be that watching TV encourages a sedentary lifestyle. Alternatively, it may be that media advertising promotes unhealthy consumption, and research has confirmed that this may be the case (Harris *et al.*, 2009).

Obesogenic environments

The term obesogenic environment was coined by Swinburn *et al.* (1999) who argued that the physical, economic, social and cultural environments of the developed world promote positive energy balance (i.e. calorie intake exceeding calorie output) and consequently weight gain and obesity. Examples of environmental influences that may encourage us to eat more than we need include the marketing of energy-dense drinks

Table 5.8 Risk of associated disease according to BMI and waist size

BMI		Waist less than or equal to 40 in. (men) or 35 in. (women)	Waist greater than 40 in. (men) or 35 in. (women)
18.5 or less	Underweight		N/A
18.5–24.9	Normal	–	N/A
25.0–29.9	Overweight	Increased	High
30.0–34.9	Obese	High	Very high
35.0–39.9	Obese	Very high	Very high
40 or greater	Extremely obese	Extremely high	Extremely high

and snacks, for example through television advertising and vending machines in schools, and the increase in portion sizes where an average meal may provide up to 2,000 kcal – almost the entire recommended daily intake for most adults. Time constraints on workers have led to an increase in demand for convenience food, pre-packaged foods with short preparation times, and in food consumption away from the home. This has also led to a decrease in structured meals and an increase in snacking which is often (although not always) densely calorific, along with the emergence of fast-food restaurants, which are associated with a high-fat diet.

Applying this to Bob

Bob works in an office spending a lot of time sitting down each day. Alongside this his work in the supermarket enables him to receive a discount on food he purchases. His sedentary behaviour and his motivation to purchase food are both environmental contributors to his poor diet and weight gain.

Psychosocial factors

Some key social factors associated with a poor diet include:

- *Low income and debt:* Healthier foods are generally more expensive than the less healthy alternatives. Fresh fruit and vegetables are less affordable.
- *Poor accessibility to affordable healthy foods:* Many local shops are closing and being replaced with larger, out-of-town stores. This is particularly an issue in deprived areas where such developments mean that there are increased costs within the local shops, poor-quality foodstuffs and less choice remaining in the locality. The out-of-town public stores may have poor transport links and consequently not be as easily accessible as the local shops with poor quality and expensive food.
- *Factors involved in food production and the food chain:* The cheap nutrient level of easily available foodstuffs such as TV dinners may contain high fat, sugar or salt content.
- *Poor literacy and numeracy skills:* These are barriers to maintaining a healthy diet, household budget, management and employment.
- *Food labelling:* The recently introduced food labelling agreement means that more information is available to the consumer. However, there is still some disagreement about the nature of the information provided and the value derived by the consumer from the information.
- *Food marketing:* Adverts to children usually focus on food that is high in fat or sugar. Consequently, the government is introducing new restrictions on what can

be advertised and marketed to young children. However, there is still doubt about the finer details of this approach and, given its recent introduction, its success is yet to be assessed.

Models of eating behaviour

One core theoretical psychological perspective of why people have unhealthy diets is the developmental approach, which suggests that food preferences are learned in childhood and can be understood in terms of exposure, social learning and associative learning.

Developmental approach

For infants and children, eating is typically a social event and others can have a considerable impact on children's food preferences and food selections. Hence, from a social learning perspective, it would be suggested that children's preferences for and consumption of disliked vegetables were enhanced when children observed peers selecting and eating foods that the observing child disliked. Parental behaviour and attitudes are central to the process of social learning; however, this association is not straightforward, as parents often differentiate between themselves and their children in terms of food-related motivations and food choice, and it has been suggested that food preferences in children are influenced more by genetic factors than acquired (Osera *et al.*, 2012). Promise of a reward is a time-honoured parental tactic for promoting consumption of healthy food. Nevertheless, it has been argued that treating food consumption in this way may actually decrease liking for that food (Birch, 1999, p. 53). This is a debated topic which has conflicting views. It has been acknowledged that the relationship between eating behaviour and rewards is not a simple one and different rewarding techniques are beneficial when considering differing outcomes i.e. consumption vs. liking (Cooke *et al.*, 2011).

The developmental model emphasises the importance of learning and focuses on the development of food preferences in childhood. From this perspective, eating behaviour is influenced by exposure, social learning and associative learning.

Applying this to Bob

Dave will develop eating behaviours partly through social learning from Bob. Therefore if Bob can change his dietary habits and eat a healthier diet this should impact upon Dave.

Cognitive approach

Cognitive models of eating behaviour explore the extent to which cognitions predict and explain behaviour. Most research from a cognitive perspective has drawn on social cognition models, and several models have been developed (see Chapter 7 for details on some of these models); the Health Belief Model (HBM: Becker and Rosenstock, 1984), Protection Motivation Theory (PMT: Rogers, 1985), Health Action Process Approach (HAPA: Schwarzer, 1992), Theory of Reasoned Action (TRA: Fishbein and Ajzen, 1975) and its descendant the Theory of Planned Behaviour (TPB: Ajzen, 1985). All five models share the assumption that attitudes and beliefs are major determinants of eating behaviour; however, they vary in terms of the cognitions they include and whether they use behavioural intentions or actual behaviour as their outcome measure.

These cognitive models of eating behaviour explore the extent to which cognitions predict and explain behaviour. Cognitive models are not only informative with regard to their ability to predict behaviour, but also provide a helpful insight into ways of influencing this behaviour (Ogden, 2007).

Improving diet

The National Institute for Health and Clinical Excellence (NICE) (2007) have published a set of generic principles that can be used as the basis for planning and delivering interventions aimed at changing health-related behaviours. The guidance is for healthcare professionals with direct or indirect responsibility for helping people to change their health behaviour. NICE recommend that practitioners working with individuals should select interventions that motivate and support people to:

- understand the short-, medium- and longer-term consequences of their health-related behaviours, for themselves and others;
- feel positive about the benefits of health-enhancing behaviours and changing their behaviour;
- plan their changes in terms of easy steps over time;
- recognise how their social contexts and relationships may affect their behaviour, and identify and plan for situations that might undermine the changes they are trying to make;
- plan explicit 'if-then' coping strategies to prevent relapse;
- make a personal commitment to adopt health-enhancing behaviours by setting (and recording) goals to undertake clearly defined behaviours, in particular contexts, over a specified time;
- share their behaviour change goals with others.

This guidance should be read in conjunction with other health guidance issued by NICE. For example, NICE (2006) have published specific recommendations on how to increase the effectiveness of interventions to improve diet and reduce energy intake. In this case, NICE recommend that dietary interventions should:

- Be multi-component (i.e. including dietary modification, targeted advice, family involvement and goal setting).
- Be tailored to the individual.
- Provide ongoing support.
- Include behaviour change strategies.
- Include awareness-raising promotional activities as part of a longer-term, multi-component intervention rather than a one-off activity.

Hence, the healthcare professional needs to be aware of the interventions that are available – whether they are structural, psychological or medical. A number of interventions have been developed and implemented to improve diet and eating behaviours. These have been at both individual and community level. Those that are most relevant to the practising healthcare professional are presented here. How they can be implemented with individuals will be described so that essential tips can be appreciated.

Applying this to Bob

If Bob started to have a wider selection of foods from which Dave could choose, and these were positively reinforced by Bob and his wife, this might lead to improved eating habits for Dave.

Box 5.1 Applying research in practice

Increasing pre-school children's consumption of fruit and vegetables. A modelling and rewards intervention (Horne et al., 2011)

This study investigated whether a modelling and rewards intervention targeted at 20 preschool children aged 2–4 years old would be effective at increasing fruit and vegetable consumption.

Rewards consisted of stickers for children who ate 1–3 pieces of the target foods, a badge and a sticker for children who ate 4–7 pieces of the target foods and for those who ate 8 pieces of the target foods they received stickers and a brick from a toy construction kit.

Modelling consisted of a video which all the children watched at the beginning of the intervention and contained two animated characters who enthusiastically modelled eating fruit and vegetables.

At the beginning of the intervention children received a different food set daily, first at snack time and again at lunchtime (each of these food sets contained two fruit and two vegetables at each time point giving a total of eight portions of fruit and vegetable overall); the consumption of these was not rewarded. Then at 32 days the intervention focused on fruit consumption, children were rewarded only at snack time and only for fruit consumption. Following this the intervention focused on vegetable consumption, again children were rewarded for vegetable consumption and again only at snack time. Follow up data was collected for fruit and vegetable consumption at six months when all of the rewards had been removed.

Findings found that the fruit and vegetable interventions produced large significant increases in fruit and vegetable consumption; these increases were maintained at follow-up after rewards had been withdrawn.

Individual level interventions

Individual level interventions provide strategies for the target population. Medical practitioners alongside health professionals can advise individuals on the strategies which impact on, and result in behaviour change.

Prescriptions for fruit and vegetables

At the level of the health practitioner, Kearney *et al.* (2005) report on a brief preventative intervention deployed in primary care consultations in a deprived area in North West England. At the centre of the scheme is a prescription for fruit and vegetables which GPs, nurses, health visitors and midwives issue to patients on an opportunistic basis. Each prescription contains four vouchers offering a £1 discount when £3 or more is spent on fruit and vegetables. As the health professionals issue the prescription they link it explicitly to key five-a-day messages. Early feedback suggested that the intervention was successful in highlighting to patients the connection between food and health. Furthermore, clinicians expressed satisfaction with having a simple preventative intervention that could be deployed quickly (1–2 minutes) and effectively during routine primary care consultations.

Primary care remains the public's preferred source of food and health information. It provides a natural setting for health promotion, which is usually long term and characterised by trust. Hence, all primary care consultations should be accompanied by some health promotion message, whether this is about diet, weight, smoking or alcohol.

Although such food prescriptions can be useful and encourage a more focused approach to dietary selection, there are psychological principles that will help explain why a person succeeds in changing their diet, and why they ask for assistance in the first place. One important concept that has been highlighted throughout this text is the concept of self-efficacy.

Self-efficacy

One of the most important concepts when looking at the success of psychological interventions is the concept of self-efficacy (French *et al.*, 1996; Dennis and Goldberg, 1996). Self-efficacy regarding weight loss (Rodin *et al.*, 1988), the ability to handle emotions, life situations (Jeffrey *et al.*, 1984) and exercise have been related to later weight loss maintenance. It is thought that the development and change in an individual's self-efficacy during an intervention phase could be a crucial aspect to weight loss (Byrne *et al.*, 2012). More information on self-efficacy is presented in Chapter 4.

Decisional balance

One way to prompt individuals into making a change is to encourage them to consider the **pros** and the **cons** of changing their behaviour. Pros and cons were originally derived from Janis and Mann's (1977) model of decision-making and have become critical constructs in the transtheoretical, or stages of change, model. The balance between the pros and cons varies depending on which stage of change the individual is in. However, change is unlikely to occur until the reasons for change outweigh the reasons for staying the same.

When thinking about change, most of us don't really consider all 'sides' in a logical way. Instead, we often do what we think we 'should' do, avoid doing things we don't feel like doing, or just feel confused or overwhelmed and give up thinking about it at all. Thinking through the pros and cons of changing or not changing is one way to help us make sure we have fully considered the consequences of our behaviour. This can help us to 'hang on' to our plan in times of stress or temptation.

Using the material in Table 5.9, a list of the pros and cons associated with changing diet or eating behaviour can be made. For most people, 'making a change' will probably mean eating healthily, but it is important to state the *specific* changes that individuals might want to make, e.g. cutting down on saturated fat and sugar, eating five portions of fruit and vegetables a day or trying to eat less salt – no more than 6g a day.

Table 5.9 Decisional balance sheet

	Benefits/pros	Costs/cons
Making a change		
Not changing		

Applying this to Bob

On the basis of the case study presented at the start of the chapter, Bob's decision balance sheet could look like this:

	Benefits/pros	Costs/cons
Making a change	Reduce weight, BMI and blood pressure.	Extra financial costs e.g. joining a gym.
	Improve general fitness – in time he will be able to return to his five-a-side football team.	Cost implications of buying fresh produce for the whole family.
	Reduce risks of developing conditions such as cancer and diabetes.	
	Increase the chances of conception (as Bob and his wife want another child).	
	Saving money – having regular takeaways will be more expensive than eating home-prepared meals.	
Not changing	Bob can eat all the foods he likes.	Health implications.
	Bob can still partake in his post-match drinking sessions.	Reduced life expectancy.
		Reduced healthy life expectancy.

Goal setting

Once the individual has made the decision that they want to change their behaviour and they want to start eating healthily, it is important for them to be given specific goals. It is of limited value if you suggest that the individual 'loses weight' or 'eats more healthily'; the guidance must be specific – 'lose two kilos', or 'start to eat five portions of fruit and vegetables per day'. In this way, the goals need to be SMART (that is, Specific, Measurable, Achievable, Realistic and Timed):

- *Specific:* Specific goals are essential to diet improvement programmes. They represent the difference in focus and motivation between 'I should lose some weight' and 'I'm going to lose a kilo a week for the next seven weeks – this means in seven weeks' time I'll be 7 kilos lighter'.
- *Measurable:* The starting point, the weight goal and milestones along the way are all required so that progress can be checked at regular intervals in order to maintain confidence and ensure the plan is on track.
- *Achievable:* It must be possible to achieve the goal; this is the key to success. If the goals are large – losing two or more stone – then the goals should be broken down into smaller steps, an initial goal of half a stone for example. A new milestone goal can then be set once you have achieved your first goal.
- *Realistic:* There's no point attempting to be half a stone lighter by the end of next week. Even if it were possible it would be setting the client up for failure in the longer term.
- *Timed:* Setting a time frame for the goal gives the client a clear target to work towards. Remember, the time frame must be measurable, achievable and realistic!

Using the case study presented at the start of the chapter, it is possible to set SMART targets for both Bob and Dave. This will help to keep them both motivated and on target.

Bob's SMART targets:
I will increase my fitness and reduce my blood pressure by walking for 45 minutes from 6.00pm–6.45pm, 3 days a week (Tuesday, Thursday and Saturday). I will do this in the park and I will take my sports clothes with me to work so I can go on my way home. On a Saturday I can take Dave with me so we both get some exercise. In two months' time I will aim to reduce my blood pressure and my weight.

Dave's SMART targets:
I will reduce the amount of fish fingers and chips that I eat. Each week for four weeks I will reduce the amount of fish finger and chip portions I eat by one. In one month's time I will have reduced that amount of fish fingers and chips that I eat to one portion a week, which I will have on a Saturday.

You need to develop these goals in conjunction with the client and the client should be asked:

What are you going to do?
How are you going to do it?
Where are you going to do it?
When are you going to do it?
With whom are you going to do it?

Once the goals are set, the process outlined in Figure 5.2 can be followed.

Changing diet through motivational interviewing

The technique described in Figure 5.2 is based on the Stages of Change model and using a motivational interviewing technique. Motivational interviewing is a directive, client-centred counselling technique for enhancing intrinsic motivation. Motivational interviewing works by helping the patient to articulate why it is important for them to change and by increasing their self-efficacy so that they have the confidence to do so. It is usually used alongside the transtheoretical model (TTM) (Prochaska and DiClemente, 1983), which is discussed in much detail throughout this text. In short, the model suggests that change proceeds through a series of stages. The model (see Figure 5.3) is

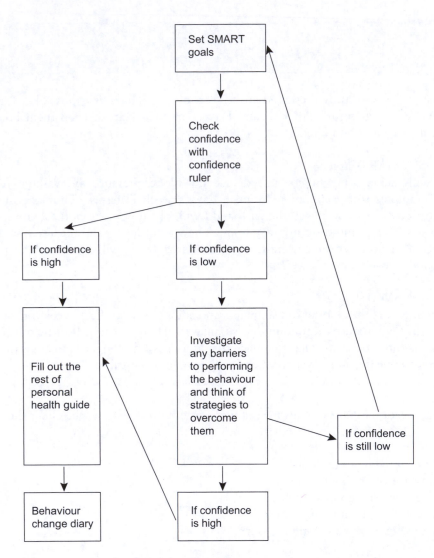

Figure 5.2 Process for encouraging weight loss

important as it allows the practitioner to identify where individuals are in their behaviour; with this in mind, appropriate interventions can be developed and implemented. The five stages of change are:

1. *Pre-contemplation:* The patient has no intention of making any changes.
2. *Contemplation:* The patient is considering making some changes.
3. *Preparation:* The patient is making small changes; has developed a plan of action and intends to initiate it in the near future.
4. *Action:* The patient is actively participating in the new behaviour.
5. *Maintenance:* The patient is continuing the new behaviour over an extended period of time.

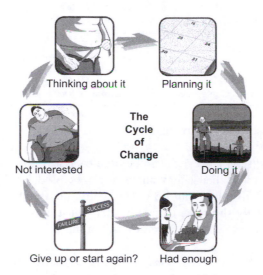

Figure 5.3 The transtheoretical Stages of Change model
Source: Prochaska *et al.*, 1992

Applying this to Bob

Bob is currently in the contemplation stage of change. He has acknowledged that he needs to change his lifestyle and with help and support changes can be made.

Dave is currently in the pre-contemplation stage. He doesn't realise that changes to his lifestyle would be beneficial.

Any intervention will require the patient to adapt their behaviour in one way or another, be it taking time to attend a hospital appointment, adapting their diet or incorporating new exercise into their daily lives. In order to adhere to such advice, the person must be ready and prepared to accept this change. One way of assessing a patient's 'readiness' to change is to use the readiness ruler (see Figure 5.4). The readiness ruler can be used at the beginning of an intervention to help target the appropriate stage of change. Alternatively, it can be used during the intervention as a way of encouraging the patient to talk about reasons for change.

Thinking that change is important is not always enough for a person to move into the action phase. Sometimes a person is ready to make a change but is not confident that they are able to do so. For this reason, both readiness and confidence are addressed in motivation-based interventions.

On a scale of 1 to 10, how certain are you that you want to change this behaviour?

1	2	3	4	5	6	7	8	9	10
Not certain at all					Not certain at all			Very certain	
Pre-contemplation			Contemplation		Preparation			Action	

Figure 5.4 Readiness ruler: improving diet

The confidence ruler (see Figure 5.5) can be used to assess how confident patients are that they are able to adapt their behaviour, or it can be used as a hypothetical question to encourage patients to talk about how they would go about making a change. It is not necessary to actually show the patient a ruler, but it may be helpful, especially for young children or patients with low literacy and numeracy skills.

On a scale of 1 to 10, how confident are you that you can change this behaviour?

1	2	3	4	5	6	7	8	9	10
Not confident at all								Very confident	

Figure 5.5 Confidence ruler

Based on the patient's confidence score, the healthcare professional might ask:

* You said your confidence was a 4, why not a 1 or a 2?
* Why not an 8 or a 9?
* What would it take to make it a 10?

The client's answers to these questions will tell you how resourceful they feel, as well as what potential barriers they have to conquer along the way. The final question will encourage the client to come up with their own solutions, tactics and ways to remove obstacles to change. It may also prove helpful to encourage the client to remember previous successes, to review obstacles and how they overcame them.

A person's belief in their ability to change is an important motivator (i.e. their self-efficacy). The healthcare professional can enhance a person's motivation to change by using open questions to elicit 'confidence talk'. Using negotiation and confidence building to persuade patients that they can change their behaviour is an important part of motivational interviewing.

Applying this to Bob

Bob could use the readiness and confidence rulers to assess his motivation to change his lifestyle and diet. For example, he could consider how important it is for him to eat more fruit and vegetables, to start doing exercise and to cut down his consumption of fatty foods.

Processes of change

While stages of change represent dimensions that allow understanding of *when* changes occur, the processes of change (Prochaska *et al.*, 1988), outlined in Table 5.10, allow understanding of *how* changes occur. Ten processes of change have been identified, and specific processes are associated with particular stages of preparation for change. There is integration between the processes of change and the stages of change. Effective self-change depends on doing the right things (processes) at the right time (stages). With a mismatch in stage and processes, a successful behavioural change is unlikely to occur. Figure 5.6 highlights how these can be integrated when attempting to change an individual's diet.

Table 5.10 The ten processes of change

Process of change	What this means	Related to diet
Consciousness raising	Increasing information about self and problem: observations, confrontations, interpretations, bibliotherapy	Look for information on improving diet. Leaflets and information guidance
Self-re-evaluation	Assessing how one feels and thinks about oneself with respect to a problem: value clarification, imagery, corrective emotional experience	Feel disappointed with self when eating something unhealthy
Self-liberation	Choosing and commitment to act or belief in ability to change: decision-making therapy, New Year's resolutions, commitment-enhancing techniques	Making a decision to quit, and making a commitment to it
Counter-conditioning	Substituting alternatives for problem behaviours: relaxation, desensitisation, assertion, positive self-statements	Rather than grabbing a chocolate biscuit, have an apple or replace eating with a form of relaxation

Process of change	What this means	Related to diet
Stimulus control	Avoiding or countering stimuli that elicit problem behaviours: restructuring one's environment (e.g. removing alcohol or fattening foods), avoiding high-risk cues, fading techniques	Remove fattening foods from the home. Replace with healthy foods
Reinforcement management	Rewarding oneself or being rewarded by others for making changes: contingency contracts, overt and covert reinforcement, self-reward	Make sure that friends and other members of the family provide reinforcement.
Helping relationships	Being open and trusting about problems with someone who cares: therapeutic alliance, social support, self-help groups	Weight watchers groups: social support from others
Dramatic relief	Experiencing and expressing feelings about one's problems and solutions: psychodrama, grieving losses, role playing	Emotional link between health and diet – worry and concern about their weight, or a recent health threat
Environmental re-evaluation	Assessing how one's problem affects the physical environment: empathy training, documentaries	How can the physical environment be improved by changing behaviour?
Social liberation	Increasing alternatives for non-problem behaviours available in society: advocating for rights of repressed, empowering, policy interventions	Wider adverts for healthy eating in society

Source: Based on Prochaska *et al.*, 1988

Applying this to Bob

Different processes of change will be useful for Bob in order to change his behaviour.

Stimulus control would be a starting point. He could remove any high fat foods and takeaway menus that he has at home. Consciousness raising would also be beneficial so he can learn about dietary composition and healthy eating. In addition Bob could also go to Weight Watchers which would give him some social support. Combining these processes of change would improve Bob's chances of not only losing weight but maintaining it.

Phase 1

Establish rapport: How's it going?
↓
Opening statement: This is what we are going to do today.
↓
Assess current eating behaviour and progress: Why do you eat your current diet, and why haven't you changed?
↓
Give feedback: Compare current diet and weight with normative graphs and forms: What do you think of the information provided?
↓
Assess readiness to change: Introduce change ruler (on a scale of 1–10 how ready are you to make any change?).

Phase 2

Tailor intervention approach		
↓	↓	↓
Stage 1	Stage 2	Stage 3
↓	↓	↓
Not ready	Unsure	Ready
↓	↓	↓
Goal: To raise awareness	Goal: To build motivation and confidence	Goal: To negotiate a plan
↓	↓	↓
Open-ended questions: 'What would need to be different for you to consider making new or additional changes in your diet?' Respect decisions Offer guidance	Explore ambivalence: 'What are the good and not so good things about making such changes?' Look to the future Refer to friends	Identify change option: 'What do you think you need to change?' Help set goals Develop action plans Summarise plan
Close the encounter: Summarise the session Support self-efficacy		

Figure 5.6 Changing diet through motivational interviewing

Community level interventions

Given the extent of the obesity problem in the UK and the potential health difficulties associated with this, it is not surprising that the UK government (along with the separate legislatures) have developed strategic plans to counteract the looming difficulties. For example, The Food and Health Action Plan and the Activity Coordination Team is a cross-government group (led by the Department of Health) to improve public health through better diet. Examples of such action include:

- Breastfeeding: action to encourage more women to breastfeed and to continue for at least six months.
- Reform of the Welfare Food Scheme: to ensure children in poverty have access to a healthy diet and increased support for breastfeeding.
- Food in Schools Programme: promoting a 'whole school approach' and encouraging greater access to healthier choices within schools.
- Work with the food industry: to address the amount of fat, salt and added sugar in the diet (with the Food Standards Agency).
- New GP contract: practices will be required to offer relevant health promotion advice to patients.
- Banning 'junk food' advertising: As of January 2007, the independent regulator for the communications industry, Ofcom, placed a total ban on adverts for foods high in fat, salt and sugar during all preschool children's programmes, all programmes on mainstream channels aimed at children, all cable and satellite children's channels, and programmes aimed at young people, such as music shows and general entertainment programmes which would appeal to a 'higher than average' number of under-16s. NICE (2010) have suggested that this might not go far enough and that advertisements between programmes for older people also have a powerful effect on children, suggesting an extension on scheduling restrictions to 9pm.

One of the largest government based interventions aimed at preventing long-term obesity is Change4Life (DOH, 2009). Based on social marketing, the intervention encourages people of all ages to change their dietary and exercise habits in an attempt to tackle the increasing obesity problem. This is done through advertising campaigns which direct you to resources and information in order to change to a healthier life. Since the launch in 2009, the programme has gained increased interest and has become effective in changing the behaviour of over 1 million families in the UK between 2009–2010 (DOH, 2010).

5 A Day programme

Devised by the Department of Health, the campaign aimed to increase the public's awareness of the government recommendations for the daily consumption of fruit and vegetables. Underpinned by the incentive to prevent illness and health inequalities an evaluation of the scheme indicates promising results. Improvements in the awareness of portion sizes, alongside the recommended daily consumption of fruit and vegetables have been seen from the latest evaluation of the scheme (Bremner et al., 2006).

The 5 A Day programme also incorporates the school fruit and vegetable scheme (SFVS). The scheme entitles children aged between 4 and 6 years old to receive a free piece of fruit or vegetables at school in an attempt to increase consumption alongside increasing awareness of healthy eating. Combined fruit and vegetable consumption was seen to increase as a result of the programme. However, effects were not seen to translate to the home setting (Teeman et al., 2010). Thus, it is imperative that dietary changes translate between environments to ensure long lasting dietary impact.

Traffic light system

In an attempt to guide individuals to make healthy choices the Food Standards Agency devised the traffic light system that gives the public an indication as to the nutritional values in food. Food products are labelled with green, red or amber coloured labels which represent low, high or medium amounts of fat, saturated fat, salt and sugar. The labels provide a quick and easy guide for individuals to make healthier dietary choices. However, it is thought that only one in four shoppers look at this information (EUFIC, 2008). Evidence has shown a consistent link between the use of nutrition labels and healthier diets, but that may be a result of healthier eaters seeking out and using the information, rather than the labels themselves promoting better diet (Campos *et al.*, 2011). With government efforts being made to address the poor diets of the nation, it is also important to understand the gap between the individuals' understanding of such healthy eating government campaigns and implementation of them.

Applying this to Bob

Bob could use all the available resources from the government campaigns to help him change his dietary habits. The Change4Life website provides information and advice on healthy eating and exercise including recipe and exercise ideas. In addition, Bob could start to use the traffic light system and start looking at the labels on the foods that he purchases in an attempt to eat a more balanced diet.

Working effectively with others

In attempting to tackle obesity, various professions such as psychologist and health professionals can provide help and support for individuals who are aiming to tackle obesity. Outlined below are examples of such professionals.

Dieticians

A dietician is a professional who advises on dietary intake and the impact on health. They offer advice to individuals to help them make health-conscious decisions. Using the science behind nutrition, they work together with an individual to draw up a dietary plan according to specific goals (weight loss) or requirements (allergies). Dieticians can also treat dietary related problems and educate individuals who require specific diets as part of a medical regime (e.g. diabetes and kidney disease).

Physiologists

Physiologists are concerned with the impact of our modern lifestyle and how this affects health and well-being. They consider external influences and the impact of that on the science within the human body. Physiologists are trained to assess the health of individuals and work together with the client to develop behaviour change strategies.

Physical training instructors

Physical training instructors work in many settings including gyms, health clubs and the NHS. Working together with their client, physical training instructors devise personal training plans, diet plans and give general advice regarding fitness. In addition, they can work together to set goals so the client reaches their target weight. The advice and input from physical training instructors can provide individuals with much needed motivation when considering weight loss.

Applying this to Bob

To help Bob address his health and weight concerns he could seek the advice of many professionals that will provide him with support in many areas. In addition, while helping him understand the impact of his diet on his health it will also advise him on ways to change his dietary behaviour. For instance, he could join a gym and, with the help of a physical training instructor, devise an exercise regime. In turn the physical training instructor could help to keep Bob motivated and on target to lose weight.

Conclusion

The consequences of a poor diet are more than just obesity. A poor diet can contribute to a range of illnesses, including coronary heart disease, cancer and type 2 diabetes. Conversely, eating the 'right' foods can prevent illness and promote health. Despite the wealth of evidence endorsing both the positive and negative impact diet can have on health, research suggests that many people do not eat a sufficiently healthy diet.

Several explanations have been put forward for why people eat what they do; these have ranged from the media, through to the social-environmental and the psychosocial. This chapter has also explored two key psychological models of eating behaviour: the developmental approach which emphasises the importance of learning and the development of food preferences, and the cognitive approach which explores the extent to which cognitions explain and predict behaviour.

Numerous interventions have been introduced to tackle the nation's poor diet; however, the effectiveness of such interventions remains poor. Future attempts to improve the nation's diet should be multi-component, include behaviour change strategies, provide ongoing support and, most importantly, be tailored to the needs of the individual; after all, one size does not fit all.

Key points

- Diet can affect health through an individual's weight but also plays a role in the development of diseases such as CHD, cancer and diabetes.
- It is estimated that food-related ill health is responsible for about 10 per cent of morbidity and mortality in the UK.
- Healthy eating can be understood in terms of five major food groups and is important for promoting health and treating ill health.
- Eating behaviour has been shown to be influenced by the media, the environment and social barriers such as availability, cost and time.
- The developmental approach emphasises the importance of learning and focuses on the development of food preferences in childhood. From this perspective, eating behaviour is influenced by exposure, social learning and associative learning.
- Research has demonstrated that self-efficacy, i.e. the belief in one's ability to exercise control over challenging demands, plays an important role in weight loss and weight maintenance.
- Decisional balance, or the individual's evaluation of the pros and cons, is a crucial component in the modification of dietary behaviours, as change is unlikely to occur until the reasons for change outweigh the reasons for staying the same.
- SMART goals are essential to diet improvement; that is, goals need to be Specific, Measurable, Achievable, Realistic and Timed.
- Motivational interviewing is a client-centred approach for eliciting behaviour change. It works by helping the patient to articulate why it is important for them to change while increasing their confidence that they are able to do so.
- According to the TTM, behaviour change can be thought of as a progression through a series of stages: pre-contemplation, contemplation, preparation, action and maintenance.
- Ten processes have been identified which explain how progression through the stages of change can occur. Effective self-change depends on doing the right things (processes) at the right time (stages).
- Community level interventions have been outlined and can be used in a combined effort as a means of long-term prevention strategy to the current obesity concern. However, the effectiveness of these is questionable.
- Health professionals such as dieticians, physiologists and physical training instructors can be useful in guiding and motivating the client to make behaviour change.

Points for discussion

- Imagine that you wanted to decrease your intake of high fat foods and maintain it in the long term. How would you do this and what interventions would be useful?
- Critically discuss the developmental model of eating behaviour.
- Compare and contrast two cognitive models of eating behaviour.
- Consider Bob's son Dave. How would you improve his diet using psychological principles?

Also consider:

- How you would assess Dave's diet;
- How Dave's environment might influence his eating behaviour.

Further resources

Conner, M. and Norman, P. (2007). *Predicting Health Behaviour*, 2nd edn. Berkshire: Open University Press.

Ogden, J. (2010). *The Psychology of Eating; From Healthy to Disordered Behaviour*, 2nd edn. Oxford: Blackwell.

Thirlaway, K. and Upton, D. (2009). *The Psychology of Lifestyle: Promoting Healthy Behaviour*. London: Routledge.

Useful web links

An online calculator for working out and interpreting a child's BMI is available at: www. healthforallchildren.co.uk on the parent's page.

Food Dudes healthy eating programme http://www.fooddudes.co.uk/

Eat well, be well – the Food Standards Agency website for consumer advice on healthy eating. It is packed with information and tips on eating a healthy balanced diet http://www. eatwell.gov.uk/

Cancer Prevention Research Centre provides a detailed overview of the Transtheoretical model, including the stages of change, processes of change, decisional balance and self-efficacy http://www.uri.edu/research/cprc/transtheoretical.htm

Motivational interviewing: resources for clinicians, researchers and trainers – provides background information on the practice of motivational interviewing http://www. motivational interview.org/

Change4Life website - http://www.nhs.uk/change4life/Pages/partners-supporters.aspx

The Food Standards Agency – Traffic Light System – http://tna.europarchive.org/ 20100910172942/http://www.eatwell.gov.uk/foodlabels/trafficlights/

References

Ajzen, I. (1985). From intention to actions: a theory of planned behaviour. In J. Kuhl and J. Beckman (eds) *Action Control: From Cognition to Behaviour*. Available at: http:// www.people.umass.edu/aizen/publications.html (accessed 20 December 2007).

Aune, D., Lau, R., Chan, D., Vieira, R., Greenwood, D., Kampman, E., and Norat, T. (2011). Nonlinear reduction in risk for colorectal cancer by fruit and vegetable intake based on meta-analysis of prospective studies. *Gastroenterology*, 141(1): 106–118.

Bates, B., Lennox, A., Bates, C., and Swan, G. (2011). *National Diet and Nutrition Survey Headline Results from Years 1 and 2 (combined) of the Rolling Programme (2008/2009 –2009/10)*. Available at: http://www.dh.gov.uk/en/Publicationsandstatistics/Publications/PublicationsStatistics/DH_128166 (accessed 30 March 2011).

Becker, M.H. and Rosenstock, I.M. (1984). Compliance with medical advice. In A. Steptoe and A. Mathews (eds) *Health Care and Human Behaviour*. London: Academic Press.

Bibbins-Domingo, K., Chertow, G., Coxson, P., Moran, A., Lightwood, J., Pletcher, M., and Goldman, L. (2010). Projected effect of dietary salt reductions on future cardiovascular disease. *New England Journal of Medicine*, 362(7): 590–599. doi:10.1056/NEJMoa 0907355

Birch, L. (1999). Development of food preferences. *Annual Review of Nutrition*, 19: 41–62.

Block, G., Patterson, B. and Subar, A. (1992). Fruit, vegetables and cancer prevention: A review of the epidemiological evidence. *Nutrition and* Cancer, 18: 1–29.

Bremner, P., Dalziel, D., and Evans. (2006) Evaluation of the 5 A Day programme, final report. Surrey: TNS Social.

Bromley, C., and Given, L. (2011) *The Scottish Health Survey 2010*, Volume 1: *Main Report*. Edinburgh: The Scottish Government. Available at: http://www.scotland.gov.uk/Publications/2011/09/27084018/914 (accessed 23 June 2012).

Brown, M., Byatt, T., Marsh, T., and McPherson, K. (2010) *Obesity Trends for Adults Analysis from the Health Survey for England 1993–2007*. Available at http://nhfshare.heartforum.org.uk/RMAssets/NHFreports/NHF_adultobese_long_170210.pdf (accessed 30 March 2012).

Boyce, T. (2007). The media and obesity. *Obesity Reviews*, 8 (1): 201–205.

Byrne, S., Barry, D., and Petry, N. M. (2012). Predictors of weight loss success. Exercise vs. dietary self-efficacy and treatment attendance. *Appetite*, 58(2): 695–698.

Campos, S., Doxey, J. and Hammond, D. (2011) Nutrition labels on pre-packaged foods: a systematic review. *Public Health Nutrition* 14: 1496–1506.

Connor Gorber, S., Tremblay, M., Moher, D. and Gorber, B. (2007). A comparison of direct vs. self-report measures for assessing height, weight and body mass index: A systematic review. *Obesity Reviews*, 8(4): 307–326.

Cooke, L. J., Chambers, L. C., Añez, E. V., and Wardle, J. (2011). Facilitating or undermining? The effect of reward on food acceptance. A narrative review. *Appetite*, 57(2): 493–497.

Dennis, K.E. and Goldberg, A.P. (1996). Weight control self-efficacy types and transitions affect weight-loss outcomes in obese women. *Addictive Behaviour*, 21: 103–116.

Department of Health (DoH) (1999). *Saving Lives: Our Healthier Nation*. London: The Stationery Office.

——(2009) *Change4Life Marketing Strategy*. London: UK: Department of Health.

——(2010) *Change4Life One Year On*. London: UK Department of Health.

——(2011a). *Change4Life Three Year Social Marketing Strategy*. Available at: http://www.dh.gov.uk/en/Publicationsandstatistics/Publications/PublicationsPolicyAndGuidance/DH_130475 (accessed 29 November 2012).

——(2011b). *Healthy Lives, Healthy People: A Call to Action on Obesity in England.* Available at http://www.dh.gov.uk/prod_consum_dh/groups/dh_digitalassets/documents/digitalasset/dh_130487.pdf (accessed 29 November 2012).

Department of Health, Social Services and Public Safety. (2011). Health Survey Northern Ireland: First results from the 2010/11 Survey. Belfast. Available at: http://www.dhsspsni.gov.uk/index/stats_research/stats-public-health.htm (accessed 10 June 2012).

Elia, M., and Russell, C. (2009) *Combating Malnutrition: Recommendations for Action – Executive Summary.* Redditch: British Association for Parenteral and Enteral Nutrition. Available at http://www.bapen.org.uk/pdfs/reports/advisory_group_report.pdf (accessed 30 March 2012).

EUFIC (2008) EUFIC Press Release from 25/09/2008: One in four UK consumers look for nutrition information on food labels. Available at: http://www.eufic.org/jpage/en/page/PRESS/fftid/Consumer-InsightsUK-results/ (accessed 23 September 2013).

Fishbein, M. and Ajzen, I. (1975). *Belief, Attitude, Intention and Behaviour. An Introduction to Theory and Research.* Available at: http://www.people.umass.edu/aizen/publications.html (accessed 20 December 2007).

French, S.A., Perry, C.L., Leon, G.R. and Faulkerson, J.A. (1996). Self-esteem and change in body mass index over 3 years in a cohort of adolescents. *Obesity Research*, 4(1): 27–33.

Harris, J. L., Bargh, J. A., and Brownell, K. D. (2009). Priming effects of television food advertising on eating behavior. *Health Psychology*, 28(4): 404–413. doi:10.1037/a0014399

Horne, P. J., Greenhalgh, J., Erjavec, M., Lowe, C., Viktor, S., and Whitaker, C. J. (2011). Increasing pre-school children's consumption of fruit and vegetables. A modelling and rewards intervention. *Appetite*, 56(2): 375–385. doi:10.1016/j.appet.2010.11.146

Janis, I.L. and Mann, L. (1977). *Decision Making: A Psychological Analysis of Conflict, Choice and Commitment.* New York: Free Press.

Jeffery, R.W., Bjornson-Benson, W.M., Rosenthal, B.S., Lindquist, R.A., Kurth, C.L. and Johnson, S.L. (1984). Correlates of weight loss and its maintenance over two years of follow-up among middle aged men. *Preventive Medicine*, 13: 155–168.

Kearney, M., Bradbury, C., Ellahi, B., Hodgson, M. and Thurston, M. (2005). Mainstreaming prevention: prescribing fruit and vegetables as a brief intervention in primary care. *Journal of the Royal Institute of Public Health*, 119: 981–986.

Key, T.J. (2011). Fruit and vegetables and cancer risk, *British Journal of Cancer,* 104 (1): 6–11.

Kushi, L.H., Doyle, C., McCullough, M., Rock, C. L., Denmark-Wahnefried, W., Bandera, E. V., Gapstur, S., Patel, A. V., Andrews, K., Gansler, T., and the American Cancer Society (2012) American cancer society guidelines on nutrition and physical activity for cancer prevention. *CA: A Cancer Journal for Clinicians,* 62(1): 30–64.

National Health Service (NHS) (2011) *5 A Day.* Available at: http://www.nhs.uk/LiveWell/5ADAY/Pages/5ADAYhome.aspx (Accessed 10 December 2012).

National Institute for Health and Clinical Excellence (NICE). (2006). *Obesity: Guidance on the Prevention, Identification, Assessment and Management of Overweight and Obesity in Adults and Children.* Available at: http://www.nice.org.uk/nicemedia/pdf/word/CG43NICE Guideline.doc (accessed 11 December 2007).

——(2007). *Behaviour Change at Population, Community and Individual Levels.* Available at: http://www.nice.org.uk/nicemedia/pdf/PH006guidance.pdf (accessed 9 July 2007).

——(2010) *Prevention of Cardiovascular Disease at Population Level.* Available at: http://www.nice.org.uk/nicemedia/live/13024/49273/49273.pdf_(accessed 9 December 2012).

NHS Live Well website (2012) http://www.nhs.uk/Livewell/Goodfood/Pages/Healthyeating.aspx (accessed 15 March 2012).

Ofcom (2006). *Annex 7 – Impact Assessment Consultation on Television Advertising of Food and Drink to Children.* Joint FSA/DoH Analysis; 2. London: Ofcom.

Ogden, J. (2007). *Health Psychology: A Textbook,* 4th edn. Buckingham: Open University Press.

Osera, T., Tsutie, S., Kobayashi, M., and Kurihara, N. (2012). Relationship of mothers' food preferences and attitudes with children's preferences. *Food and Nutrition*, 3: 1461–1466.

Pan, A., Sun, Q., Bernstein, A. M., Schulze, M. B., Manson, J. E., Stampfer, M. J., Willett, W. C., Hu, F. B. (2012) Red meat consumption and mortality. *Archives of Internal Medicine*, March 12. DOI: 10.1001/archinternmed.2011.2287.

Parkin, D. (2011). 1. The fraction of cancer attributable to lifestyle and environmental factors in the UK in 2010. *British Journal of Cancer*, 105 Suppl: 2S2–S5. doi:10.1038/bjc.2011.474

Pilátová, M., Chripková, M. and Mojžiš, J. (2011). Cruciferous vegetables in cancer prevention, *ActaFacultatisPharmaceuticaeUniversitatisComenianae*, 53(1): 62–71.

Powell, L. H., Calvin, J. E., and Calvin, J. E. (2007). Effective obesity treatments. *American Psychologist*, 62: 234–246.

Prochaska, J.O. and DiClemente, C.C. (1983). Stages and processes of self-change smoking: towards and integrative model of change. *Journal of Consulting and Clinical Psychology*, 51: 390–395.

Prochaska, J.O., DiClemente, C.C. and Norcross, J. C. (1992). In search of how people change: application to addictive behaviors. *American Psychologist*, 47(9): 1102–1114.

Prochaska, J.O., Velicer, W.F., DiClemente, C.C. and Fava, J. (1988). Measuring processes of change: Applications to the cessation of smoking. *Journal of Consulting and Clinical Psychology*, 56: 520–528.

Rodin, J., Elias, M., Silberstein, L.R. and Wagner, A. (1988). Combined behavioural and pharmacologic treatment for obesity: predictors of successful weight maintenance. *Journal of Consulting and Clinical Psychology*, 56: 399–404.

Rogers, R.W. (1985). Attitude change and information integration in fear appeals. *Psychological Reports*, 56: 179–182.

Routen, A., Edwards, M., Upton, D., Peters, D (2011). The impact of school-day variation in weight and height on National Child Measurement BMI determined weight category in Year 6 Children. *Child Care Health Development*, 37(3): 360–367.

Scarborough, P., Bhatnagar, P., Wickramasinghe, K. K., Allender, S., Foster, C., and Rayner, M. (2011). The economic burden of ill health due to diet, physical inactivity, smoking, alcohol and obesity in the UK: an update to 2006–07 NHS costs. *Journal of Public Health*, 33(4): 527–535.

Scarborough, P., Morgan, R., Webster, P., and Rayner, M. (2011). Differences in coronary heart disease, stroke and cancer mortality rates between England, Wales, Scotland and Northern Ireland: the role of diet and nutrition. *BMJ Open*, 1(1), e000263.

Scientific Advisory Committee on Nutrition (SACN) (2008) *The Nutritional Wellbeing of the British Population.* Available at: http://www.sacn.gov.uk/pdfs/nutritional_health_of_the_population_final_oct_08.pdf (accessed 5 December 2012)

Schwarzer, R. (1992). Self-efficacy in the adoption and maintenance of health behaviours: Theoretical approaches and a new model. In R. Schwarzer (ed.) *Self-efficacy: Thought Control of Action.* Washington, DC: Hemisphere.

Sodhi MK. (2010). TV Viewing versus play – trends and impact on obesity. *Online Journal of Health and Allied Sciences*, 9(2): 6.

Swinburn, B.A., Egger, G.J. and Raza, F. (1999). Dissecting obesogenic environments: the development and application of a framework for identifying and prioritising environmental interventions for obesity. *Preventative Medicine*, 29: 563–570.

Tanaka, T., Shnimizu, M. and Moriwaki, H. (2012) Cancer chemoprevention by carotenoids, *Molecules (Basel, Switzerland)*, 17(3): 3202–3242.

Teeman, D., Lynch, S., White, K., Scott, E., Waldman, J., Benton, T., Shamsan. Y., Stoddart, S., Ransley, J., Cade, J. and Thomas, J. (2010). *The Third Evaluation of the School Fruit and Vegetable Scheme*. London: Department of Health.

The Health and Social Care Information Centre, NHS. (2011). Statistics on obesity, physical activity and diet: England. Available at http://www.ic.nhs.uk/webfiles/publications/003_Health_Lifestyles/opad11/Statistics_on_Obesity_Physical_Activity_and_Diet_England_2011_revised_Aug11.pdf (accessed 4 April 2012).

Wang, Y., McPherson, K., Marsh, T., Gortmaker, S., and Brown, M. (2011). Health and economic burden of the projected obesity trends in the USA and the UK. *Lancet*, 378(9793): 815–825. doi: 10.1016/S0140-6736(11)60814-3.

Welsh Government (2011) Welsh Health Survey 2010. Available at: http://www.wales.gov.uk/statistics (accessed 13 January 2013).

Whitlock, G., Lewington, S., Sherliker, P., Clarke, R., Emberson, J., Halsey, J., and Peto, R. (2009). Body-mass index and cause-specific mortality in 900 000 adults: collaborative analyses of 57 prospective studies. *Lancet*, 373(9669), 1083–1096.

World Cancer Research Fund. (2007). *Food Nutrition, and the Prevention of Cancer: A Global Perspective*. Washington, DC: American Institute for Cancer Research.

World Health Organization (WHO). (2004). *Report 916: Diet, Nutrition and the Prevention of Chronic Diseases*. Geneva: World Health Organization.

World Health Organization. (2009). Global Health Risks: *Mortality and Burden of Disease attributable to selected major risks*. Available at: http://www.who.int/healthinfo/global_burden_disease/GlobalHealthRisks_report_full.pdf (accessed 30 March 2012).

6 Being active

Learning objectives

At the end of this chapter you will:
- understand what being physically active means
- recognise how much physical activity is required to remain healthy
- understand physical activity patterns in the UK at present
- appreciate why some people do not achieve the recommended level of physical activity to remain healthy
- have explored available interventions to help people increase their levels of physical activity.

Case study

George is a 40-year-old manager of a bank call centre. He is responsible for the performance of his call centre and the line management of a number of staff. He works long hours since money is tight and commutes about 10 miles to and from work every day. George is married with three small children. His wife finds caring for three young children tiring and is very keen for George to get home promptly to help with the bedtime routine, although this is not always possible. They have only one car and it is needed in the evenings to take the older children to their various leisure activities. Whilst he enjoyed playing football at school, George stopped playing in his 20s due to a persistent knee injury. He has taken no exercise since, other than occasionally going swimming with his children. Over the past decade his weight has crept up and he is now over the recommended weight for his height, although not yet in the obese range.

Recently, George has been under a lot of pressure at work. He went to the GP reporting difficulty in sleeping and heart palpitations. After ensuring that George had no underlying severe physiological condition that was responsible for his symptoms, George's doctor diagnosed stress and depression and prescribed an anti-depressant together with beta blockers to control the heart palpitations.

George does not want to take either of the medications prescribed by the doctor. He comes to see you in your clinic to discuss alternative strategies to manage his symptoms. When he realises that exercise can be an effective treatment for stress and depression he is initially very enthusiastic about it but soon becomes despondent when he realises that it may mean him spending longer away from his wife and family. He feels that his wife will not support any activity that means he gets home any later and cannot see how he could incorporate an appropriate level of physical activity into his already busy day.

Applying this to George

George needs to build a sustainable physical activity routine if he is to alleviate his stress and anxiety without recourse to drug therapy.

Introduction

There are many opportunities for people to be physically active during the day, because physical activity in its broadest sense includes any movement. Formally, physical activity can be defined as: 'Any bodily movement produced by the skeletal muscles that results in energy expenditure and is usually measured in kilocalories (kcal) per unit of time' (Casperen *et al.*, 1985, cited in Biddle and Mutrie 2008, p. 9)

For many people in Western societies, including the UK, their normal daily occupations no longer require even moderate levels of physical activity. The amount of non-leisure physical activity in the UK has declined consistently over the past few decades (Department for Transport, 2010). Consequently, many health professionals find themselves attempting to encourage clients to increase the physical activity they do in their leisure time through sport or exercise.

Applying this to George

George's occupation is mostly sedentary so any physical activity he achieves will be leisure-based or active transport.

Sport includes an element of competition that is not present in exercise activities. Rejeskis and Brawley 1988, cited in Biddle and Mutrie (2008, p. 10) define sport as: 'Rule-governed, structured and competitive and involves gross motor movement characterised by physical strategy, prowess and chance.'

The relationship between physical activity, exercise and sport can be conceptualised as a range of overlapping activities as illustrated in Figure 6.1.

At first, government strategies to increase physical activity in the population focused on encouraging more people to take up sport as a leisure-time activity: 'Sport for all' (www.olympic.org, accessed July 2009). However, more recently, the focus has moved away from sport towards exercise and then away from exercise towards occupational physical activity, because significant uptake of sport or exercise has not been achieved. Consequently, the emphasis of public health initiatives in the twenty-first century has been on encouraging non-sporting physical activity such as walking, cycling, gardening or housework (Department of Health, 2011; Department of Health, Physical Activity, Health Improvement and Protection, 2011; Scottish Government, 2011; Welsh Government, 2011b; National Institute for Health and Clinical Excellence, 2006; 2007; 2008a; 2008b; 2010; 2011).

Increasingly the importance of sedentary time in relationship to health is being acknowledged (Department of Health, 2010). Sedentary behaviours have been described by the Department of Health, Physical Activity, Health Improvement and Protection (2011, p. 10) as:

> Multi-faceted and might include behaviours at work or school, at home, in transit and in leisure time. Typically, sedentary behaviours include watching TV; using a computer; travelling by car, bus or train; and sitting to read, talk, do homework or listen to music.

People who spend less time in sedentary activities accrue additional health benefits over and above the benefits that accrue from meeting the physical activity recommendations. Encouraging activities such as gardening, walking and cycling, even if they are not meeting the criteria for moderate physical activity still has the potential to reduce time spent in sedentary activities.

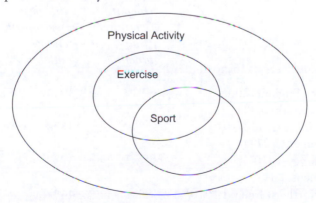

Figure 6.1 The relationship between physical activity, exercise and sport
Source: Thirlaway and Upton, 2009, p. 87. Reproduced with permission

Well over a decade after the Department of Health (1999) published their recommended physical activity levels of 30 minutes of moderate physical activity five times a week, and after many years of policy and interventions to encourage the population to meet these recommendations, still only 40 per cent or less of the populations of England, Wales, Scotland and Northern Ireland are meeting these criteria (Table 6.1). Scottish men are the most likely to meet the weekly target but still less than half are physically active.

The impact of over a decade of interventions to increase physical activity is not impressive (Table 6.1). In 2011 the Welsh Government published a report 'Health Trends in Wales (Welsh Government, 2011a). There was no evidence of any change in physical activity levels over this period with the percentage of Welsh men and women who are physically active remaining largely static at about 30 per cent overall, the lowest across the four home countries. A similar picture of static levels of physical activity is reported by the Scottish Health Survey 2010 (Scottish Government, 2011) over the period 2008 to 2010, although they report consistently higher levels of physical activity than are found in Wales. Other surveys of activity report similar findings.

The Department of Health in 2004 reported that over the past two or three decades there had been a small increase in the proportion of people in England engaging in leisure activity but a reduction in routine physical activity, such as that achieved through necessary tasks of work, travel or running a home. More recently, the Department for Transport (2010) reported in their Active Transport Strategy document that the number of people in England walking and cycling has dropped significantly

Table 6.1 The percentages of men and women living in the UK achieving the government guidelines for weekly physical activity as set out in Start Active, Stay Active (Department of Health, Physical Activity, Health Improvement and Protection, 2011)

Source of data	% of people achieving government activity guidelines	% of men achieving government activity guidelines	% of women achieving government activity guidelines
Health Survey for England 2008 (Department of Health 2011)	34%	39%	29%
Health Survey for Scotland 2010 (Scottish Government 2011)	39%	45%	33%
Welsh Health Survey 2010 (Welsh Government, 2011)	30%	37%	24%
Health Survey Northern Ireland 2010/11 (Department of Health, Social Services and Public Safety 2011)	38%	44%	35%

over the past 30 years and that the UK has some of the lowest levels of walking and cycling in Europe. The Office of National Statistics in 2010 released figures that showed that the annual miles walked per person had dropped by 22 miles in the 15-year period from 1995 to 2010 (Office of National Statistics, 2010). This is a very disappointing decline in what is probably the most common, easiest and safest form of physical activity. More positively, the distance cycled per person remained static in the same time frame but unfortunately far fewer people cycle than walk. It has been argued that active transport could be a key factor in the achievement of healthy levels of physical activity (Department for Transport, 2010; Jones et al., 2007). Recently there have been a number of interventions aimed at increasing levels of cycling and walking that report some encouraging findings and these will be considered later in the chapter (Department for Transport, 2010; Sloman et al., 2010).

Physical activity is currently the only lifestyle behaviour where men are more likely to achieve government guidelines than women (Table 6.1). Sport is often seen as a traditional male activity, which may contribute to this finding. The Scottish Health Survey 2010 (Scottish Government, 2011) reported far more men engaged in team sports than women who are more likely to participate in exercise classes such as aerobics.

Applying this to George

George would appear to follow a typical male trend of sports participation whilst young and a rapid decline into sedentary behaviour once middle-aged.

As both men and women get older their activity levels decline (Welsh Government, 2011b; Scottish Government, 2011; Department of Health, Social Services and Public Safety, 2011; Department of Health, 2010). The age-related decline in activity is more marked in men than women, but fewer women are active initially so by the time men and women are in their sixties their activity levels are similar. This supports the notion that men are achieving higher physical activity levels because they play more sport. Sporting participation decreases with age more markedly than any other physical activity (Scottish Government, 2011). The relationship between physical activity and social class as measured by the National Statistics Socio-Economic Classification (NS-SEC) is complex and can be best described by an inverted U-shaped curve, with those at either end of the social class scale being the least likely to be active. The Health of Minority Ethnic Groups Survey (Joint Health Surveys Unit, 2004) measured participation in physical activity among the main minority groups in England. Compared to the general population, South Asian and Chinese men and women were much less likely to participate in physical activity of any kind. Bangladeshi men and women were the most inactive and were almost twice as likely as the general population to be classified as sedentary.

Government recommendations for physical activity

In the 1999 Department of Health document *Saving Lives: Our Healthier Nation*, the government recommended that adults took: '30 minutes of moderate exercise 5 times a week.'

Similarly to the 5 A Day fruit and vegetable message, 5 times a week is now a well-known recommendation. In 2011 the Chief Medical Officers of England, Wales, Scotland and Northern Ireland launched their new UK-wide physical activity strategy 'Start Active, Stay Active' (Department of Health, Physical Activity, Health Improvement and Protection, 2011). Whilst remaining broadly the same in terms of amount of activity it now has a much more detailed set of physical activity recommendations including separate recommendations for the under 5s, young people aged 5 to 18, adults aged 19 to 64 and older adults aged 65 and over. The adult recommendations are set out in Table 6.2.

ADULTS (19–64 years):
1. Adults should aim to be active daily. Over a week, activity should add up to at least 150 minutes (2.5 hours) of moderate intensity activity in bouts of 10 minutes or more – one way to approach this is to do 30 minutes on at least 5 days a week.
2. Alternatively, comparable benefits can be achieved through 75 minutes of vigorous intensity activity spread across the week or a combination of moderate and vigorous intensity activity.
3. Adults should also undertake physical activity to improve muscle strength on at least two days a week.
4. All adults should minimise the amount of time spent being sedentary (sitting) for extended periods.

Older adults (65+ years)
1. Older adults who participate in any amount of physical activity gain some health benefits, including maintenance of good physical and cognitive function. Some physical activity is better than none, and more physical activity provides greater health benefits.
2. Older adults should aim to be active daily. Over a week, activity should add up to at least 150 minutes (2.5 hours) of moderate intensity activity in bouts of 10 minutes or more – one way to approach this is to do 30 minutes on at least 5 days a week.
3. For those who are already regularly active at moderate intensity, comparable benefits can be achieved through 75 minutes of vigorous intensity activity spread across the week or a combination of moderate and vigorous activity.
4. Older adults should also undertake physical activity to improve muscle strength on at least two days a week.
5. Older adults at risk of falls should incorporate physical activity to improve balance and co-ordination on at least two days a week.
6. All older adults should minimise the amount of time spent being sedentary (sitting) for extended periods.

Table 6.2 UK recommendations for adult levels of physical activity

	Total recommended amount of physical activity	Intensity moderate	Muscle strengthen exercise	Physical activity for balance and co-ordination
Adults 19–64 years	150 minutes (2.5 hours) per week	30 minutes, 5 days a week	On at least 2 days a week	N/A
Older adults 65+ years	150 minutes (2.5 hours) per week	30 minutes, 5 days a week	On at least 2 days a week	On at least 2 days a week

Source: Adapted from *Start Active, Stay Active* (Department of Health, Physical Activity, Health Improvement and Protection, 2011, p. 7)

The updated advice clearly indicates that the recommendations are for a minimum level of activity and that 'more is better'. For the first time the difference between physical activity levels and levels of sedentary time are acknowledged. Reducing sedentary time, regardless of whether the alternative activity reaches the threshold for moderate activity, has benefits for health over and above those achieved by performing moderate to vigorous physical activity for 2.5 hours or more a week (Department of Health, Physical Activity, Health Improvement and Protection, 2011; Sedentary Behaviour and Obesity Expert Working Group, 2010).

An important issue in these recommendations is the use of the word 'moderate'. What is moderate for one person may be either intense or light for the next. *Start Active, Stay Active* (Department of Health, Physical Activity, Health Improvement and Protection, 2011) provides some useful guidance about what constitutes light, moderate and vigorous activity and their advice is based on the Department of Health 2004 publication *At Least Five A Week* and summarised in Table 6.3.

Table 6.3 Intensities and energy expenditure for common types of physical activity

Activity	Intensity	Energy expenditure (kcal equivalent of a person of 60 kg doing activity for 30 minutes)
Ironing	Light	69
Cleaning and dusting		75
Walking – strolling at 2 mph		75
Painting/decorating	Moderate	90
Walking – 3 mph		99
Vacuuming		105
Golf – walking and pulling clubs	Moderate	129

Activity	Intensity	Energy expenditure (kcal equivalent of a person of 60 kg doing activity for 30 minutes)
Badminton – social		135
Tennis – doubles		150
Walking – brisk 4 mph	Moderate	150
Mowing lawn – walking		165
Cycling – 10–12 mph		180
Aerobic dancing	Vigorous	195
Cycling – 12–14 mph		240
Swimming – slow crawl		240
Tennis – singles	Vigorous	240
Running – 6 mph (10 minutes/mile)		300
Running – 7 mph (8.5 minutes/mile)		345
Running – 8 mph (7.5 minutes/mile)		405

Source: Adapted from *At Least 5 a Week*, Department of Health (Department of Health 2004), © Crown Copyright 2004. Crown Copyright material is reproduced with permission under the terms of the Click-Use Licence

The recent UK-wide physical activity strategy document *Start Active, Stay Active* (Department of Health, Physical Activity, Health Improvement and Protection 2011, p. 7) recommends higher levels of physical activity for children than are recommended for adults (Table 6.4).

Early years (under 5s):
1. Physical activity should be encouraged from birth, particularly through floor-based play and water-based activities in safe environments.
2. Children of pre-school age who are capable of walking unaided should be physically active daily for at least 180 minutes (3 hours), spread throughout the day.
3. All under 5s should minimise the amount of time spent being sedentary (being restrained or sitting) for extended periods (except time spent sleeping).

Children and young people (5–18 years):
1. All children and young people should engage in moderate to vigorous intensity physical activity for at least 60 minutes and up to several hours every day.
2. Vigorous intensity activities, including those that strengthen muscle and bone, should be incorporated at least three days a week.
3. All children and young people should minimise the amount of time spent being sedentary (sitting) for extended periods.

Table 6.4 UK recommendations for levels of physical activity in
individuals aged 18 and under

	Total recommended amount of physical activity	Intensity moderate to vigorous	Muscle strengthen exercise	Physical activity for balance and co-ordination
Early years under 5s	180 minutes (3 hours) per day		N/A	N/A
Children and young people 5–18 years	At least 60 minutes each day	At least 60 minutes each day	N/A	N/A

Source: Department of Health, Physical Activity, Health Improvement and Protection 2011, p. 7

Applying this to George

It is important when communicating with George about his plans to increase his physical activity that what is meant by light, moderate and vigorous is clearly explained and agreed by both parties.

All policy documents acknowledge that the appropriate level of physical activity for good health is not definitive. For weight loss and prevention of weight regain after weight loss there is evidence that higher levels of physical activity are required (Department of Health, Physical Activity, Health Improvement and Health Protection, 2011; Saris *et al.*, 2003). Furthermore, *Start Active, Stay Active* acknowledges that there is clear evidence, particularly for coronary heart disease and type 2 diabetes, that greater participation brings greater benefits (Department of Health, Physical Activity, Health Improvement and Health Protection, 2011). In the past there have been strong calls in Britain for the advice to change from 'moderate' to 'vigorous', perhaps in recognition that a practitioner understanding of the term 'moderate' may be more demanding than a lay understanding of it (BBC News, 2007). The counterargument is that even small increases in physical activity can improve health (Wen *et al.*, 2011) and setting more challenging targets may deter sedentary individuals from attempting to take up physical activity. As is discussed in depth later in the chapter, and in Chapter 4, setting achievable goals is a cornerstone of effective behavioural change (Ajzen, 1998). From a public health perspective the greatest benefits are perceived to be achieved from moving the sedentary to light or moderate activity levels (Department of Health, 2009).

Applying this to George

Any increases in physical activity that George can make are likely to bring some health benefits regardless of whether he actually reaches the government recommendations for activity.

Mental health

Whilst the government's physical activity recommendations are clearly aimed at improving physical health, there is increasing awareness and associated recommendations about the use of physical activity to improve psychological well-being (Crone *et al.*, 2009; National Institute of Clinical Excellence, 2008c). It is clear that physical activity can help maintain general well-being and can also be effective in the treatment of mental health problems (Department of Health, Physical Activity, Health Improvement and Protection, 2011; National Institute of Clinical Excellence, 2009; Government Office for Science, 2008). It is not clear what is the best level of physical activity for well-being and/or treatment of mental health conditions but the current evidence suggests that lower levels of physical activity may be effective in improving psychological well-being than are required to improve physical health (Crone *et al.*, 2009).

Applying this to George

George is sedentary and looking to reduce his stress and depression. He is not currently obese. Setting him a goal of moderate physical activity should deliver the mental health benefits that he requires and may offer additional protective benefits against further weight gain. Setting too hard a target may be unrealistic and potentially detrimental to his self-efficacy.

Health consequences of low physical activity

If you are physically active you are likely to live longer than your sedentary colleagues regardless of whether you are young or old, male or female and regardless of ethnicity or social class (US Department of Health and Human Services, 2008; Department of Health, 2009; Department of Health, Physical Activity, Health Improvement and Protection, 2011; Wen *et al.*, 2011). Indeed, it has been suggested that adults who keep physically fit through activity are 50 per cent less likely to die prematurely than sedentary adults (Warburton *et al.*, 2006). Others are more conservative in their estimates of benefits. The Department of Health (2009) estimated that adults who are physically active have a 20–30 per cent reduced risk of premature death.

Physical activity influences a wide range of health conditions. For example, people who are physically active can achieve up to a 40 per cent reduced risk of developing coronary heart disease, stroke, diabetes and some cancers (Department of Health, Physical Activity, Health Improvement and Health Protection, 2011). Physical activity can also play a role in reducing mental health problems such as depression, stress and anxiety (Crone *et al.*, 2009; National Institute of Clinical Excellence, 2008c, 2009). Newly diagnosed individuals with such chronic diseases face not only a reduction in life expectancy but also a potential reduction in quality of life for the remainder of their lives. Whilst the relationship of physical activity to each disease is valuable, what makes physical activity particularly important is that it can prevent so many different diseases. Physical activity has an important role in treatment but it is its potential to prevent or delay disease onset that is so impressive.

Applying this to George

George has multiple issues of stress, depression and weight gain so one benefit of utilising physical activity as an intervention is that he can tackle them all simultaneously, whereas the medical option involves two different types of medication. Furthermore, stress and depression, if untreated, are both related to weight gain and cardiovascular problems. Consequently, taking physical activity to relieve stress and depression will also serve a preventative function for George, reducing his risk of obesity, cardiovascular disease and type 2 diabetes.

Weight maintenance

Levels of obesity are rising throughout the Western world and the UK is no exception to this trend. In 2011 the Department of Health in England described overweight and obesity as: 'Probably the most widespread threat to health and wellbeing in this country' (Department of Health, 2011, p. 5).

Across all four home countries there has been a threefold increase in obesity from 1980 to 2011 (Department of Health, 2011; Department of Health, Physical Activity, Health Improvement and Protection, 2011; Scottish Government, 2011; Welsh Government, 2011b; Department of Health, Social Services and Public Safety, 2011). Obesity is often associated with physical inactivity leading the Department of Health in 2004 to conclude that: 'Obesity is the main visible sign of inactivity' (Department of Health, 2004, p. 20).

However, it is important to recognise that it is possible to be obese and still achieve high levels of physical activity that will have benefits for health regardless of whether or not recommended body weight is maintained.

Maintaining a healthy body weight should be easy. At its simplest, energy input simply has to equal energy output and weight will remain constant. If your energy intake exceeds your energy output, you will gain weight. Physical activity increases energy output and so decreases the likelihood that an individual will gain weight. However, moderate physical activity is unlikely to make a major contribution to weight loss. Physical activity, at the level suggested by the government, by itself can result in modest weight loss of between 1 to 3 per cent (Pate *et al.*, 2010). Higher levels of physical activity can have more dramatic effects on body weight, but suggesting that obese individuals take even higher levels of physical activity than those recommended by the government is potentially dangerous and probably too challenging for currently sedentary individuals to achieve. Nevertheless, many health professionals and academics have called for new guidelines for weight-loss physical activity to be established. However, recent policy has not developed separate activity recommendations for the overweight other than commenting that more than the recommendations are probably required for weight loss and weight maintenance (Department of Health, 2011; Department of Health, Physical Activity, Health Improvement and Protection, 2011). Previously, the Chief Medical Officer for England did make additional recommendations in his 2004 report, saying:

> 45–60 minutes of moderate activity per day may be needed to prevent the development of obesity … and people who have been obese and have managed to lose weight may need to do as much as 60–90 minutes activity a day in order to avoid regaining weight.
>
> Department of Health, 2004, p. 5

Applying this to George

If George were to achieve an increase in his physical activity levels on its own it is unlikely to result in weight loss but it will help to prevent further weight gain.

Assessment of physical activity

It is beyond the scope of this text to provide a comprehensive review of all the available tools to measure physical activity – over 30 different measures have been reported – but there are a number of good textbooks where this can be obtained (e.g. Buckworth and Dishman, 2002; Thompson *et al.*, 2009). To report the physical activity levels of different groups in the population you will need a measure that is quick and easy to administer to a large number of people. To measure physical activity as part of an individualised fitness programme, you might want a very detailed and accurate measure.

When you are thinking about measuring physical activity you need to consider whether you simply want to know the total time spent physically active in a given period or whether you wish to explore the physical activity in more depth. You may wish to know the time spent at different intensities of physical activity. You may wish to understand the impact that the physical activity is having on the physical state of an individual. You may wish to know the amount of energy a person is using, which might be particularly useful if you are interested in weight control or weight loss. You can measure levels of physical activity in one of four ways, described in Table 6.5.

The first three methods are objective assessments of activity whereas observation is a more subjective assessment (Table 6.5). Objective measures of energy expenditure are more precise, giving reliable information about the duration and intensity of activity, but they can be costly and often not practical for large-scale studies. Furthermore, objective measures cannot tell you much about the type of activity undertaken. The most usual form of observation is to use a questionnaire. The more complex questionnaires can provide detailed information about the type of activities undertaken and good information about duration and frequency but only imprecise information about the intensity of the activity (Table 6.5).

If you are going to use a questionnaire-based assessment of physical activity it is very important to use an established questionnaire that has been tested for reliability and validity. The best questionnaires will have been validated by an objective measure of physiological response to physical activity (such as heart-rate monitoring) or an objective measure of energy expenditure, such as doubly labelled water (Shepard, 2003). Shepard (2003) draws attention to the limited reliability and validity of physical activity questionnaires in general and advises that questionnaires can only be used for simple classification of activity levels and not to estimate individual overall energy expenditure.

Table 6.5 Categories of physical activity measurement

Method of measurement	Assessment	Information available
Measuring a physiological response to physical activity	Objective	Duration Intensity
Calculating the energy expenditure of physical activity	Objective	Duration Intensity
Assessing physiological adaptations to physical activity	Objective	Duration Intensity
Observing (either directly or indirectly) physical activity	Subjective	Duration Intensity Type Frequency

Why are people physically inactive?

The government guidelines for physical activity are not daunting and indeed many health professionals would like them to be more challenging, yet the majority of the population remain sedentary (Department of Health, Physical Activity, Health Improvement and Protection, 2011). The reasons why are undoubtedly complex and not simply down to individual choices. In physical activity, perhaps more than any other lifestyle choice, the role of the physical environment is increasingly recognised as important (Jones *et al.*, 2007; Department for Transport, 2010; Department of Health, 2010; National Institute of Clinical Excellence, 2008a). Environmental, social, demographic, psychological and biological factors have all been implicated in physical activity and the relationship between these factors has been usefully conceptualised by Jones *et al.* (2007) as shown in Figure 6.2.

Obesogenic environments

Health promotion and education in the past tended to be on the individual and persuading the individual to change, but the unsupportive nature of the modern

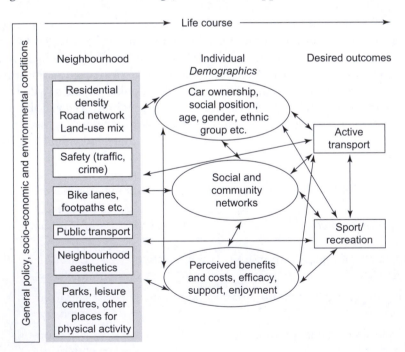

Figure 6.2 Evidence-informed model of the potential determinants of sport/physical activity

Source: Adapted from *Tackling obesities: future choices – obesogenic environments – evidence review,* Government Office for Science (Jones, A., Bentham, G. Foster, C., Hillsdon, M. and Panter, J. 2007), © Crown copyright 2007. Reproduced under the terms of the Click-Use Licence.

environment is now increasingly recognised to play a role in the low levels of physical activity in Western societies (National Institute of Clinical Excellence, 2008a; Department for Transport, 2010; Department of Health, Physical Activity, Health Improvement and Protection, 2011; Jones *et al.*, 2007). The term obesogenic has been adopted by policy makers and refers to an environment that is both supportive of high-calorie intake and unsupportive of physical activity (Foster *et al.*, 2006; Jones *et al.*, 2007).

So what is an obesogenic environment? It has not been clearly characterised, but certainly includes cultural, social and physical characteristics. A robust evidence-base evaluating the impact of the environment on physical activity is starting to accrue. A review of interventions that used the environment to encourage physical activity included 25 studies, 19 of which were studies aimed at encouraging the use of stairs (Foster *et al.*, 2006). Whilst encouraging the use of stairs is undoubtedly a worthwhile venture, it is unlikely to increase the physical activity of any single individual by more than 10 minutes a day. The initial focus on encouraging stair use, often by decisional prompts, may reflect the difficulties with both instigating and evaluating more major changes to the environment. For instance, changing the environment to facilitate walking or cycling to work might require the building of cycle paths and the provision of showers, lockers and bicycle sheds. Such major changes to the built environment have not been well evaluated in the past but more recent developments are beginning to be instigated and evaluated (Department of Health, Physical Activity, Health Improvement and protection, 2011; Sloman *et al.*, 2010).

Whilst the physical environment is clearly a factor in physical activity and particularly in active transport, Jones *et al.* (2007) have concluded that the influence of the environment is probably small and the mechanisms are unclear. One thing is clear: the actual environment is less important than the way people perceive it (Maddison *et al.*, 2009). Jones *et al.* (2007) raise concerns that improving the environment by building more cycle paths, safe places to walk etc. may have its main effects on those who are already active rather than the sedentary. It doesn't matter how many cycle paths you build if people do not see themselves as able to use them. We need to understand why some people feel able to use good environmental resources to be physically active and some people do not. It is clear that interventions that both improve the environment and provide psychological support for change are more effective than a standalone change in the environment (National Institute for Health and Clinical Excellence, 2006; Yang *et al.*, 2010).

Applying this to George

George currently uses his car to commute to work and to transport his children to extra curricular activities. In this way the obesogenic environment that makes car use the easiest method of transport is negatively impacting on his lifestyle. Environmental and work-place initiatives to encourage cycling to work could enable George to achieve the recommended levels of physical activity.

Psychological factors

Many different individual factors have been postulated to underpin physical activity behaviours; some of the key factors are presented in Table 6.6. The basic tenet of most traditional health promotion campaigns is to present either the risk of an unhealthy behaviour and/or the benefits of a healthy behaviour. Traditionally health promotion has been based on the assumption that individuals will weigh up the costs and benefits of physical activity and make a decision about whether to take up physical activity. However, understanding that lack of physical activity is bad for your health has not been found to predict physical activity (Harrison *et al.*, 2002).

It would appear that perceptions and beliefs about the health risks and benefits of physical activity play only a small part in explaining variations in physical activity behaviours. Some authors have argued that they may be necessary but are not sufficient to promote physical activity change. However, studies such as Blue (2007), which found no relationship between risk perception and activity levels, raise the question as to whether a perception of risk is necessary at all. It would seem that investing time or money in informing people about the costs of being sedentary and the benefits of being physically active is unlikely to generate widespread increases in physical activity.

Barriers to performing physical activity, such as lack of access to resources or lack of time, have some relationship to whether people are active but perceived behavioural control over such barriers has been found to be a better predictor of physical activity than the actual barriers themselves (Ayotte *et al.*, 2010). Individuals often cite a list of barriers to physical activity as an explanation for remaining sedentary. Working with them to look at how they can overcome these barriers and increase confidence in their own ability to control these external factors is more likely to generate change than changing the barriers. If barriers are removed, perhaps by improving leisure

Table 6.6 Psychosocial factors implicated in behavioural change

Psychosocial factor	Potential to increase physical activity
Perception of the risk of physical inactivity	Minimal
Belief in the effectiveness of physical activity to improve health	Minimal
Objective barriers to physical activity	Minimal
Perceived behavioural control – perceived ability to overcome recognised barriers	Good
Social norms	Minimal as currently measured, but may be more useful if measured as perceived peer levels of activity
Self-efficacy	Good
Self-regulation	Good
Social support	Good

facilities in the local area, such strategies are more likely to be utilised if their implementation is supported by psychological support for uptake of the new behaviour.

Applying this to George

If George is to engage in active transport he will need to believe that he can overcome any perceived barriers.

Social norms refer to what is both acceptable and practised behaviour in the majority of an individual's peer group. Measures of social norms for physical activity have consistently predicted little variation in physical activity, but usually measure perceptions of what significant others think is acceptable behaviour (injunctive social norms) rather than perceptions of peer behaviour itself (Priebe and Spink, 2011). This has led some authors to argue that social influences on intentions to exercise and exercise behaviour are less important than individual factors. However, recently Priebe and Spink (2011) reported that descriptive norms were highly correlated with individual physical activity. Currently an accurate perception of peer physical activity for most groups in the population will be one of low levels of physical activity. Jones et al. (2007 p. 38), in their extensive review of obesogenic environments for the influential Foresight project remain convinced that 'capturing the concept of social norm and modifying that norm is one of the major public health challenges'.

There is considerable evidence to suggest that social support plays an important role in adherence to physical activity (Kouvonen et al., 2011). The Whitehall II Study, which followed over 5,000 working people from a baseline assessment between 1997 and 1999 to a follow-up assessment between 2002 and 2004, found that high emotional and practical social support could help individuals remain physically active. High levels of practical social support also supported positive changes in physical activity (Kouvonen et al., 2011). The Whitehall II study is important because it is one of the few longitudinal studies reporting factors that can make a positive and sustained impact on levels of physical activity. A recent systematic review of reviews by Greaves et al. (2011) evaluating factors associated with increased effectiveness of physical activity interventions also found that social support was a consistent factor in successful physical activity interventions. Consequently, the evidence for social support being a key factor in both increasing and maintaining physical activity levels is extremely robust. Greaves et al. (2011) recommend, based on their review, that future interventions should encourage participants to engage others who are important to them (such as family, friends and colleagues) in planned changes in physical activity.

Applying this to George

George has a clear idea of what the benefits of activity would be for him. Currently, he perceives that he lacks social support for taking up exercise and he sees both the lack of support from his wife and his long working day as barriers to undertaking physical activity. Generating social support from his wife and also from his workplace for George's planned changes to his physical activity will significantly increase his likelihood of making a change and sustaining it.

Probably, the most important psychological factor to emerge from research into physical activity behaviour is the concept of self-efficacy (Maddison *et al.*, 2009; Ashford *et al.*, 2010; Ayotte *et al.*, 2010). Self-efficacy refers to internal aspects of control such as perceived ability and self-confidence for specific activities. Ayotte *et al.* (2010), in one of the more recent of a number of studies reporting similar findings, found that both middle-aged and young-old individuals who reported higher levels of exercise self-efficacy were more likely to be physically active. Self-efficacy predicts both the adoption and maintenance of physical activity (Ashford *et al.*, 2010). Self-efficacy has been argued to be enhanced by personal accomplishment or mastery, vicarious experience or verbal persuasion. According to Ayotte *et al.* (2010) people with high self-efficacy are more likely to utilise self-regulatory strategies, which in turn exert a large total effect on physical activity. Self-regulatory strategies include: goal setting, self-monitoring, planning and problem solving. The impact of self-regulatory strategies on self-efficacy is likely to be through the positive feedback achieved from setting and achieving goals, highlighting the importance of setting short-term, challenging but achievable targets. The value of effective self-regulatory techniques has been firmly established by Greaves *et al.* (2011) in their review of reviews of effective physical activity interventions which concluded that using self-regulatory techniques was associated with increased intervention effectiveness. Self-efficacy is not unrealistic optimism as it is based on experience, so in consequence realistic goals and plans that an individual can achieve are essential to increase self-efficacy (Ashford *et al.*, 2010).

Applying this to George

George has low self-efficacy about his ability to increase his physical activity. Helping him increase his self-efficacy through self regulatory techniques such as specific goal setting, prompting self monitoring and providing feedback on performance will increase his chances of achieving his goals.

Stages of change

A key concept that has emerged from process models of change such as the transtheoretical model (TTM) is the idea that changing lifestyle behaviours is not a one-off decision but a continuous process and that people move between different motivational states (see Chapter 4). Identifying where individuals are in terms of stages of change may well result in more effective interventions to support the uptake of physical activity (Table 6.7).

Different types of psychological support are more likely to be effective at different stages. When individuals are in the pre-contemplation stage they may need education and motivational interventions to encourage them to move into the contemplation stage. Individuals who are contemplating or preparing to change may need to be helped to build self-efficacy for the proposed change. Individuals who are in the action or maintenance stage will need support to stay motivated, again through increases in self-efficacy and in self-regulation. They need to ensure that their new physical activity behaviour becomes a habitual behaviour that they can maintain without constant cognitive effort (Verplanken and Melkevik 2008).

Habitual behaviour

The powerful influence of past behaviour over future behaviour (Verplanken and Melkevik, 2008) adds support to the argument that being physically active is an ongoing process. Consistent patterns of past behaviours are often referred to as habits. The reasons why people take up physical activity may be different from the reasons

Table 6.7 The stages of change in relation to achieving the government recommendations for physical activity

Stages of change	Behavioural and motivational characteristics
Pre-contemplation	Individuals are sedentary and have no intention of doing 30 minutes of physical activity five times a week in the next six months
Contemplation	Individuals are sedentary but intend to take up physical activity to the level of the government recommendations within six months
Preparation	Individuals are taking some physical activity and intend to achieve acceptable levels of activity within six months
Action	Individuals have taken up physical activity and are exercising for at least 30 minutes five times each week. This is the least stable stage and relapse is likely
Maintenance	Individuals have been regular exercisers for six months or more and are unlikely to relapse

why people maintain the behaviour. Starting something new is a conscious choice but maintaining the behaviour may be habitual. Habits are those behaviours that we do automatically in response to a situation, rather than behaviours we think about. Past physical activity is an important predictor of future physical activity (Hirvensalo and Lintunen, 2011; Verplanken and Melkevik, 2008) which suggests that developing physical activity habits is key to promoting long-term positive changes in physical activity. So what supports the development of a habit? Aarts *et al.* (1997) suggested that enjoyment is an essential aspect of habit formation. Traditional approaches to health behaviours have been negatively focused, looking predominantly at why people don't exercise. Consequently, enjoyment as a moderator of physical activity choices is seldom investigated. Nevertheless, studies that do consider enjoyment report that individuals who are regular long-term exercisers report positive emotions during and following physical activity (Hagberg *et al.*, 2009; Schneider and Cooper, 2011).

Interventions to increase physical activity

Interventions to increase physical activity have been many and varied in many different settings with many different sections of society (Greaves *et al.*, 2011; Department of Health, Physical Activity, Health Improvement and Protection, 2011). It is increasingly acknowledged that to make a significant impact on physical activity levels, interventions will need to be both at the level of the community and individualised (Department of Health, Physical Activity, Health Improvement and Protection, 2011; Department of Health, 2009).

Individual level interventions

Individualised interventions for the purposes of this text refer to interventions to increase physical activity that are aimed at an individual or at a small group of individuals. Interventions such as these can be delivered in primary care and are frequently provided by public and commercial leisure centres and gyms. Walking and cycling groups are run by most councils and there are a plethora of independent groups that organise group level physical activities. Recently there has been a rapid growth in personal trainers who offer support for physical activity to both individuals and small groups. Individualised interventions are usually either information, or behavioural or frequently a combination of both. Unfortunately, in terms of evaluation, research often only evaluates short-term interventions of between 8 to 12 weeks which frequently demonstrate changes in physical activity behaviours immediately after the intervention which are not sustained in the long term (Pavey *et al.*, 2011). It is clear that behavioural change requires long-term support if it is to be sustained (Hardcastle and Hagger, 2011). Strategies for providing long-term support for physical activity are required if we are going to achieve any longer term population changes in physical activity levels. Referring people into short-term exercise programmes that then cease is not an effective strategy as individuals then have to locate and integrate into another activity group, which they may or may not have the psychological, practical or financial resources to achieve.

It should be noted that many individualised interventions are delivered at the individualised level but are part of a wider-scale community wide initiative to increase physical activity. So for example the exercise referral scheme is a UK-wide intervention to increase physical activity but it is delivered through individualised programmes (Pavey et al., 2011). Many pedometer studies are highly individualised in that individuals get given a pedometer, advice and any follow-up feedback on a one-to-one basis but are frequently part of a wide-scale scheme to encourage walking within an organisation or community (Naylor and McKay, 2009).

Exercise referral schemes

Exercise referral schemes are very popular in the UK, with an estimated 600 schemes currently running. These schemes have the opportunity to provide many of the psychological support strategies described earlier, such as social support and goal setting which are known to promote physical activity. A recent randomised controlled trial (RCT) of the Welsh National Exercise Referral Scheme (NERS) found that all participants in the scheme had higher levels of physical activity than those in the control group, with this difference being significant for those patients referred for coronary heart disease risk factors. They also reported positive effects on depression and anxiety, particularly in those referred for mental health reasons. A particularly interesting aspect of this trial was that it included an economic evaluation which concluded for those who adhere to the full programme the scheme is likely to be marginally cost saving (Murphy et al., 2010). In 2011 a systematic review with meta-analysis of exercise referral schemes was published in the British Medical Journal (Pavey et al., 2011) which concurred with the findings from the Murphy et al. (2010) RCT trial. The review found some evidence of a short-term increase in physical activity and a reduction in levels of depression in sedentary individuals who participated in the scheme compared with usual care but no evidence of sustained increases in physical activity. Pavey et al. (2011) concluded that there was support for the potential role of exercise referral schemes to increase physical activity and consequently improve public health but that one of the major limitations of the referral scheme is its focus on short-term interventions (typically 10 to 16 weeks) and the predominance of referrals into gym-based programmes. As mentioned earlier referring individuals into short-term programmes with no transition into long-term programmes is not effective. Participants need long-term support to sustain changes in physical activity. This is an issue of resourcing with many exercise referral schemes lobbying for funds for longer term support schemes (Personal communication, Wyatt-Williams, 2013). Exercise referral schemes are also expanding their repertoires of activities with 'green' exercise opportunities now available and also links with walking schemes that are permanent programmes (Personal communication, Wyatt-Williams, 2013). The current evidence for the value of the exercise referral scheme is encouraging and plans to expand and develop are more encouraging still.

Pedometers

One thing that has emerged from work on goal setting and physical activity is that positive feedback about the successful achievement of goals is key to continued success (Nigg *et al.*, 2008; Watkinson *et al.*, 2010). Regular professional feedback requires significant input from a health professional, so the possibility of feedback through self-monitoring using a relatively cheap monitoring system such as a pedometer has generated a lot of interest. Pedometers have recently become commonplace and the target of 10,000 steps a day is well known (Slack, 2006; Bennett *et al.*, 2006). Research has demonstrated that pedometers can be used successfully as part of a goal-setting programme to increase both the number of steps taken daily (Normand, 2008; Baker *et al.*, 2008: Fitzsimons *et al.*, 2012) and the pace at which individuals walk (Johnson *et al.*, 2006). However, the problem of setting goals that are both challenging and realistic remains, and the general goal of 10,000 steps a day would appear to have been too challenging for many individuals and resulted in failure to meet the daily target, loss of self-efficacy and giving up on the walking programme. In 2006 the National Institute for Health and Clinical Excellence (NICE, 2006) concluded that there was no evidence that the general use of pedometers increases physical activity levels either in the long or short term. However, more recently in the 'Walking for Well-being in the West Study' pedometers were found to be an effective intervention with step counts increased and maintained over 12 months (Fitzsimons *et al.*, 2012) (see Box 6.1).

Box 6.1 Applying research in practice

Does physical activity counselling enhance the effects of a pedometer-based intervention over the long-term: 12-month findings from the Walking for Wellbeing in the West study (Fitzsimons *et al.*, 2012)

This community-based walking intervention was set in the west of Glasgow and it was designed to evaluate the effectiveness of pedometer use either with or without additional cognitive or behavioural support.

Seventy-nine low active men and women (predominantly women) were randomly assigned to receive either a pedometer-based walking programme plus physical activity consultations or the same programme and minimal advice.

Both interventions successfully increased and maintained step counts over 12 months but the physical activity consultations may encourage individuals to be active in other ways beyond walking.

This study is important because it was methodologically rigorous; participants were randomised to the intervention and because it is one of the few pedometer studies to assess impact in the long term (at 12 months).

Some of the limitations of the study were the drop out rate; only 61 per cent of the original sample was available at 12 month follow-up and also the participants were predominantly white, well educated and middle class.

Informational interventions

Hillsdon *et al.* (2005) in their evidence briefing to the Health Development Agency reported that brief advice from a health professional supported by written materials was likely to produce modest short-term (12 weeks or less) increases in physical activity. Information given on an individual basis can be seen as directly relevant to the individual, who cannot ignore their own susceptibility as easily as they can information from media-based campaigns. However, Kinmonth *et al.* (2008) reported no change in physical activity behaviour in sedentary individuals with a family history of type 2 diabetes in response to a motivational advice leaflet when assessed at six months and one year post intervention. They conclude that personal education alone is unlikely to increase physical activity in an environment when there are plentiful inducements to keep still. It is to be hoped as active transport and other wider public health strategies embed themselves into society over the coming years that personal interventions will have more chance of success.

Behavioural and psychosocial interventions

Behavioural and psychosocial interventions include strategies such as persuasion, motivational interviewing, self-regulation and social support. In 2005 Hillsdon *et al.* concluded that interventions that taught behavioural skills and were tailored to individual needs were associated with more long-term changes than interventions without such psychological support. More recently Greaves *et al.* (2011) in their review of reviews concluded that intervention effectiveness was increased by using well-defined/established behavioural change techniques. Further support for the value of psychologically based behavioural change programmes comes from Ogilvie *et al.* (2007), who found that targeted behavioural change programmes were the most effective way to promote walking. Psychologically orientated behavioural change programmes can work through a number of different psychological mechanisms. Perhaps most importantly they can provide regular contact with a health or physical activity practitioner who, seen regularly, can provide social support. Greaves *et al.* (2011) found that increased contact with the intervention provider was associated with increased effectiveness. Furthermore, an exercise specialist can set appropriate goals that foster and develop self-efficacy. Good behavioural change interventions include advice and help with goal setting, overcoming obstacles and developing social support, which facilitate uptake and maintenance of physical activity by increasing self-efficacy (Greaves *et al.*, 2011; Ayotte *et al.*, 2010).

Motivational interviewing

Motivational interviewing (MI) aims to increase an individual's motivation to consider change rather than showing them how to change. If a person doesn't want to change then it is irrelevant if they know how to do it or not. However, if a person is motivated to change then the interventions aimed at changing behaviour can begin. MI can therefore be viewed as the first stage of a process that moves people towards being physically active. The key aspects of MI are presented in Chapter 4. Hardcastle and Hagger (2011) found that participants in an MI intervention to increase physical activity found regular consultations with the MI practitioner helped facilitate lifestyle change. The participants also felt that on-going monitoring and continued support was paramount in their maintenance of any physical activity changes. This requirement for on-going support resonates throughout the literature and suggests that regardless of the intervention, be it one-to-one MI or exercise referral interventions, it must be long-term, perhaps not at initial intensity but nevertheless sustained (Greaves *et al.*, 2011; Hardcastle and Hagger, 2010).

Applying this to George

Working with George in a client-centred way, using motivational interviewing techniques, is more likely to result in increased physical activity than giving him advice about the risks of inactivity and benefits of physical activity.

Goal setting

The key to successful goal setting is setting challenging but realistic goals that enable people to feel they have achieved a goal and giving them confidence that they can achieve the next sub-goal on their way to a healthy level of physical activity. Getting goals right is a tricky task and requires understanding the physical capacities of an individual, their level of skill and their self-efficacy for the various activities that may be involved. Consequently, it requires the skilled input of a health or exercise specialist. It is not enough to set appropriate individualised goals – individuals need to get regular feedback, which may be provided by the health professional or alternatively it may be possible for an individual to self-monitor performance and receive feedback in that way. The key strategies for successful goal setting in relation to physical activity are presented in Table 6.8.

It has been argued that setting behavioural goals, such as attending an exercise class, rather than physiological goals, such as weight loss, are more effective goals to set because the individual has more direct control over behaviour. Furthermore, Segar *et al.* (2008) found that middle-aged women who had weight loss goals participated in less physical activity than their contemporaries who had physical activity goals focused on well-being and stress reduction. It may be sensible when working with people who wish to lose weight to encourage them to set interim goals around well-being in order for them to achieve the physical activity levels that they require.

Table 6.8 Effective strategies in goal setting to increase physical activity

Strategy	Example
Explore client motivation. This might be done using the stages of change paradigm. Pre-contemplation clients are not ready for goal setting	A middle-aged women refers herself to you to increase her physical activity levels to help her lose weight. Clearly, she is motivated to be more physically active. You need to explore the overarching goal. A weight loss goal may be less achievable than a stress reduction goal
Break down long-term goal into a series of short-term sub-goals and create an action plan	You might set the client a series of short-term goals, such as increasing weekly steps or getting off the bus two stops earlier to walk to work
Attempt where possible to set behavioural goals rather than physiological goals	If your client has an overarching aim of weight loss you should nevertheless encourage them to set behavioural goals rather than physiological 'pounds lost' targets
Evaluate client self-efficacy for the various behaviours involved in goal achievement	There are many different types of physical activity and the more confident the client is about performing an activity the more likely they are to achieve it
Tailor sub-goals to client to ensure they are challenging but realistic and perceived as such by the client	Your client may wish to set goals that are unrealistic; rapid weight loss is attractive to most individuals wishing to lose weight. You need to negotiate a goal for which you are likely to be able to deliver positive feedback
Provide regular feedback to the client or provide a mechanism for the client to self-monitor performance and receive feedback	Feedback needs to be regular, supportive and reflect behavioural achievements and physiological achievements if appropriate
Goal adaptation	For long-term complex change the short-term sub-goals may need to be reviewed and renegotiated as the client's physiological status and self-efficacy change in response to behavioural adaptation

Applying this to George

To increase George's self-efficacy about his ability to be more active, he needs to be encouraged to set himself challenging but achievable goals that he can review regularly.

Social support

One advantage of goal setting, as described previously, is that it requires sustained input from a health specialist and this in itself can provide social support for physical activity. Such behavioural-specific social support has also been demonstrated to support physical activity when provided by friends and peers (Greaves *et al.*, 2011, Kouvonen *et al.*, 2011). Exercise groups can also provide social support for maintaining physical activity (Gruber, 2008). Furthermore, there is evidence from older women that exercise groups can develop over time to provide not only specific social support for maintaining physical activity, but also more general emotional support as the relationships made within the group develop (Bidonde *et al.*, 2009). Consequently, encouraging individuals to participate in exercise groups has the potential to benefit health both through the increased levels of physical activity and also through the social support networks that individuals may develop over time.

Applying this to George

George's social support network is mainly based on his family. Will their general emotional support provide the support for his proposed change in physical activity or will he require further specific social support?

Community level interventions

Community based interventions can involve environmental changes to remove barriers to physical activity; they can be informational or behavioural (Table 6.9). Many interventions at the level of the community are complex, involving a range of strategies. Consequently, evaluating complex and often simultaneous community level interventions can be difficult. However, evidence is emerging about effective ways to evaluate complex interventions that mean more recent interventions such as 'Smarter Choice Programmes in Sustainable Transport Towns' have been more effectively evaluated (Sloman *et al.*, 2010).

Environmental interventions

Public health policy addressing physical activity is increasingly focused on the obesogenic environment by integrating health and transport strategies to promote active transport (Department for Transport, 2010; National Institute for Clinical Evidence, 2008b; Department for Health, Physical Activity, Health Improvement and Protection, 2011). Evidence is just starting to emerge that such policies and associated interventions can make an impact.

Table 6.9 Physical activity interventions in community settings

Type of intervention	Aims
Information-based	To change knowledge and attitudes about the benefits and opportunities for physical activity within a community
Behavioural	To assist people in the development of behavioural management skills that enable them to adopt and maintain behavioural change and/or to create social environments that facilitate and enhance behavioural change
Environmental/policy	To change the structure of physical and organisational environments to provide safe, attractive and convenient places for physical activity

In 2004 the Department for Transport launched its sustainable transport towns project to see whether intensive town-wide smarter choice programmes could significantly influence travel behaviour and traffic. The projects involved changes to the infrastructure, informational and persuasive communications. Three towns were selected to run the projects; Darlington, Peterborough and Worcester. All three programmes aimed to increase use of non-car options, specifically bus travel, cycling and walking, but did not necessarily all use the same strategies. In their review of the projects Sloman et al. (2010) report that cycling increased substantially by between 26 and 30 per cent compared to a decline in similar medium-sized towns. Walking also increased, although not as dramatically, by between 10 and 13 per cent. Again this should be seen in the light of a decline in walking elsewhere. Sloman et al. (2010) conclude that the evidence supports expanding the project wider in the UK. It is important to recognise that these sustainable town projects whilst making changes to the infrastructure and environment also included a range of other informational and supportive strategies. Yang et al. (2010) add further weight to the evidence that active transport interventions can be effective. Their review of interventions to promote cycling conclude that community-wide promotional activities and improving the infrastructure for cycling have the potential to increase cycling by modest amounts. However, they also conclude that changing the environment should always be accompanied by advice and support if substantial changes in travel behaviour are to be gained (Yang et al., 2010).

In the first edition of this book we commented that there was no evidence that active transport schemes were impacting positively on physical activity levels but that this may have reflected the time it takes for such schemes to be implemented and take effect. The first edition concluded that we may see a reversal of the decline in active transport over the next decade. This early evidence is promising, however the UK still has the lowest levels of cycling and walking in Europe. It is important therefore that these localised interventions and strategies are sustained and implemented more widely.

Since the first edition of this book there has been a growth of interest in 'green' activities. There is increasing evidence that taking part in outdoor physical activity in natural or 'green' environments is particularly beneficial for health and well-being (Hawkins *et al.*, 2011). Such environments include nature reserves, woodlands and gardens, but health benefits have also been found from physical activity conducted in more urban green spaces such as inner city parks. Walking in green environments, gardening at home, allotment gardening and community gardening are all physical activities that are receiving increasing attention as potential health-giving activities as a result of the synergistic benefits of exercising and interacting with nature. Common gardening tasks have been shown to involve both moderate and low levels of physical activity for sustained periods (Park *et al.*, 2008, 2011), so the impact of gardening on sedentary time can be considerable. Recently, it has been suggested that allotment gardening is particularly beneficial for health and this may be because of the social interaction opportunities that the allotment site provides as well as the physical activity in a green environment (Hawkins *et al.*, 2011).

All the research indicates that environmental adaptations need to be supported by behavioural interventions to support adaptation to the environment and positive changes in physical activity or we run the risk of supporting only the physical activity behaviours of the currently active (Jones *et al.*, 2007).

Information interventions

Community level information interventions can be as short and simple as point-of-decision prompts at the bottom of where a choice of the lift or the stairs is available, or a more complicated media campaign to encourage people to take up more leisure time activity (Lewis and Eves, 2012; Sloman *et al.*, 2010). Decisional prompts at the base of buildings with a number of floors have been found to be effective in increasing the decision to take the stairs rather than the lift (Lewis and Eves, 2012) (see Box 6.2). Information can be provided through the media in written form or through radio and television campaigns. Increasingly, information is provided through the internet, such as the Change4Life campaign (Department of Health, 2009). In social cognitive terms an information intervention usually attempts to increase people's perception of risk from inactivity. Alternatively, or as well as, an information campaign may highlight the benefits of exercise for health. Most physical activity campaigns will take such a health-orientated focus, although reference to social benefits or enjoyment is not uncommon. Wakefield *et al.* (2010) in their review of informational campaigns found no evidence that informational-only media-based campaigns were effective, which is what we would have predicted from the research evidence about communicating risk and benefits (Thirlaway and Upton, 2009). Multi-component interventions, such as the sustainable transport town projects, where media-based information plays a central part, are more likely to be successful at increasing physical activity (Sloman *et al.*, 2010; Department for Transport, 2010).

Box 6.2 Applying research in practice

Prompt before the choice is made: effects of a stair-climbing intervention in university buildings (Lewis and Eves, 2012)

This paper investigated the effectiveness of volitional and motivational components of a stair-climbing intervention in the workplace during three stages: baseline; a motivational component; and a motivational plus volitional component.

Baseline observations were followed by a motivational intervention which was placed in each of the buildings. This was followed by a volitional intervention, which consisted of a point-of-choice prompt, supplemented by the motivational one.

A total of 14,138 observations were recorded finding that motivational components did not increase stair climbing. However when a volitional component was added (point-of-choice prompt) at the time and place individuals choose their method of ascent, stair climbing increased significantly. It was concluded that the visibility of a prompt at the time a behavioural choice is made appears necessary to change actual behaviour.

Working effectively with others

Physical activity has not traditionally had practitioners embedded into the health service. Dieticians are established professionals allied to medicine whereas physical activity has remained firmly in the remit of local authorities and increasingly private gyms and personal trainers. The Welsh national exercise referral scheme (NERS) is the first wide-scale government scheme that attempts to provide a clear pathway from primary (and sometimes secondary care) into supportive physical activity outside of the health service. NERS comprises two distinct but inter-related elements:

1. Generic NERS sessions for 'low risk' population groups that need some support to increase fitness and reduce general risks of developing chronic conditions; these are 16 week programmes.
2. Specialist NERS sessions for population groups deemed to be 'higher risk' and needing to undertake tailored exercise sessions as part of their rehabilitation; these can be 16 to 48 week programmes depending on the condition.

Many exercise referral schemes (not only NERS) are now expanding their range of activities and individuals can be referred not only to gyms but to increasing diverse activities, including outdoor activities such as Nordic walking. This is often the first port of call for practice nurses, doctors and other specialists such as community diabetic nurses who are trying to encourage physical activity as a preventative strategy. The downside of the scheme is that for some groups in the population uptake and adherence were low. For example the evaluation of the NERS found that those who owned a car were twice as likely to join the scheme than non-car owners (Murphy *et al.*, 2010). Adherence to the scheme in different areas of Wales ranged from 11 per cent and 62 per cent suggesting that the scheme is not reaching all sectors in society equally (Murphy *et al.*, 2010); although this has improved following a Motivational Interviewing Training Programme for the exercise professionals and the development of sustainable exit route opportunities within local communities (Personal communication, Wyatt-Williams, 2013). The scheme is in its early days and is expanding its range of activities through collaborative working with Let's Walk Cymru, Age Cymru and other Green Exercise Opportunities which leads individuals towards sustainable exercise within their local communities. Participants continue to receive encouragement to exercise through goal setting and motivational interviewing for a year post referral. For health professionals interested in promoting physical activity in their clients and patients exercise referral schemes offer a safe route into physical activity. Outside of exercise referral the interested health professional will need to work with the local community physical activity networks and local authorities to understand what is available to support individuals into physical activity.

Conclusion

Educational campaigns to increase physical activity have had little impact on population levels of physical activity. We live in an obesogenic environment which discourages physical activity. People need psychological support to enable them to become more physically active and this support will need to be long term if they are both to adopt and maintain healthy levels of physical activity. Currently, evidence suggests that self-regulation through goal setting, self-monitoring and feedback is the most effective way to promote physical activity. Well-set goals can build self-efficacy and support physical activity in the long term. It is clear that enjoyment is central to the long-term maintenance of physical activity but it is not clear why some people enjoy physical activity and others do not. This is an area worthy of further research.

Applying this to George

George is one of the majority of people who understands that physical activity would improve his health and he would like to be more active but he cannot see how he can overcome the barriers he perceives to being more physically active. He doesn't need any more information about his risk or the benefits of physical activity. He needs support in finding a solution that is appropriate to his personal situation. He needs to be encouraged to make small changes to his activity that will give him a sense of achievement and the self-efficacy to attempt further changes. If he wishes to utilise active transport as a strategy he will need to understand the habitual nature of activities such as driving to work and attempt to break the bad habit of driving to work and establish the good habit of cycling to work. He is far more likely to achieve this if his local community invest in supporting cycling. He will lack social support for physical activity if it reduces his time in the home, so utilising active transport will minimise the impact of increasing his physical activity on his family and increase the likelihood that his wife will be supportive. Furthermore, if cycling to work means the car is more available to his wife she may be more supportive.

Key points

- Only a minority of the population achieve the government recommendations for physical activity.
- What makes physical activity so important for health outcomes is the strength of its effect over such a wide range of conditions.
- People generally understand the risks of being sedentary and the benefits of physical activity but still do not get active.
- Self-efficacy is one of the best predictors of successful increases of physical activity and can be built through the encouragement of self-regulatory techniques in individuals.
- Individuals attempting to increase their physical activity levels are most likely to succeed if they get practical and emotional social support from friends, family and/ or the exercise programme.
- The establishment of good physical activity habits may be crucial in the promotion of physical activity.
- Perceptions of the environment may be more important than the objective environment for physical activity.

Points for discussion

- As with other lifestyle activities physical activity interventions are not accessed equally by all members of a community. How can we promote physical activity in those experiencing high levels of deprivation?
- Being sedentary is associated with poorer health and well-being. Should we be encouraging people to reduce their sedentary time, with any level of physical activity or should we remain focused on at least moderate physical activity?
- How would you encourage a person who is currently overweight/obese to become more physically active? Which psychological factors must you be aware of when planning an intervention to promote a more active lifestyle for them and why?

Further resources

Dugdill, L., Crone, D. and Murphy, R. (2009). *Physical Activity and Health Promotion*. Oxford: Wiley-Blackwell.

Bouchard, C., Blair, S. & Haskell, W. (2012). *Physical Activity and Health*, 2nd edn. Leeds: Human Kinetics.

Change for life 0300 123 4567 http://www.nhs.uk/Change4Life

British Heart Foundation http://www.bhfactive.org.uk

Diabetes UK http://www.diabetes.org.uk

References

Aarts, H., Paulussen, T. and Schaalma, H. (1997). Physical exercise habit: on the conceptualisation and formation of habitual health behaviours. *Health Education Research*, 21: 363–374.

Ajzen, I. (1998). Models of human social behaviour and their application to health psychology. *Psychology and Health*, 13: 735–739.

Ashford, S., Edmunds, J. & French, D.P. (2010). What is the best way to change self-efficacy to promote lifestyle and recreational physical activity? A systematic review with meta-analysis. *British Journal of Health Psychology*, 15: 265–288.

Ayotte, B. J., Margrett, J., A. & Hicks-Patrick, J. (2010). Physical activity in middle-aged and young-old adults: the roles of self-efficacy, barriers, outcome expectancies, self-regulatory behaviours and social support. *Journal of Health Psychology*, 15(2): 173–185.

Baker G., Gray, S.R., Wright, A., Fitzsimons C., Nimmo M., Lowry R., and Mutrie N. (2008). The effect of a pedometer-based community walking intervention 'Walking for Wellbeing in the West' on physical activity levels and health outcomes: a 12-week randomized controlled trial. *International Journal of Behavioural Nutrition and Physical Activity*, 5, 44

BBC News. (2007). Exercise 'must be tough to work'. To be healthy, you really do need to break into a sweat when you exercise, say experts. Available at: www.bbc.co.uk (accessed September 2007).

Bennett, G.G., Wolin, K.Y., Viswanath, K., Askew, S. Puleo, E. and Emmons, K.M. (2006). Television viewing and pedometer-determined physical activity among multi-ethnic residents of low income housing. *American Journal of Public Health*, 96: 1681–1685.

Biddle, S.J.H. and Mutrie, N. (2008). *Psychology of Physical Activity. Determinants, Wellbeing & Interventions*, 2nd edn. Oxon: Routledge.

Bidonde, J.M., Goodwin, D.L. and Drinkwater, D.T. (2009). Older women's experiences of a fitness program: The importance of social networks. *Journal of Applied Sport Psychology*, 21(1): S86–S101.

Blue, C.L. (2007). Does the theory of planned behaviour identify diabetes-related cognitions for intention to be physically active and eat a healthy diet? *Public Health Nursing*, 24(2): 141–150.

Buckworth, J. and Dishman, R. (2002). *Exercise Psychology*. London: Human Kinetics.

Caspersen, C. J., Powell, K. E., & Christenson, G. M. (1985). Physical activity, exercise, and physical fitness: definitions and distinctions for health-related research. Public health reports, 100(2): 126.

Crone, D., Heaney, L. and Owens, C.S. (2009). Physical activity and mental health. In L. Dugdill, D. Crone and R. Murphy (eds) *Physical Activity and Health Promotion*. London: Wiley-Blackwell.

Department of Health (1999). *Saving Lives: Our Healthier Nation*. London: The Stationery Office.

——(2004). *At Least Five a Week*. London: The Stationery Office.

——(2009). *Be Active, Be Healthy*. London: HM Government.

——(2010). *Health Survey for England, 2010*. The NHS Information Centre, 2011. Available at: http://www.ic.nhs.uk/pubs/hse10report (accessed 11 January 2013).

——(2011). *Healthy Lives, Healthy people: A Call to Action on Obesity in England*. London: HM Government.

Department of Health, Physical Activity, Health Improvement and Protection (2011). *Start Active, Stay Active*. London: DoH.

Department of Health, Social Services and Public Safety (2011). *Health Survey Northern Ireland: First Results from the 2010/11 Survey*. Belfast: Department of Health, Social Services and Public Safety.

Department for Transport (2010). *Active Transport Strategy*, London: DfT Publications.

Fitzsimons C.F., Baker G., Gray S.R., Nimmo, M.A., Mutrie N. (2012). Does physical activity counselling enhance the effects of a pedometer-based intervention over the long-term: 12-month findings from the Walking for Wellbeing in the west study. *BMC Public Health*, 12: 206.

Foster, C., Hillsdon, M., Cavill, N., Bull, F., Buxton, K. and Crombie, H. (2006). *Interventions that Use the Environment to Encourage Physical Activity: Evidence Review*. London: NICE.

Government Office for Science (2008). *Mental Capital and Wellbeing: Making the Most of Ourselves in the 21st Century*. Final project report. London: Government Office for Science.

Greaves, C. J., Sheppard, K. E., Abraham, C., Hardeman, W., Roden, M., Evans, P.H. & Schwartz, P., The IMAGE Study Group (2011). Systematic review of reviews of intervention components associated with increased effectiveness in dietary and physical activity interventions. *Biomedical Central Public Health*, 11, 119.

Gruber, K.J. (2008). Social support for exercise and dietary habits among college students. *Adolescence*, 43(171): 557–575.

Hagberg, L.A., Lindahl B., Nyberg L., Hellenius L. (2009). Importance of enjoyment when promoting physical exercise. *Scandinavian Journal of Medicine and Science in Sport*, 19(5): 740–747.

Hardcastle, S., & Hagger, M., S. (2011). 'You can't do it on your own': Experiences of a motivational interviewing intervention on physical activity and dietary behaviour. *Psychology of Sport and Exercise*, 12: 314–323.

Harrison, J.W., Mullen, P.D and Green, L.W. (2002). A meta-analysis of studies of the health belief model with adults. *Health Education Research*, 7: 107–116.

Hawkins JL., Thirlaway K. Backx, K, & Clayton D (2011). Allotment gardening and other leisure activities for stress reduction and healthy aging. *HortTechnology*, 21: 577–585.

Hirvensalo M. and Lintunen T. (2011). Life-course perspective for physical activity and sports participation. *European Review of Aging and Physical Activity*, 8: 13–22.

Hillsdon, M., Foster, C., Cavill, N., Crombie, H. and Naidoo, B. (2005). *The Effectiveness of Public Health Interventions for Increasing Physical Activity among Adults: A Review of Reviews*, 2nd edn. London: Health Development Agency.

Johnson, S.T., McCargar, L.J., Bell, G.J., Tudor-Locke, C., Harber, V.J. and Bell, R.C. (2006). Distilling a complex prescription for type 2 diabetes management through pedometry. *Diabetes Care*, 29(7): 1654–1655.

Joint Health Surveys Unit (2004). *Health Survey for England. The Health of Minority Ethnic Groups*. London: The Stationery Office.

Jones, A., Bentham, G., Foster, C., Hillsdon, M. and Panter, J. (2007). *Tackling Obesities: Future Choices – Obesogenic Environments – Evidence Review*. London: United Kingdom Government Foresight Programme, Office of Science and Innovation.

Kinmonth, A., Wareham, N., J., Hardeman, W., Sutton, S., Prevost, T., A., Fanshawe, T., Williams, K., M., Ekeland, U., Speigilhalter, D. & Griffin, S., J. (2008). Efficacy of a theory-based behavioural intervention to increase physical activity in an at-risk group in primary care (ProActive UK): a randomized trial. *Lancet*, 371: 41–48.

Kouvonen, A., De Vogli, R., Stafford, M., Shipley, M., Marmot, M., G., Cox, T., Vahtera, J., Vaananen, A., Heponiemi, T., Singh-Manoux, A. & Kivimaki M (2011). Social support and the likelihood of maintaining and improving levels of physical activity: the Whitehall II Study. *European Journal of Public Health*, 22: 514–518.

Lewis, A. and Eves, F. (2012). Prompt before the choice is made: effects of a stair-climbing intervention in university buildings. *British Journal of Health Psychology*, DOI: 10.1111/j.2044-8287.2011.02060.

Maddison, R., Vander Hoorn, S., Jiang, Y., Ni Mhurchu, C., Exeter, D., Dorey, E., Bullen, C., Utter, J., Schaaf, D. & Turley M. (2009). The environment and physical activity: the influence of psychosocial, perceived and built environmental factors. *International Journal of Behavioural Nutrition and Physical Activity*, 6: 19.

Murphy, S., Raisanen, L., Moore, G., Tudor Edwards, R., Linck, P., Hounsome, N., Williams, N., Ud Din, N. & Moore, L. (2010). *The Evaluation of the National Exercise Referral Scheme in Wales*. Cardiff: Welsh Government.

National Institute for Health and Clinical Excellence. (2006). Four commonly used methods to increase physical activity: brief interventions in primary care, exercise referral schemes, pedometers and community-based exercise programmes for walking and cycling. London: NICE.

——(2007). *Behavioural Change at Population, Community and Individual Levels*. London: NICE.

——(2008a). *Promoting and Creating Built or Natural Environments that Encourage and Support Physical Activity*. London: NICE.

——(2008b). *Workplace Health Promotion: How to Encourage Employees to be Physically Active*. London: NICE.

——(2008c). *Occupational Therapy Interventions and Physical Activity Interventions to Promoting the Mental Well-being of Older People in Primary Care and Residential Care*. London: NICE.

——(2009). *Depression: The Treatment and Management of depression in Adults*. London: NICE.

——(2010). *Prevention of Cardiovascular Disease at Population Level*. London: NICE.

——(2011). *Preventing Type 2 Diabetes: Population and Community Level Interventions in High Risk Groups and the General Population*. London: NICE.

Naylor, P.J. and McKay, H.A. (2009). Prevention in the first place: schools a setting for action on physical inactivity. *British Journal of Sports Medicine*, 43: 10–13.

Nigg, C.R., Borrelli, B., Maddock, J. and Dishman, R.K. (2008). A theory of physical activity maintenance. *Applied Psychology: An International Review*, 57(4): 544–560.

Normand, M.P. (2008). Increasing physical activity through self-monitoring, goal setting and feedback. *Behavioural Interventions*, 23: 227–236.

Office of National Statistics (2010). National Travel Survey. London: The Stationery Office.

Ogilvie, D., Foster, C., E., Rothnie, H., Cavell, N. Hamilton, V., Fitzsimons, C., F.M. and Mutrie, N. (2007). Interventions to promote walking: systematic review. *British Medical Journal Online*, DOIi: 10.1136/bmj.39198.722720.BE.

Park, S. A., Shoemaker, C. A., & Haub, M. D. (2008). Can older gardeners meet the physical activity recommendation through gardening? *HortTechnology*, 18, 639–643.

Park, S., Lee, K., & Son, K. (2011). Determining exercise intensities of gardening tasks as a physical activity using metabolic equivalents in older adults. *HortScience*, 46: 1706–1710.

Pate, R.R., Yancey, A.K. and Kraus, W.E (2010). The 2008 physical activity guidelines for Americans: implications for clinical and public health practice. *American Journal of Lifestyle Medicine*, 4 (3): 209–217

Pavey, T.G., Taylor, A.H., Fox, K.R., Hillsdon, M., Anokye, N., Campbell, J.L., Taylor, R.S. *et al.* (2011). Effect of exercise referral schemes in primary care on physical activity and improving health outcomes: systematic review and meta-analysis. *BMJ: British Medical Journal*, 343.

Priebe, C.S. & Spink, K.S. (2011). When in Rome: descriptive norms and physical activity. *Psychology of Sport and Exercise*, 12: 93–98.

Rejeski, W. J., & Brawley, L. R. (1988). Defining the boundaries of sport psychology. *The Sport Psychologist*. 2(3): 231–242.

Saris, W.H.M., Blair, S.N., van Baak, M.A., Eaton, S.B., Davies, P.S.W., Di Pietro, L., Fogelholm, M., Rissanen, A., Schoeller, D., Swinburn, B., Tremblay, A., Westerterp, K.R. & Wyatt, H (2003). How much physical activity is enough to prevent unhealthy weight gain? Outcome of the IASO 1st Stock Conference and consensus statement. *Obesity Reviews*, 4: 101–114.

Schneider, M. and Cooper, D.M. (2011). Enjoyment of exercise moderates the impact of a school-based physical activity intervention. *International Journal of Behavioural Nutrition and Physical Activity*, 8: 64.

Scottish Government (2011). *The Scottish Health Survey 2010, Volume 1: Main Report*. Edinburgh: The Scottish Government. Available at: http://www.scotland.gov.uk/Publications/2011/09/27084018/91 (accessed 11 January 2013).

Sedentary Behaviour and Obesity Expert Working Group (2010). *Sedentary Behaviour and Obesity: Review of the Current Scientific Evidence*. London: Department of Health.

Segar, M.L., Eccles, J.S. and Richardson, C.R. (2008). Type of physical activity goal influences participation in healthy midlife women. *Women's Health Issues*, 18: 281–291.

Shepard, R.J. (2003). Limits to the measurement of habitual physical activity by questionnaires. *British Journal of Sports Medicine*, 37: 197–206.

Slack, M.K. (2006). Interpreting current physical activity guidelines and incorporating them into practice for health promotion and disease prevention. *American Journal of Health System Pharmacy*, 63: 1647–1653.

Sloman, L., Cairns, S., Newson, C., Anable, J., Pridmore, A. and Goodwin, P. (2010). *The Effects of Smarter Choice Programmes in the Sustainable Travel Towns: Summary Report*. London: DfT.

Thirlaway, K.J. and Upton, D. (2009). *The Psychology of Lifestyle: Promoting Healthy Behaviour*. London: Routledge.

Thompson, W.R., Gordon, N.F. and Pescatello, L.S (2009). ACSM's guidelines for exercise testing and prescription. Lippincott: Williams & Wilkins.

US Department of Health and Human Services (2008). *Physical Activity Guidelines Advisory Committee Report*, from the Physical Activity Guidelines Advisory Committee. US Department of Health and Human Services.

Verplanken, B. and Melkevik, O. (2008). Predicting habit: the case of physical exercise. *Psychology of Sport and Exercise*, 9: 15–26.

Wakefield M.A., Loken B. and Hornik (2010). Use of mass media campaigns to change behaviour. *Lancet*, 367: 1261–1271.

Warburton, D.E.R, Whitney, N.C. and Bredin, S.S.D. (2006). Health benefits of physical activity: the evidence. *Canadian Medical Association Journal*, 174: 801–809.

Watkinson, C., van Sluijs, E.M.F., Sutton, S., Marteau, T. and Griffin, S.J. (2010) Randomised controlled trial of the effects of physical activity feedback on awareness and behaviour in UK adults: the FAB study protocol, *BMC Public Health*, 10: 114.

Welsh Government (2011a). *Health Trends in Wales 2011*. Cardiff: WAG

——(2011b). *Welsh Health Survey 2010*. Available at: http://www.wales.gov.uk/statistics (accessed 11 January 2013).

Wen, C.P., Wai, J.P.M., Tsai, M.K., Yang, Y.C., Cheng, T.Y.D., Lee, M., Chan, H.T., Tsao, C. K., Tsai, S. P. and Wu, X. (2011). Minimum amount of physical activity for reduced mortality and extended life expectancy: a prospective cohort study. *Lancet*, 378: 1244–53.

Wyatt-Williams J (2013). *National Exercise Referral Coordinator, Welsh Local Government Association*. Personal communication.

Yang L., Sahlqvist S., McMinn, A., Griffin, S.J. and Ogilvie D (2010). Interventions to promote cycling: systematic review. *British Medical Journal*, 341: c5293.

7 Sensible drinking

Learning objectives

At the end of this chapter you will:
- have recognised the extent of harmful, hazardous and binge drinking in the UK
- understand the government recommendations for sensible drinking
- have reviewed the health and economic consequences of drinking alcohol
- have evaluated the role of psychological factors in drinking too much
- have evaluated the available interventions to help people reduce their drinking.

Case study

Charlotte is a 35-year-old marketing executive who works in a large advertising company. She has worked in the firm since graduating from college and has been regularly promoted. Much of her work involves networking with clients. Charlotte drank heavily as a student and, unlike many of her contemporaries, has not reduced her drinking. Drinking is part of her work culture. Charlotte often travels with her work, staying in expensive hotels and drinking late with colleagues and clients. Charlotte is proud of her ability to drink on a par with her male colleagues and to get up early after a long night and work well. Charlotte takes a lot of exercise and considers that the exercise she takes offsets the alcohol she consumes.

Charlotte and her partner are considering starting a family but have so far been unable to conceive. They have come to see you for advice about assisted conception. Charlotte's partner is clearly concerned about her drinking and thinks she should cut down. Charlotte is less concerned and thinks she will be able to 'cut down a bit' once she is pregnant. Charlotte says she doesn't drink all that much, probably around the government guidelines unless there is a special occasion! She goes on to imply that she thinks government recommendations are rather stringent and that on the continent they are far more relaxed about drinking. You suspect that Charlotte drinks well over the weekly recommended limits and is probably a dependent drinker.

Introduction

Alcohol is a chemical compound, ethyl alcohol, often called ethanol. Ethanol produces intoxication through its action on the brain and is a legal psychoactive drug. Intoxication leads to impairments in psychomotor control, reaction time and judgement. Intoxication also influences mood and reduces social inhibitions (Babor *et al.*, 2010).

In the UK the alcoholic content of drinks is usually stated on the container as percentage volume but it can also be measured as fluid ounces, millilitres, grams or units. One unit of liquid contains 8 grams of pure alcohol. It is generally understood that one drink contains one unit of alcohol, which can sometimes be true. However, many beers and wines are stronger, having higher percentage volumes of alcohol than those cited in Table 7.1. Furthermore, many servings are larger than the standard measures (Table 7.1).

Applying this to Charlotte

If Charlotte is counting each drink as a unit, drinking large glasses of wine, or strong lagers, then she could easily be underestimating her alcohol consumption by at least half.

People can easily be categorised as smokers or non-smokers but categorising people as drinkers or non-drinkers, although just as straightforward, is not as useful. Smoking is bad for you, with no positive aspects whatsoever. The majority of the UK population, similarly to all Western societies, do not smoke. However, the picture is very different

Table 7.1 Drinks containing 1 unit of alcohol

Single (25 ml) pub measure of spirits (40% alcohol)
Small glass (125 ml) of wine (9% alcohol)
Half a pint of standard strength beer/lager/cider (3.5% alcohol)

Source: www.alcoholandyou.org

when it comes to alcohol. Ninety per cent of people in the UK drink alcohol and the relationship between alcohol and health is complicated (HM Government, 2007). Whereas most smokers wish to quit only 18 per cent of people who drink in the lower risk ranges wish to change their behaviour (HM Government, 2012). Drinking a lot is bad for you but drinking moderately has some health benefits, particularly for men. Moderate drinkers have lower mortality rates than non-drinkers (Lee *et al.*, 2009). Some countries ban alcohol or promote total abstinence but the policy in the UK is to promote 'sensible drinking', not total abstinence (HM Government, 2007, 2012). Sensible drinking has been defined by the government as: 'drinking in a way which is unlikely to cause yourself or others significant risk of harm' (HM Government, 2007, p. 3).

In contrast, hazardous drinking has been defined as *'an established pattern of drinking which brings the risk of physical and psychological harm'* (McManus *et al.* (2009).

Whereas, harmful drinking is:

> drinking at levels that lead to significant harm to physical and mental health and at levels that may be causing substantial harm to others. Examples include liver damage or cirrhosis, dependence on alcohol and substantial stress or aggression in the family.
>
> HM Government, 2007, p. 3

Recently, the phrase 'binge drinking' has been adopted by the media. Originally the term binge was used by health professionals to describe a prolonged drinking spree lasting at least two or three days. However, the term is now more broadly applied to describe a single drinking session that leads to drunkenness (Plant and Plant, 2006; HM Government, 2007, 2012). Binge refers to the time frame of drinking. It reflects the importance of the pattern in which alcohol is consumed for health and social outcomes. In 2007 binge drinking was described by the government as:

> drinking too much alcohol over a short period of time, e.g. over the course of an evening and it is typically drinking that leads to drunkenness. It has immediate and short-term risks to the drinker and to those around them.
>
> (HM Government, 2007, p. 3)

However, in the government's latest alcohol strategy document the definition of binge drinking is more objective: 'Measured by those who self-report drinking on their heaviest drinking day in the previous week more than 8 units per day for men and more than 6 units per day for women' (HM Government, 2012, p. 5).

Alcohol dependence and volitional drinking

Alcohol dependence is a recognised syndrome and the criteria for alcohol dependence are shown in Table 7.2. People learn to become dependent on alcohol, although there is evidence that some people are more susceptible to become dependent than others

(Grant *et al.*, 2009; Kalsi *et al.*, 2009; Barr *et al.*, 2010). Alcohol interacts with neurotransmitter systems, which reinforces drinking behaviour through their influence on the positive outcomes from drinking – feeling euphoric, relaxed etc. So, psychological and physiological processes both contribute to the risk of developing a dependency. Individuals differ greatly in their neurophysiological and psychological responses to alcohol and therefore in their risk of developing a clinical dependency. Most people who drink alcohol do not become dependent drinkers. In 2001 Orton reported that 7.5 per cent of men and 2.1 per cent of women in Britain in the 1990s could be classified as having a clinical dependency on alcohol. Eight years later McManus *et al.* (2009) reported that 8.7 per cent of men and 3.3 per cent of women could be classified as being dependent on alcohol, indicating a slight increase in dependency levels. Interestingly, they also report that levels of dependency in young men (aged between 16 and 24) who have the highest dependency levels in the population had dropped from 11.5 per cent in 2000 to 9.3 per cent in 2007. The data all point to drinking patterns changing in the UK. However, dependency is not all or nothing, and many people have lesser degrees of dependency or habit.

Many people, health professionals included, believe that the only serious problems with drinking arise in dependent drinkers or binge drinkers. However, epidemiological studies have made it clear that there is a host of problems related to drinking that are not associated with excessive and dependent drinking, including an increased risk of developing a range of chronic diseases (Rehm *et al.*, 2009; French and Zavala, 2007).

Table 7.2 ICD-10 diagnostic criteria for alcohol dependence

Evidence of tolerance to the effects of alcohol, such that there is a need for markedly increased amounts to achieve intoxication or desired effect, or that there is a markedly diminished effect with continued use of the same amount of alcohol.

A physiological withdrawal state when alcohol use is reduce or ceased, or use of a closely related substance with the intention of relieving or avoiding withdrawal symptoms.

Persisting with alcohol use despite clear evidence of harmful consequences as evidenced by continued use when the person was actually aware of, or could be expected to have been aware of, the nature and extent of harm.

Preoccupation with alcohol use, as manifested by important alternative pleasures or interests being given up or reduced because of alcohol use; or a great deal of time being spent in activities necessary to obtain alcohol, consume it or recover from its effects.

Impaired capacity to control drinking behaviour in terms of its onset, termination or level of use, as evidenced by alcohol being often taken in larger amounts or over a longer period than intended or any unsuccessful effort or persistent desire to cut down or control alcohol use.

A strong desire or compulsion to use alcohol.

Source: Adapted from WHO, 2010

Since the publication of the first edition of this book there has been increasing media interest in the impact of alcohol on our health. A 25 per cent increase in liver disease deaths in England between 2001 and 2009 was widely reported and discussed in the UK media (Effiong *et al.*, 2012; *Guardian*, 2012). Furthermore intoxication is a major factor in many social problems such as disorderly behaviour, violence and crime. Intoxication is possible without dependence (Babor *et al.*, 2010).

Applying this to Charlotte

Based on the ICD-10 diagnostic criteria (Table 7.2) it is unlikely that Charlotte would be classified as a dependent drinker. She is probably best defined as someone who engages in harmful drinking as defined by HM Government (2007).

In 2007 the government paper 'Safe. Sensible. Social' reported that 35 per cent of men and 20 per cent of women exceeded the daily benchmarks on at least one day in the previous week. Other studies have reported levels somewhat higher than these (Table 7.3). Self-report is known to be inaccurate, and people are generally understood to be optimistic about lifestyle behaviours, underestimating drinking and overestimating fruit and vegetable consumption (Scottish Government, 2010).

People drink more when they are young (Welsh Government, 2011; Scottish Government, 2010; Department of Health, Social Services and Public Safety, 2011; Department of Health, 2010). Men traditionally drink more alcohol than women and remain more likely to exceed government recommended guidelines even though those guidelines are higher than those recommended for women. There is evidence that young women are starting to drink more. Emslie *et al.* (2009) reported, in their cross-sectional study of three generations from the west of Scotland, that across the generations the youngest cohort had had the smallest difference between levels of drinking in men and women. Drinking patterns are fluid and subject to a myriad of physiological, psychological cultural and economic influences which makes the picture of gender-related drinking in the UK difficult to interpret. In 2006/7 concerns were articulated about the increased levels of drinking in young British women compared to previous generations (Plant and Plant, 2006; HM Government, 2007; News, 2007). However, further longitudinal evaluation is required to determine whether this is an acute feature of young adult life in women who will then reduce their drinking in later life or whether this trend of increased drinking in young women will persist through the life course (Emslie *et al.*, 2009).

There is evidence in the UK that drinking levels have stabilised and in Scotland that the proportions of both men and women drinking in excess of weekly limits declined between 2003 and 2010 (Scottish Government, 2010). However, too many people still drink more than is healthy. Even in England, where the lowest levels of drinking are reported, more than one-third of men report drinking over the daily recommended units on at least one day a week and for men in Scotland and in Wales that proportion is closer to or above 50 per cent respectively (Table 7.3).

Table 7.3 Drinking prevalence rates in men and women in the UK

Source of data	% of men reporting > 4 units of alcohol on at least one day in the previous week	% of women reporting > 3 units of alcohol on at least one day in the previous week	% of men reporting binge drinking in the previous week	% of women reporting binge drinking in the previous week	% of men reporting exceeding weekly limits	% of women reporting exceeding weekly limits
Statistics on Alcohol: England (NHS, 2012	35%	28%	19%*	12%*	26%	17%
Health Survey for Scotland 2010 (Scottish Government, 2011)	43%	33%	26%*	16%*	27%	18%
Welsh Health Survey (Welsh Assembly Government 2011)	51%	37%	34%*	21%*	No data available	No data available
Health Survey Northern Ireland 2010/2011 (Department of Health, Social Services and Public Safety, 2011)	No data available	No data available	No data available	No data available	27%	16%

*these figures reflect the percentage of men and women who reported that they drank more than twice the recommended daily limit of alcohol on at least one day of the week (for men > 8 units and for women > 6 units daily).

> ## Applying this to Charlotte
>
> Charlotte clearly thinks it is acceptable for her to drink a lot and has not yet reduced her drinking as she ages. She does acknowledge that she should reduce her drinking if she were to become pregnant. The average age of pregnancy has risen considerably, so if pregnancy does trigger a reduction in drinking in women it will be coming far later for the current generation of women.

Hurcombe *et al.* (2010) reviewed the research on alcohol and ethnicity in the UK since 1995 and concluded that, despite diversity within and between ethnic groups, most minority ethnic groups had higher levels of abstinence and lower levels of drinking than those reported by people from white backgrounds. In particular abstinence is high in people from Pakistani, Bangladeshi and Muslim backgrounds. What is interesting is that when people from these generally abstinent groups do drink they tend to drink heavily; these groups have similar levels of alcohol dependency and are less likely to seek support and advice from professionals for their drinking problems (Hurcombe *et al.*, 2010). In many minority ethnic groups, being in a high income group is associated with lower likelihood of abstinence and higher levels of drinking. It is possible that drinking is under-reported in some young people and women from ethnic minorities where their drinking is proscribed (Hurcombe *et al.*, 2010).

Unlike smoking, no straightforward linear socio-economic patterns in drinking emerge. We see different socio-economic effects on patterns of drinking in men and women. Whereas men at the lower end of the socio-economic scale are more likely to 'binge' drink than their professional or managerial counterparts, in women there is either no socio-economic influence on drinking reported or professional/managerial women are found to drink more. Only in ethnic minority groups is drinking clearly a high income group activity (Hurcombe *et al.*, 2010).

Government recommendations

Sensible drinking

Since 2007 the government has recommended that:

- Adult women should not regularly drink more than 2–3 units of alcohol a day;
- Adult men should not regularly drink more than 3–4 units of alcohol a day; and
- Pregnant women or women trying to conceive should avoid drinking alcohol. If they do choose to drink, to protect the baby they should not drink more than 1–2 units of alcohol once or twice a week.

HM Government, 2007, p. 3; 2012, p. 5

These daily guidelines replace the original weekly guidelines of 14 units a week for women and 21 units a week for men and were conceived to highlight the importance of avoiding 'binge drinking' (Moss *et al.*, 2009). In 2011 the UK parliament Science and Technology Committee (Science and Technology Committee, 2011) advised that the evidence on alcohol and health needed reviewing but that in the meantime the public should be advised to take at least two alcohol-free days a week and the sensible daily limits should not be increased.

Harmful drinking

The government defines harmful drinking for women as drinking more than six units a day or over 35 units a week. Harmful drinking for men is defined as more than eight units a day or over 50 units a week (HM Government, 2007).

Hazardous drinking

Intakes between the upper sensible limits of 3 and 4 units per day for women and men, respectively, and harmful drinking levels are considered hazardous (Anderson, 1993).

Binge drinking

There is much debate about what binge drinking is. Is it the number of units you consume, the alcohol content of your blood or the degree of drunkenness you experience that best defines binge drinking? Units consumed is usual in most policy documents and drinking more than double the daily safe limits in one session is usually considered a 'binge'. However, it must be acknowledged that many individuals would not consider 6–8 units in an evening to constitute binge drinking, particularly if it doesn't result in them feeling particularly drunk (Plant and Plant, 2006). On the other hand, more than six or eight units (depending on your sex) are enough to significantly increase your risk of cardiovascular events (O'Keefe *et al.*, 2007).

> Trends in binge drinking are usually identified in surveys by measuring those drinking over 6 units a day for women or 8 units a day for men. In practice, many binge drinkers are drinking substantially more than this level or drink this amount rapidly, which leads to the harm linked to drunkenness.
>
> HM Government, 2007, p. 3

Applying this to Charlotte

In common with many other people, Charlotte considers the government recommendations for sensible drinking to be rather stringent and probably erring on the side of caution.

Health consequences of drinking

The relationship between drinking and health is complicated. Viewed overall, the effects of alcohol on health are predominantly negative. However, alcohol can have positive effects on health outcomes when consumed moderately (Balakrishnan et al., 2009; O'Keefe et al., 2007; French and Zavala, 2007).

Indirect health consequences of drinking

People under the influence of alcohol are more likely to be aggressive and behave violently, hurting other people and themselves (HM Government, 2007 & 2012; Hughes et al., 2007; Room et al., 2005; Plant and Plant, 2006). Almost half of the incidences of domestic violence are caused by people under the influence of alcohol. In 2007 the HM Government (2007) reported that amongst young people who binge drink a quarter become involved in anti-social or disorderly behaviour (HM Government, 2007; McManus et al., 2009). More recently in 2012 the HM Government recognized the role that 'pre loading' plays in binge drinking and anti-social behaviour. Individuals who drink before going out were found to be 4 times more likely to drink in excess of 20 units on one night out and 2.5 times more likely to have been involved in a fight (HM Government, 2012, Hughes et al., 2007). Drinking also has the potential to make people more vulnerable to crime (Nicolas et al., 2008). Fifteen per cent of rape victims recorded by the 2001 British Crime Survey were raped when they were under the influence of alcohol. Heavy drinking has also been linked to increased numbers of sexual partners (see Chapter 9), which increases the risk of sex-related infections.

People who are intoxicated are also more likely to have accidents. Car accidents are the most common form of unintentional alcohol-related injury (Room et al., 2005). The World Health Organisation (WHO, 2002) estimate that 20 per cent of car accidents worldwide are alcohol related. In the UK in 2011, 5 per cent of road casualties and 15 per cent of all road deaths occurred when someone was drink-driving (Department of Transport, 2012). In the UK, where drink-driving laws are relatively stringent, from 1980 to 1999 the number of people killed or seriously injured annually in drink-driving incidents fell from 9,000 to fewer than 3,000, which is a significant reduction in alcohol-related incidents. However, the number of people killed or seriously injured in drink-driving incidents over the past 10 years has stabilised and new strategies to reduce such unnecessary fatalities may be needed (HM Government, 2007).

Direct consequences of drinking

Alcohol has been found to increase the risk of over 60 medical conditions (Room *et al.*, 2005). The relationship between alcohol consumption and cardiovascular health is not linear; often it is the pattern of drinking that is important. Patterns of drinking, especially irregular, heavy drinking, have been linked to an increase risk of coronary heart disease, stroke and diabetes even when the overall volume of alcohol intake is low (Room *et al.*, 2005; O'Keefe *et al.*, 2007). Conversely, regular low to moderate alcohol consumption is associated with a reduced risk of cardiovascular disease. Another drinking pattern that appears positive for cardiovascular disease is drinking with meals (Room *et al.*, 2005; O'Keefe *et al.*, 2007). French and Zavala (2007) reported that there is a J-shaped relationship between drinking and total mortality, with moderate drinkers having the lowest mortality rates, heavy drinkers the highest and abstainers/light drinkers somewhere in between.

In some diseases a linear relationship between alcohol consumption and disease does exist. Breast cancer risk increases linearly with increased alcohol consumption, with 10 grams of alcohol a day increasing the relative risk of breast cancer by 9 per cent. A daily consumption of between 30 and 60 grams a day increases the relative risk by 41 per cent (Chen *et al.*, 2011). Depression, epilepsy and alcohol addiction can all be caused by excessive drinking (Room *et al.*, 2005; Balakrishnan *et al.*, 2009; HM Government, 2007; Plant and Plant, 2006). Furthermore, drinking can make existing psychological conditions such as depression or anxiety worse.

The disorders most people think of as being caused by alcohol are liver diseases, but many people who have liver disorders are not heavy drinkers. In 2001 there were 9,231 deaths from liver diseases and in 2009 there were 11,575, a rise of 25 per cent. Although not all these deaths are alcohol related, alcoholic liver disease is the most common cause of liver disease death (Effiong *et al.*, 2012).

In England and Wales, alcohol-related injury or illness accounts for 180,000 hospital admissions a year (HM Government, 2007). Alcohol-related deaths in the UK have more than doubled between 1991 and 2006, from 6.9 per cent to 13.4 per cent per 100,000 (Office of National Statistics, 2008). A summary of the major disease and injury conditions related to alcohol and the percentage of incidents that are attributable to alcohol is presented in Table 7.4.

One area of concern is the number of people living with chronic diseases who regularly drink above the sensible drinking guidelines. Many people with diseases such as diabetes, coronary heart disease and hypertension where alcohol is implicated in the aetiology and progression of the disease continue to drink beyond their diagnosis (see Table 7.5).

Table 7.4 Major disease and injury conditions related to alcohol. Diseases are listed in order, with those with the highest percentage of alcohol involvement listed first

Disease or injury
Alcohol use disorders
Cirrhosis of the liver
Oesophageal cancer
Liver cancer
Homicide
Motor vehicle accidents
Mouth and oropharynx cancers
Epilepsy
Poisonings
Self-inflicted injuries
Drownings
Haemorrhagic stroke
Breast cancer
Falls
Ischaemic heart disease
Unipolar depressive disorders
Diabetes
Ischaemic stroke

Table 7.5 Percentage of people not drinking sensibly despite diagnosis

Condition	Men	Women
Hypertension	42	10
CHD	34	6
Stroke	33	7
Diabetes	35	8
Kidney disease	26	6
Depression	42	16

Source: *Safe. Sensible. Social. The Next Steps in the National Alcohol Strategy*, Department of Health and The Home Office (2007), © Crown copyright 2007. Reproduced under the terms of the Click-Use Licence

Measuring drinking

Population levels of drinking can be estimated from per capita consumption, which is basically an estimate of all the alcohol produced (minus all alcohol exports) and imported into a country divided by the number of adults living there. Per capita consumption is a crude measure that is useful for international comparisons and for monitoring population consumption over time. However, it tells us little about who is drinking within that population or anything about how they drink. Collecting data from individuals provides more useful information about drinking. Physiological measures such as a urine test provide an objective measure of alcohol levels and some indication about drunkenness, but individual differences in alcohol tolerance will influence the levels of drunkenness displayed. Surveys are probably both the most common and also the most problematic way to collect data about drinking. Surveys can tell us a lot about who is drinking and on patterns and volume of consumption, and can enable comparisons over time. They are a useful way of evaluating the effectiveness of alcohol intervention strategies. However, non-response bias is a potential problem for drinking surveys, which usually achieve response rates of about 60 per cent. It is plausible that the types of people who do not complete surveys about drinking are different in their drinking from the types of people who do complete surveys and this introduces a serious bias. Furthermore, it is well established that people completing surveys about their drinking tend to underestimate the amount of alcohol that they consume (Plant and Plant, 2006). Nevertheless, survey estimates of alcohol consumption do predict alcohol-related conditions, which suggest that they do at least place people in an appropriate place in the drinking continuum (Room *et al.*, 2005). A summary of the strategies available to measure drinking is provided in Table 7.6.

Table 7.6 Methods to measure drinking

Method	Advantages	Disadvantages
Per capita consumption	Enables international comparisons and monitoring of population drinking over time	Crude, subject to error and fails to identify who is drinking
Breathalyser tests	An objective, acute measure of alcohol levels	Needs to be immediate, gives only limited data about drunkenness
Urine tests	An objective, acute measure of alcohol levels	Needs to be immediate, gives only limited data about drunkenness
Blood samples	An objective, acute measure of alcohol levels	Needs to be immediate, gives only limited data about drunkenness

Method	Advantages	Disadvantages
Questionnaire surveys of drinking habits	A quick and easy way of accessing data from a large sample. Can provide information about drinking patterns over time	Prone to response biases. People tend to underestimate their drinking in surveys. Response rates to drinking surveys are usually about 60%, so information cannot be said to be representative
Interviews about drinking habits	Provides in-depth data about drinking habits	Prone to response biases. Not practical for large-scale surveys
Direct observation	Free from response biases. Unlikely to provide data about drinking patterns over time	Difficult to achieve reliable results in drinking situations. Not practical for large-scale surveys

Applying this to Charlotte

It would be possible to get an accurate measure of how much Charlotte drank at any one point by taking a blood sample whilst she was drunk. However, this is not likely to occur unless she is arrested. Asking Charlotte to self-report on her drinking is likely to be biased as she may well adapt her answers to reflect what she knows are recommended drinking levels.

Why do people drink more alcohol than is sensible?

People in the UK have always drunk alcohol, sometimes sensibly and sometimes stupidly, so fundamentally nothing has changed. Overall, the majority of adults drink at least occasionally and most people drink moderately with few harmful effects. There are many reasons why people drink: because they enjoy the taste, because they like the disinhibiting effects of alcoholic drinks and because consuming them is a sociable thing to do in our culture (HM Government, 2012). Young people often start to drink as part of their transition into adulthood (Measham and Ostergaard, 2011). In the UK, drinking is a symbolic behaviour that facilitates social bonding and peer status in adolescents. Some authors have argued that alcohol can provide young people with a seemingly adult status (Paglia and Room, 1999). More recently Kuntsche and Cooper (2010) reported that enhancement motives (seeking fun and excitement) predict weekend drinking behaviour in young people more than other psychosocial factors. Alcohol consumption at any age can be functional, providing pleasure, alleviating boredom, satisfying the desire for sensation seeking or acting as a coping or escape mechanism.

Alcohol serves an important social function. It enhances social integration and facilitates the development of relationships (Kuther and Timoshin, 2003). It is hardly surprising that people drink most at a period in their lives which is normally associated with the development of stable adult relationships (Paglia and Room, 1999). Increased levels of drinking in newly divorced people may in part be due to the breakdown of stable relationships and the desire to establish new relationships (HM Government, 2007). Social isolation is a key factor in poor health outcomes (York Cornwell and Waite, 2009), so the positive social function of alcohol in enabling people to develop social relationships should not be overlooked.

Applying this to Charlotte

Charlotte started to drink a lot at college, where drinking enabled her to make friends and cope with the transition from adolescence to adulthood.

Socio-economic factors

The relationship between socio-economic factors and drinking is not simple. There is some evidence that people from the most deprived walks of life are more likely to binge drink, develop alcohol dependency and to die from conditions caused by excessive drinking (HM Government, 2007). However, regular consumption at levels above the recommended limits is more likely in people from higher socio-economic groups, particularly in women (Craig and Mindell, 2008; Welsh Assembly Government, 2009). Alcohol in our culture can be considered to have no class boundaries.

Applying this to Charlotte

Charlotte is one of the new generations of professional women who drink to excess regularly, illustrating that excess drinking, unlike smoking, is not class related.

Psychological factors

Many different psychological factors have been used to explain why people drink. Initially, it was believed that educating people about the risks of excessive alcohol consumption would change their behaviour. However, similarly to other lifestyle behaviours, there is little evidence that perceptions of risk can explain much if any of the variation in drinking behaviour (Moss *et al.*, 2009).

Kuther and Timoshin (2003) investigated the role of social cognitive variables in predicting alcohol use. They found that self-efficacy for controlling drinking predicted self-reported drinking. Those who believed they could control their drinking drank less. Gilles *et al.* (2006) demonstrated that alcohol expectancies and self-efficacy are related to drinking behaviour. Williams *et al.* (2007) found that self-efficacy was a key factor in predicting improved drinking habits in individuals identified as drinking unhealthily in the primary care setting. Similarly, Murgraff *et al.* (2007) found that improving self-efficacy for the ability to control their drinking resulted in a reduction in binge drinking in young women.

Applying this to Charlotte

As a woman working in a traditionally male environment Charlotte may not feel able to refuse a drink when she is out with clients and colleagues.

Social norms are consistently related to drinking behaviour. Studies that report strong relationships between social norms and drinking behaviour ask individuals how much they think their peers are drinking (descriptive norms). Kuther and Timoshin (2003) looked at both descriptive peer norms and descriptive parental norms, and found that both were associated with levels of drinking in students, although the relationship was stronger for peer norms. The impact of descriptive social norms represented through virtual social networks rather than traditional social networks has also been demonstrated in recent research (see Box 7.1). It is clear that for young people at least we establish what is typical and appropriate group normative behaviour from both actual and virtual interactions (Litt and Stock, 2011). Both McAlaney *et al.* (2007) and Bertholet *et al.* (2011) have demonstrated that college students typically over-estimate the amount of alcohol consumed by their peers. Similarly, in the workplace the descriptive drinking norms within that organisation and among colleagues were strongly associated with drinking behaviours both within and outside the working environment (Barrientos-Gutierrez *et al.*, 2007). The relationship between perceptions of peer drinking norms and individual drinking has influenced interventions to reduce drinking. An individual could overestimate the acceptability of drinking among his or her peers or may underestimate the practice of health behaviours (Ramos and Perkins, 2006). Consequently, a number of interventions have attempted to challenge individual perceptions of normative drinking behaviours amongst their peers and have met with some success (Ramos and Perkins, 2006; Delong *et al.*, 2006).

However, it can be argued that drinking plays a valuable role in establishing social relationships and networks. Kuther and Timoshin (2003) found that students who reported higher levels of drinking were significantly more likely to report high levels of social support. High levels of social support are important for the well-being of people and protect against a range of health conditions (Cohen and Janicki-Deverts, 2009). It is important to recognise the value of drinking to young people who are embarking on the difficult job of establishing secure adult relationships.

The evidence that understanding stage of change is useful or important in changing drinking behaviours is not conclusive with some authors arguing that the transtheoretical model (TTM) cannot help in predicting drinking behaviour (Callaghan *et al.*, 2007; Williams *et al.*, 2007). Williams *et al.* (2007) found that measures of readiness to change did not predict either future heavy episodic drinking or future overall consumption in 312 primary care patients who drank unhealthily. They found that self-efficacy for controlled drinking predicted lower consumption and less heavy episodic drinking and concluded that interventions that support self-efficacy, such as motivational interviewing, might have greater utility than stage-based interventions for promoting behavioural change in people who drink unhealthily. Conversely, Heather *et al.* (2009) argue that if you measure the stage of change accurately then the model does predict 'getting better' which lends support to systematic treatment approaches based on the concept of stages of change.

In conclusion, there is some evidence that social cognitive factors can predict sensible drinking in populations. In particular, social norms, measured as descriptive social norms, are important in understanding drinking behaviour. As with other lifestyle behaviours, risk perception appears to have little or no value in predicting drinking behaviour. Similarly to other lifestyle behaviours, the role of self-efficacy in promoting drinking behavioural change looks promising.

Applying this to Charlotte

The drinking culture in Charlotte's job clearly plays a large role in her drinking choices.

Box 7.1 Applying research in practice

Adolescent alcohol-related risk cognitions: the roles of social norms and social networking sites (Litt and Stock, 2011)

This paper examined the impact of socially based descriptive norms on willingness to drink alcohol, prototype favourability, perceived vulnerability for alcohol related consequence, and affective-based attitudes towards alcohol use.

Descriptive norms were manipulated by having 189 young adolescents view experimenter-created profile pages from the social networking site Facebook, which either showed older peers drinking or not.

Findings found that Facebook profiles portraying alcohol use as normative among older peers significantly impacted on willingness to use, attitudes towards use, and perceived vulnerability.

The authors concluded that adolescents who perceive that alcohol use is normative, as evidenced by Facebook profiles, are at higher risk for cognitions shown to predict alcohol use than adolescents who do not see alcohol use portrayed as frequently on Facebook. This research is important because it demonstrates how perceptions of peer normative behaviour are influenced by virtual social network, at least in young people. Young people who use social network sites will usually be 'friends' with a far larger number of individuals than they regularly interact with in 'real' settings.

Interventions to reduce drinking

The Nuffield Council on Bioethics (2007) have argued that public health policies should be about enforcement and they propose an 'intervention ladder' as a useful way of conceptualising public health interventions and their impact on an individual's choice (Table 7.7).

Until recently, for drinking, current government policies have been firmly focused on strategies from the final two rows of the table, guiding choices and enabling choices, although certain limited strategies from higher in the table, such as taxation on alcohol and limited legal restrictions on drinking in some contexts (driving), have been in place for some time. However, the latest government alcohol strategy (HM Government, 2012) does commit to tackling the availability of cheap alcohol by introducing a minimum unit price which is believed by many practitioners to be (if set high enough) a highly cost-effective strategy to reduce harm from alcohol (Anderson *et al.*, 2009; Wagenaarr *et al.*, 2009). The Chief Medical Officer for England in 2009 suggested that a minimum price of 50 pence per unit of alcohol would generate a reduction in health and social harm (Black *et al.*, 2010).

Many interventions to encourage sensible drinking are aimed at adolescents and young people with the goal of preventing the establishment of unhealthy drinking habits. The rationale for a predominance of interventions for this age group includes

Table 7.7 The intervention ladder

Level	Description	Drinking example
Eliminate choice	Introduce laws that entirely eliminate choice	Prohibition
Restrict choice	Introduce laws that restrict the options available to people	Remove alcohol from supermarkets
Guide through disincentives	Introduce financial or other disincentives to influence behaviour	Increase taxes of alcohol via taxation
Guide through incentives	Introduce financial or other incentives to influence people's behaviour	Fund alcohol-free events
Guide choices	Change the default policy	Recommend sensible levels of alcohol consumption
Enable choice	Help individuals to change their behaviour	Provide drinking cessation schemes

Source: Adapted from Nuffield Council on Bioethics, 2007

the indisputable fact that young people are the heaviest drinkers in society (HM Government, 2012). Furthermore, there is an assumption that 'bad leads to bad' as studies indicate that alcohol misuse in adolescence places individuals at increased risk for adult alcohol abuse and related problems (Fiellen *et al.*, 2013); although it should be remembered that it only increases the risk and bad beginnings do not always have bad ends. Many people who experiment with excessive drinking in their youth are not excessive drinkers in their mid-to-late twenties (Masten *et al.*, 2008). Nevertheless, it is indisputable that it is in adolescence that drinking begins, so encouraging sensible drinking in this cohort continues to be high on public health agendas.

Individual level interventions

Early drinking interventions

There are a great many school, university and community-based programmes focused on preventing the early onset of drinking and promoting sensible drinking (Anderson *et al.*, 2009). In 2003 Foxcroft *et al.* reviewed the effectiveness of programmes designed to prevent excessive drinking in young people and, worryingly, found very little evidence that any of these programmes were effective. What they did find was that several studies did reduce drinking in the short term (12 weeks or less) but that drinking had returned to baseline levels when re-assessed later.

More recently, and in line with increased confirmation from genetic studies that certain individuals have an increased genetic risk for developing addictions to alcohol and/or other substances (Barr *et al.*, 2010; Grant *et al.*, 2009; Kalsi *et al.*, 2009), the efficacy of personality-targeted interventions has been investigated (see Box 7.2). It is encouraging to see that initial research indicates that personality targeted interventions may be useful (O'Leary-Barrett *et al.*, 2010; Conrod *et al.*, 2011). However, it also raises ethical issues as the genetic underpinning of these 'at risk personality factors' start to be understood (Barr *et al.*, 2010; Clarke and Thirlaway, 2011; Grant *et al.*, 2009; Kalsi *et al.*, 2009). Dependency and addiction are complex conditions and are multi-factorial, undoubtedly influenced by a number of different genes and also by a range of environmental factors. Genetic risk is highly personal, sensitive, complex and potentially discriminating information. As we start to understand genetic risk for complex multi factorial behaviours such as drinking alcohol, the potential benefits of using such information will have to be carefully considered in light of the considerable costs (Clarke and Thirlaway, 2011).

Box 7.2 Applying research in practice

Personality-targeted interventions delay uptake of drinking and decrease risk of alcohol-related problems when delivered by teachers (O'Leary-Barrett *et al.*, 2010)

This large scale, multi-school trial examined the efficacy of teacher-delivered personality targeted interventions for drinking over a six-month period.

The study was a randomised controlled trial with schools allocated either to the intervention arm or the control arm. Over 2000 students were assessed for elevated personality risk factors for substance misuse such as sensation seeking, impulsivity, anxiety sensitivity and hopelessness. There were 696 adolescents invited to participate in teacher-led personality targeted interventions and 463 were assigned to the non-intervention control group.

At six months post intervention the students who had participated in the intervention were drinking significantly less overall and had a 55 per cent decreased risk of binge drinking compared to students in the control group.

As is common with all lifestyle intervention research the follow-up period is short and longer-term evaluations are necessary. Nevertheless, it is encouraging to see that interventions to reduce drinking can be effective in individuals assessed as at a higher risk for developing hazardous or harmful drinking behaviours. This trial is important because it demonstrates that trained professionals can deliver personality-targeted programmes; they do not always need to be facilitated by a clinical practitioner. This research is also important because it indicates a different way of identifying 'at risk' individuals whereas traditionally we have used social demographic factors to identify 'at risk' groups.

Family-based interventions

There have been some promising family-based interventions, including the Iowa Strengthening Families (ISF) Programme and the Preparing for Drug Free Years (PDFY) Programme (Spoth *et al.*, 2004). Both programmes aimed to develop prosocial bonds within the family and coping skills of the adolescent. Spoth *et al.* (2004) reported that both interventions delayed the initiation of drinking and reduced current use compared to the control group and that these differences persisted for four years past baseline. Interventions like this with long term effects are reassuring and suggest that it is possible to intervene positively in adolescent drinking. However, great care must be taken to identify the active ingredient in successful interventions, given the very many programmes that fail to deliver long-term change. It would seem that increasing the skills of young people (an efficacy-based intervention) and improving their social support networks are key to enabling them to resist peer pressure to take up drinking. Foxcroft *et al.* (2003) raise a note of caution when interpreting these findings in a British context. The different legal position and promotion of abstinence until 21 in the US compared to the promotion of sensible drinking in the UK may mean that successful strategies in the US may not be successful in the UK. Indeed, Percy *et al.* (2011) suggest in their report for the Joseph Rowntree Foundation that parental attempts to restrict teenagers' contact with alcohol are seldom effective, although the parental attempts they describe are predominantly around injunctive norms, i.e. the setting of rules and expectations. Interestingly in the Joseph Rowntree Foundation report the most effective parental strategy was not to drink or to drink very little themselves (Percy *et al.*, 2011). In this way the Rowntree study supports the growing body of literature which suggests that injunctive norms and expectations about what is acceptable drinking behaviour do not influence drinking, whereas descriptive norms (what people believe their peers are actually drinking) are important. Whilst adolescents are living at home their parents will form part of their regular social circle and provide evidence about what is acceptable drinking for their children.

Student interventions

In 2007 Carey *et al.* published a review of individual-level interventions to reduce college student drinking which included 62 studies and nearly 14,000 participants. They reported that participants in risk reduction interventions drank significantly less relative to controls over follow-up intervals of up to six months. Whilst this is a review of a very specific group of young people it is nevertheless very positive that interventions to reduce drinking in this group, where drinking is endemic, can reduce the amount of alcohol consumed. The review indicates that individual, face-to-face interventions using motivational interviewing and personalised normative feedback result in the greatest reductions in alcohol-related problems.

Face-to-face individualised interventions are a resource intensive intervention and young people do not often seek help for their drinking behaviour (Bewisk *et al.*, 2010). The internet has the potential to provide some level of personalised feedback and interaction whilst being a less resource intensive intervention. It may also be a more acceptable way for young people to look for help with their drinking. A multi-centred study in four universities in the UK demonstrated that web-based interventions for student drinking can be effective (Bewick *et al.*, 2010). In this instance, similarly to the study with adolescents described in Box 7.1, the intervention was based in social normative theory with participants receiving both personalised feedback and social norms information. Interestingly, the control group in this study were monitored on their drinking without receiving the intervention but their drinking still reduced. This indicates that monitoring has an impact on drinking, possibly because it encourages self-regulation (see Chapter 4 for more on self-regulation).

Established drinking interventions

Intervening in primary care is the most common way for behavioural interventions to reach their audience of established drinkers (Mulvihill *et al.*, 2005). In Britain, brief counselling interventions in primary care settings are the most common way that people who volitionally drink too much will receive support (Mulvihill *et al.*, 2005). It is likely that many people who are clinically dependent on alcohol and who perhaps warrant more intense intervention are also treated in this way, and so the effectiveness of these interventions for volitional drinkers may be underestimated if participants with a serious addictive disorder are included.

Brief interventions

There are two main types of brief intervention: structured brief advice or extended brief intervention. Nearly all of the latter are based on the principles and practice of 'motivational interviewing' (see Chapter 4, psychology in practice).

Brief interventions for alcohol use are well researched. They have many advantages. They are acceptable to individuals with less severe drinking problems for whom more intensive treatment would not be acceptable. They can be administered by a wide range of health professionals in many settings and are inexpensive (NICE, 2010). Brief interventions, although varied, have been described by Moyer *et al.* (2002) as having the six features linked in Table 7.8. Such a format for brief interventions is also recognised by Williams *et al.* (2007) who state that brief alcohol counselling interventions generally include assessment, feedback, advice and goal setting.

Level of motivation derives from the stage of change concept which acknowledges the importance of the individual's motivational state (Table 7.8). Self-efficacy is another key social-cognitive variable which has been consistently found to predict behavioural change. Consequently, the theoretical underpinnings of such an approach are clear. Interestingly, Williams *et al.* (2007) found that readiness to change did not predict reduction of drinking in their cohort of people identified in primary care as drinking unhealthily, whereas levels of self-efficacy did predict a reduction in drinking. Williams *et al.* (2007) argue that in the busy primary care setting, formal assessment of readiness to change may not be necessary.

Table 7.8 Key features of brief interventions

1   A goal of reduced or non-problem drinking rather than abstinence
2   Delivered by a health professional as opposed to an addiction specialist
3   Directed at volitional rather than dependent drinkers
4   Addressing individuals' level of motivation to change drinking habits
5   Being self (as opposed to professionally) directed, and/or
6   Having the following ingredients: feedback of risk; encouraging responsibility for change; advice; menu of options; therapeutic empathy; enhancing self-efficacy

Brief interventions, while following this basic framework, can vary, and, in particular, the length of a brief intervention, although intuitively short, can range from one 5-minute session to brief multi-contact interventions. Many studies have found that brief interventions can reduce drinking (Nilsen *et al.*, 2008; Mulvihill *et al.*, 2005; Williams *et al.*, 2007; NICE, 2010). However, Mulvihill *et al.* (2005) in their comprehensive review conclude that multi-contact brief interventions are more effective than single very brief sessions. Moyer *et al.* (2002) raise a note of caution that many studies report only short-term follow-up of a year or less. Given that Foxcroft *et al.* (2003) in their review of interventions aimed at young people found that most of the short-term effectiveness of interventions had disappeared at medium-term follow-up, the lack of long-term follow-up of brief interventions needs to be addressed.

As brief interventions for drinking become to be an established method of addressing hazardous drinking, the settings in which the intervention is delivered have started to be considered. In particular, the efficacy of the intervention within accident and emergency departments is being considered (NICE, 2010; Nilsen *et al.*, 2008). Intervening when individuals are in the NHS as a result of their hazardous drinking may capture more people for whom the intervention is appropriate than is achieved within primary care settings. There is some evidence that intervening with a brief intervention within accident and emergency settings can be effective and reduce drinking levels (Nilsen *et al.*, 2008). However, the capacity for accident and emergency staff to deliver such brief interventions as a regular part of their role has not been established (NICE, 2010). Other settings that have been explored as suitable for brief interventions for drinking include the workplace (Webb *et al.*, 2009).

Cognitive behavioural therapy

Cognitive behavioural therapy has also been found to reduce drinking in some studies (Mulvihill *et al.*, 2005). The cognitive behavioural therapy approach emphasises the ability to exercise control, and the physiological cravings for alcohol can undermine the therapeutic approach. Furthermore, the therapist and the client have to agree on the level of control they are aiming for: total abstinence or controlled drinking (Westbrook *et al.*, 2007).

Community level interventions

There are certain groups in the UK who would support prohibition and the criminalisation of alcohol (elimination or restriction of choice in the intervention ladder, see Table 7.7) but these are a minority voice and there is no likelihood of prohibition becoming policy in the UK. However, alcohol is illegal for certain age groups in various countries. In the US, you cannot legally drink alcohol before you are 21, whereas in the UK you may drink alcohol in private from the age of 5 but may not purchase or drink alcohol in a public place until you are 18. Consequently, some interventions, particularly school-based interventions in the US, have a goal of total abstinence. The rationale for such a stance is not only to limit damaging drinking in young people in the 'here and now' but also to reduce the risk of problem drinking later, because the earlier a person starts to drink, smoke or use illegal drugs the higher the risk of later abuse (Masten *et al.*, 2008; Saunders and Rey, 2011). In the UK, where young people are legally allowed to drink before the age of 21, there is more of a problem with binge drinking in young people. However, many countries with equally lax laws about the age of drinking do not report the same incidence of binge drinking that is reported in Britain (HM Government, 2012). Nevertheless, there is evidence that increasing the minimum drinking age would reduce drinking in young people (Kaestner and Yarnoff, 2011).

Taxation as a public health measure is a familiar practice in smoking (Guidance through disincentives, Table 7.7). It is only effective if people drink less in response to rising price. Some people have argued that it would only be worthwhile to increase taxes if people who are currently drinking hazardously or dangerously drank less in response to the rise in tax. In 1995 Manning *et al.* (1995) argued that moderate drinkers are more affected by price changes than heavy drinkers so taxation would not decrease the risk of alcohol-disorders. However, in 2010 Black *et al.* reported that amongst their cohort of individuals with serious alcohol problems the lower the price paid per unit the more units a patient consumed. Wagenaar *et al.* (2009) also report that price affects drinking across the whole population of drinkers from light drinkers to heavy drinkers. Xu and Chaloupka (2011) suggest that adolescents are particularly responsive to the price of alcohol and that increasing the price of alcohol would be effective in reducing heavy drinking and related harm among this cohort. Finally, in 2012 there is a move towards using alcohol taxation as a public health measure (HM Government, 2012).

Early drinking interventions

Many community level drinking interventions aimed at young people are educational in nature. In essence these are risk communication messages and the evidence from psychological research is that improving risk perceptions will have little impact on levels of drinking. Unsurprisingly then, there is little evidence that alcohol education and health promotion have any positive effect on drinking habits in the UK (Plant and Plant, 2006) or the US (Anderson *et al.*, 2009). These campaigns are heard and understood because knowledge about UK drinking guidelines in heavy and binge drinkers has been reported to be as high as 98 per cent (Moss *et al.*, 2009) so it is not that the message is failing to reach the designated audience, rather that the message has no impact on behaviour. Worryingly in the past, there has been some evidence that educational programmes to reduce drinking can have the opposite effect and increase drinking (Duryea and Okwumabua, 1988: Hopkins *et al.*, 1988; Wechsler *et al.*, 2003). More recently, Anderson *et al.* (2009) reported that industry-funded educational programmes tend to lead to positive views about alcohol and the alcohol industry. It is possible that young people who may be attracted to unconventionality or rebelliousness could be attracted by the described risks that are intended to prevent initiation of drinking.

Wechsler *et al.* (2003) evaluated a social marketing based intervention in two colleges in the US. The intervention involved a poster campaign that stated that most students had five drinks on a night out. The result of this was that students drinking fewer than five drinks increased their consumption whilst there was no impact on the drinking of those originally drinking more than five drinks. Wechsler *et al.* (2003) conclude that whilst social marketing strategies are an attractive solution to the problem of heavy drinking for the alcohol industry, they are at best ineffective and at worst counter-productive and tougher measures aimed at limiting access to alcohol and controlling the marketing practices of the beverage industry are more likely to be effective in reducing drinking.

Established drinking interventions

Many interventions to challenge established drinking are aimed at addictive drinkers. Nevertheless, community level interventions to challenge less serious drinking exist. As predicted by psychological research, health promotion messages that inform people about the risks of drinking are as ineffective in established drinkers as they are in early drinkers (Room, 2004; Babor *et al.*, 2010; Plant and Plant, 2006). However, there is evidence that informational campaigns and, in particular, mass media campaigns and health warning labels do have a role to play in the promotion of sensible drinking. In multi-level campaigns where an informational message is supported by programmes to support sensible drinking, decreases in drinking levels have been reported (Paglia and Room, 1999).

There is a significant body of work on workplace drinking norms that suggests that changing workplace drinking norms to support sensible drinking could be key in changing drinking behaviours both in work and non-work contexts (Barrientos-Gutierrez *et al.*, 2007). The challenge will be to develop interventions that can successfully change group-based norms. Challenging descriptive social norms in interventions with young people has been utilised with some success but usually as part of a more individualized intervention (Paglia and Room, 1999; Prochaska *et al.*, 2004). Similar work-based interventions may well be a useful additional strategy for established drinkers. Webb *et al.* (2009) carried out a systematic review of work-place interventions and found 10 studies that reported on work-place alcohol interventions but all had methodological problems. The various study designs, types of interventions, measures employed and types of work-places varied considerably, making comparison of results difficult. However, it appears from the evidence that brief interventions, interventions contained within health and lifestyle checks, psychosocial skills training and peer referral have potential to produce beneficial results. Whilst tackling drinking in the workplace may be identifying a particularly useful community setting in which to work, the interventions that appear to work are more individualised.

Applying this to Charlotte

A work-based intervention would be particularly useful for Charlotte as it is through work that most of her drinking occurs. A change in work culture would support her if and when she decides to change her drinking.

Working effectively with others

Sensible drinking advice ranges from universal prevention messages to specialist treatment. It is increasingly acknowledged that there is a wide-scale need for support with sensible drinking that goes further than public health-based health promotion but is not specialist addiction treatment. Alcohol screening and brief interventions provide a middle level intervention to fill this gap (Burrell *et al.*, 2006) and there are now a number of established brief interventions available and training packages for health professionals to deliver these interventions (Burrell *et al.*, 2006; NICE, 2010). Unlike physical activity or weight reduction, where primary care professionals can direct individuals to out of health care settings for support, supporting sensible drinking remains very much a health care led activity. However, there is increasing interest in delivering brief interventions for drinking in sites outside of primary care and GP surgeries such as accident and emergency settings and also out of health care settings completely and into workplace settings (NICE, 2010). The move to intervening in emergency service settings is in response to evidence that brief interventions for drinking are most productive at a 'moment of crisis' (Burrell *et al.*, 2006, p. 8). The idea is to carry out both the screening and the brief intervention within the same setting, although it is possible that individuals who are screened outside of primary care may also be referred to their GP for intervention.

Regardless of the move to deliver brief interventions in a range of non GP settings, the GP surgery is likely to remain the first port of call for individuals who are actively looking for help with reducing their drinking. Consequently, many health professionals in primary care will require training in order to deliver such programmes and also in identifying when more specialist treatment from their colleagues in alcohol and addiction services is required.

Conclusion

Many people drink more alcohol than is good for them. Drinking is most prevalent in the young, where peer group drinking has been postulated to encourage and support excessive drinking. Similarly, workplace drinking cultures in adults have been found to play a significant role in supporting excessive drinking. It has been argued that reducing the availability and increasing the cost of alcohol are the best ways to reduce excess drinking, and after resisting the calls to increase the cost or limit the sale of alcohol for many years, in 2012 the government agreed to consider introducing minimum cost per unit of alcohol legislation. Interventions that attempt to build self-efficacy for reducing drinking and that challenge perceived social norms for drinking are the best way to help people change their drinking habits within a culture that is generally complicit in excess drinking.

Applying this to Charlotte

It is going to be difficult to help Charlotte until she recognises that she is drinking too much and is motivated to change. The stages of change concept would define her as at the pre-contemplation stage. Introducing her to the idea that many women of her age drink considerably less than she does might be a good way to start.

Motivational interviewing may be effective for Charlotte. On the one hand she has the social support from her partner for change, on the other the challenges of a very pro-drinking culture at work. Removing Charlotte from a working culture that supports excessive drinking would increase the chances of successfully motivating Charlotte to reduce her drinking. However, this is an unlikely scenario. If Charlotte becomes motivated to reduce her drinking then she will need to build her refusal self-efficacy so that she can continue to network with clients and colleagues without drinking to excess.

Charlotte is in the habit of drinking a lot. If she were to succeed in becoming pregnant this would be an ideal time to change this habit and develop new, healthier habits. A major life event such as becoming pregnant upsets routines and provides an opportunity to change habits.

Key points

- Alcohol contributes to a wide range of lifestyle diseases.
- Many people in the UK drink more alcohol than is good for their health.
- Young people are the most likely to drink heavily and to binge drink.
- Young women are drinking more than they did in previous generations.

- Many people will have established drinking habits that are difficult to overcome without being strictly clinically dependent.
- The availability and low cost of alcohol have been implicated in the early establishment of drinking in young people.
- Perceived social norms within university and workplace environments have been found to support hazardous drinking.
- Brief interventions for alcohol use that have a goal of sensible drinking, rather than abstinence, can be delivered by non-addiction specialists and usually include assessment, feedback, advice and goal setting.
- Brief interventions for alcohol use have been found to reduce drinking in the short term, although long-term effects on drinking have not been established.
- Interventions that develop self-efficacy for reducing drinking have been found to be effective.

Points for discussion

- What are the benefits and costs associated with identifying individuals with a genetic risk becoming addicted to alcohol?
- Delaying the onset of drinking in adolescents and young people has been found to reduce the incidence of alcohol-related problems in later life. Should we consider raising the legal drinking age in public places to 21?
- Should we be introducing brief interventions to reduce problem drinking for everyone who visits an accident and emergency unit or is admitted to hospital due to a drink-related incident?

Further resources

Alcoholics Anonymous 0845 769 7555 http://www.alcoholicsanonymous.org.uk/
Talk to FRANK 0800 77 66 00 www.talktofrank.com
Drinkaware Trust http://www.drinkaware.co.uk/
Down your Drink http://www.downyourdrink.org.uk/
NHS: Units of alcohol calculator http://units.nhs.uk/links.html

References

Anderson, P, Chisholm, D & Fuhr, D. C. (2009). Effectiveness and cost-effectiveness of policies and programmes to reduce the harm caused by alcohol. *Lancet,* 373(9682): 2234–2246.
Babor, T., Caetano, R., Casswell, S., Edwards, G., Giesbrecht, N., Graham, K., Grube, J., Gruenewald, P., Hill, L., Holder, H., Homel, R., Osterberg, E., Rehm, J., Room, R., Rossow, I. (2010). *Alcohol: No Ordinary Commodity,* 2nd edn. Oxford: Oxford University Press.

Balakrishnan, R., Allender, S., Scarborough, P., Webster, P. and Rayner, M. (2009). The burden of alcohol-related ill health in the United Kingdom. *Journal of Public Health,* 31(3): 366–373.

Barrientos-Gutierrez, T., Gimeno, D., Mangione, T.W., Harrist, R.B. and Amick, B.C. (2007). Drinking social norms and drinking behaviours: a multilevel analysis of 137 workgroups in 16 worksites. *Occupational and Environmental Medicine,* 64: 602–608.

Barr, C.S. Chen, S.A., Schwandt, M.L., Lindell, S.G., Sun, H., Suomi, S.J. and Heilig, M. (2010). Suppression of alcohol preference by naltrexone in the rhesus macaque: a critical role of genetic variation at the μ-opioid receptor gene locus. *Biological Psychiatry* 67: 78–80.

Bertholet, N., Gaume, J., Faouzi, M., Daeppen, J.B., and Gmel, G. (2011). Perception of the amount of drinking by others in a sample of 20-year-old men: the more I think you drink, the more I drink. *Alcohol and Alcoholism,* 46 (1): 83–87.

Bewick, B., M., West, R., Gill, J., O'May, F., Mulhern, B., Barkham, M. & Hill, A., J. (2010). Providing web-based feedback and social norms information to reduce student alcohol intake: a multisite investigation. *Journal of Medical Internet Research* 12(5): e59.

Black, H., Gill, J., and Chick, J. (2010). The price of a drink: levels of consumption and price paid per unit of alcohol by Edinburgh's ill drinkers with a comparison to wider alcohol sales in Scotland. *Addiction,* 106: 729–736.

Burrell, K., Sumnall, H., Witty, K. & McVeigh, J. (2006). *Preston Alcohol Brief Intervention Training Pack: Evaluation Report.* Centre for Public Health John Moores University.

Callaghan, R.C., Taylor, L. and Cunningham, J.A. (2007). Does progressive stage transition mean getting better? A test of the Transtheoretical Model in alcoholism recovery. *Addiction,* 102(10): 1588–1596.

Carey, K.B., Scott-Sheldon, L.A.J., Carey, M.P. and DeMartini, K.S. (2007). Individual-level interventions to reduce college student drinking: a meta-analytic review. *Addictive Behaviour,* 32(11): 2469–2494.

Chen, W.Y., Rosner, B., Hankinson, S.E., Colditz, G.A. and Willnett, W.C. (2011). Moderate alcohol consumption during adult life, drinking patterns, and breast cancer risk. *JAMA,* 306(17): 1884–1890.

Clarke, A. and Thirlaway, K. (2011). Genetic counselling for personalised medicine. *Human Genetics,* 130(1): 27–31.

Cohen, S. and Janicki-Deverts, D. (2009). Can we improve our physical health by altering our social networks? *Perspectives on Psychological Science,* 4, 375–378.

Conrod, P.J., Castellanos-Ryan, N. and Mackie, C.J. (2011). Long-term effects of a personality-targeted intervention to reduce alcohol use in adolescents. *Journal of Consulting and Clinical Psychology,* 79(3): 296–306.

Craig, R. and Mindell, J. (2008). *Health Survey for England 2006. Volume 1: Cardiovascular Disease and Risk Factors in Adults.* London: The Information Centre.

Delong, W., Schneider, S.K., Towvim, L.G., Gomberg, L., Murphy, M.J., Doerr, E.E., Simonen, N.R., Mason, K.E. and Scribner, R.A. (2006). A multi-site randomized trial of social norms marketing campaigns to reduce college student drinking. *Journal of Studies on Alcohol,* 67(6): 868–879.

Department of Health (2010). *Health Survey for England, 2010.* The NHS Information Centre, 2011. Available at: http://www.ic.nhs.uk/pubs/hse10report (accessed 11 January 2013).

Department of Health, Social Services and Public Safety (2011). *Health Survey Northern Ireland: First Results from the 2010/11 Survey.* Belfast: Department of Health, Social Services and Public Safety.

Department of Transport (2012). *Reported Road Casualties in Great Britain: 2011 Annual Report.* Newport: Office of National Statistics.

Duryea, E.J. and Okwumabua, J.O. (1988). Effects of a preventive alcohol education programme after 3 years. *Journal of Drug Education*, 18, 23–31.

Emslie, C., Lewars, H., Batty, G.D. and Hunt, K. (2009). Are there gender differences in levels of heavy, binge and problem drinking? Evidence from three generations in the west of Scotland. *Public Health*, 123: 12–14.

Effiong, K. Osinowo A., Pring A., & Verne J. (2012). *Deaths from Liver Disease: Implications for End of Life Care in England*. London: National End of Life Care Intelligence Network.

Fiellin, L.E., Tetrault, M., Becker, W.C., Fiellin, D.A. and Hoff, R.A. (2013). Previous use of alcohol, cigarettes, and marijuana and subsequent abuse of prescription opioids in young adults. *Journal of Adolescent Health* 52, (2): 158–163.

Foxcroft, D.R., Ireland, D., Lister-Sharp, D.J., Lowe, G. and Breen, R. (2003). Longer-term primary prevention for alcohol misuse in young people. *Addiction*, 98: 397–411.

French, M.T. and Zavala, S.K. (2007). The health benefits of moderate drinking revisited: alcohol use and self-reported health status. *American Journal of Health Promotion*, 21, 484–491.

Gilles, D.M., Turk, C.L. and Fresco, D.M. (2006). Social anxiety, alcohol expectancies, and self-efficacy as predictors of heavy drinking in college students. *Addictive Behaviour*, 31: 388–398.

Grant JD., Agrawal A., Bucholz K., Madden P. *et al.* (2009). Alcohol consumption indices of genetic risk for alcohol dependence. *Biological Psychiatry*, 66(8): 795–800.

Heather, N., Honekopp, J. and Smailes, D. (2009). Progressive stage transition does mean getting better: a further test of the Transtheoretical Model in recovery from alcohol problems. *Addiction*, 104(6): 949–58.

HM Government. (2007). *Safe. Sensible. Social. The Next Steps in the National Alcohol Strategy*. London: Department of Health and The Home Office.

——(2012). *The Government's Alcohol Strategy*. London. The Home Office.

Hopkins, R.H., Mauss, A.L., Kearney, K.A. and Weisheit, R.A. (1988). Comprehensive evaluation of a model alcohol education curriculum. *Journal of Studies on Alcohol and Drugs*, 49(01): 38.

Hughes, K., Quigg, Z., Bellis, M.A., van Hasselt, N., Calafat, A., Kosir, M., Juan, M., Duch, M. and Voorham, L. (2007). Alcohol, nightlife and violence: the relative contributions of drinking before and during nights out to negative health and criminal justice outcomes. *Addiction*, 103: 60–65.

Hurcombe, R., Bayley, M. and Goodman, A. (2010). *Ethnicity and Alcohol: A Review of the UK Literature*. York: Joseph Rowntree Foundation.

Kaestner, R. and Yarnoff, B. (2011). Long term effects of minimum legal drinking age laws on adult alcohol use and driving fatalities. *The Journal of Law and Economics*, 54(2): 325–363.

Kalsi, G., Prescott, C.A., Kendler, K. and Riley, B. (2009). Unravelling the molecular mechanisms of alcohol dependence. *Trends in Genetics*, 25(1): 49–55.

Kuntsche, E., and Cooper, M.L. (2010). Drinking to have fun and to get drunk: motives as predictors weekend drinking over and above usual drinking habits. *Drug and Alcohol Dependence*, 110(3): 259–262.

Kuther, T.L. and Timoshin, A. (2003). A comparison of social cognitive and psychosocial predictors of alcohol use by college students. *Journal of College Student Development*, 44: 143–154.

Lee, S.J., Sudore, R.L., Williams, B.A., Lindquist, M.S., Chen, H.L. and Covinsky, K.E. (2009). Functional limitations, socioeconomic status and all-cause mortality in moderate drinkers. *Journal of the American Geriatrics Society*, 57(6): 955–962.

Litt, D.M. and Stock, M.L. (2011). Adolescent alcohol-related risk cognitions: the roles of social norms and social networking sites. *Psychology of Addictive Behaviors*, 25(4): 708–13.

Manning, W.G., Blumberg, L. and Moulton, L.H. (1995). The demand for alcohol: the differential response to price. *Journal of Health Economics*, 14: 123–148.

Masten, A.S., Faden, V.B., Zucker, R.A. and Spear, L. P. (2008). Underage drinking: a developmental framework. *Pediatrics*, 121(Supplement 4): S235–S251.

McAlaney, J. and McMahon, J. (2007). Normative beliefs, misperceptions and heavy episodic drinking in a British student sample. *Journal of Studies on Alcohol and Drugs*, 68(3): 385–392.

McManus, S., Meltzer, H., Brugha, T., Bebbington, P. and Jenkins, R. (2009). *Adult Psychiatric Morbidity in England, 2007. Results of a Household* Survey. Leeds: The NHS Information Centre for Health and Social Care.

Measham F. and Ostergaard J. (2011). *Emerging Drug Trends in Lancashire: Night Time Economy Surveys: Phase One Report*. Lancashire: Lancashire drug and alcohol action team.

Moss, A.C., Dyer, K.R. and Albery, I.P. (2009). Knowledge of drinking does not equal sensible drinking. *Lancet*, 374: 1242.

Moyer, A., Finney, J.W., Swearingen, E. and Vergun, P. (2002). Brief interventions for alcohol problems a meta-analytic review of controlled investigations in treatment seeking and non-treatment seeking populations. *Addiction*, 97: 279–292.

Mulvihill, C., Taylor, L., Waller, S., Naidoo, B. and Thom, B. (2005). *Prevention and Reduction of Alcohol Misuse: Evidence Briefing*, 2nd edn. London: Health Development Agency.

Murgraff, V., Abraham, C. and McDermott, M. (2007). Reducing Friday alcohol consumption among moderate women drinkers: evaluation of a brief evidence-based intervention. *Alcohol and Alcoholism*, 42: 37–41.

News (2007). Alcohol, breast and colorectal cancer. *European Journal of Cancer*, 43: 1225.

NHS (2012). *Statistics on Alcohol: England 2012*. Health and Social Care Information Centre.

NICE (2010). *Alcohol-use Disorders: Preventing Harmful Drinking: NICE Public Health Guidance 24*. London: NICE.

Nicolas, S., Kershaw, C. and Walker, A (2008). *Crime in England and Wales 2007/2008*. London: Home Office. Available at: www.homeoffice.gov.uk/rds/pdfs08/hosb0708.pdf. (accessed 10 January 2013).

Nilsen, P., Baird, J., Mello, M.J. et al. (2008). A systematic review of emergency care brief alcohol interventions for injury patients. *Journal of Substance Abuse Treatment*, 35(2): 184–201.

Nuffield Council on Bioethics. (2007). *Public Health Ethical Issues*. London: Nuffield Council. Available at: www.nuffieldbioethics.org (accessed 15 January 2013).

Office of National Statistics (ONS). (2008). *News Release: Alcohol-related Death Rates Continue to Rise*. London: Office of National Statistics.

O'Keefe, J.H., Bybee, K.A. and Lavie, C.J. (2007). Alcohol and cardiovascular health. The razor-sharp double-edged sword. *Journal of the American College of Cardiology*, 50(11): 1009–1014.

O'Leary-Barrett, M., Mackie, C.J., Castellanos-Ryan, N., Al-Khudhairy, N. and Conrod, P.J. (2010). Personality-targeted interventions delay uptake of drinking and decrease risk of alcohol-related problems when delivered by teachers. *Journal of the American Academy of Child and Adolescent Psychiatry*, 49(9): 954–963.

Orton, J. (2001). *Excessive Appetites*, 2nd edn. Chichester: John Wiley & Sons.

Paglia, A. and Room, R. (1999). Preventing substance use problems among youth: a literature review and recommendations. *Journal of Primary Prevention*, 20: 3–50.

Percy, A., Wilson, J., McCartan, C. and McCrystal, P. (2011). Teenage drinking cultures. York: Joseph Rowntree Foundation.

Plant, M. and Plant, M. (2006). *Binge Britain*. Oxford: Oxford University Press.

Prochaska, J.M., Prochaska, J.O., Cohen, F.C., Gomes, S.O., Laforge, R.G. and Eastwood, B.S. (2004). The Transtheoretical model of change for multi-level interventions for alcohol abuse on campus. *Journal of Alcohol and Drug Education*, 47: 34–50.

Ramos, D. and Perkins, D.F. (2006). Goodness of fit assessment of an alcohol intervention program and the underlying theories of change. *Journal of American College Health*, 55: 57–64.

Rehm, J., Mathers, C., Popova, S., Thavorncharoensap, M. *et al.* (2009). Global burden of disease and injury and economic cost attributable to alcohol use and alcohol-use disorders. *Lancet*, 373: 2223–2233.

Room, R. (2004). Disabling the public interest: alcohol strategies and policies for England. *Addiction*, 99: 1083–1089.

Room, R., Babor, T. and Rehm, J. (2005). Alcohol and public health. *Lancet*, 365: 519–530.

Saunders, J. and Rey, J. (2011). *Young People and Alcohol: Impact, Policy Prevention, Treatment*. London: Wiley.

Science and Technology Committee (2011). *Science and Technology Committee – Eleventh Report. Alcohol Guidelines*. Available at: http://www.parliament.uk/business/committees/committees-a-z/commons-select/science-and-technology-committee/inquiries/parliament-2010/alcohol-advice/ (Accessed 15 January 2013).

Scottish Government (2011). *The Scottish Health Survey 2010, Volume 1: Main Report*. Edinburgh: The Scottish Government. Available at: http://www.scotland.gov.uk/Publications/2011/09/27084018/91 (accessed 23 January 2013).

Spoth, R.L., Redmond, C., Shin, C. and Azevedo (2004). Brief family interventions effects on adolescent substance initiation: school-level growth curve analysis 6 years following baseline. *Journal of Consulting and Clinical Psychology*, 72: 534–542.

The Guardian (2012). Alcohol abuse contributes to big rise in deaths from liver disease. Available at: http://www.theguardian.com/society/2012/mar/22/alcohol-rise-deaths-liver-disease (accessed 5 February 2013).

Wagenaar, A.C., Salois, M.J., and Komro, K.A. (2009). Effects of beverage alcohol price and tax levels on drinking: a meta-analysis of 1003 estimates from 112 studies. *Addiction*, 104: 179–190.

Webb, G., Shakeshaft, A., Sanson-Fisher, R. and Havard, A. (2009). A systematic review of work-place interventions for alcohol-related problems. *Addiction*, 104(3): 365–377.

Welsh Assembly Government. (2009). *Welsh Health Survey 2008: Initial Headline Results*. Cardiff: Welsh Assembly Government.

Welsh Government (2011). Welsh Health Survey 2010. Available at: http://www.wales.gov.uk/statistics (accessed 23 January 2013).

Wechsler, H., Nelson, T., Lee, J.E., Seibring, M., Lewis, C. and Keeling, R.P. (2003). Perceptions and reality: a national evaluation of social norms marketing interventions to reduce college students heavy alcohol use. *Journal of Studies of Alcohol*, 64: 484–494.

Westbrook, D., Kennedy, H. and Krik, J. (2007). *An Introduction to Cognitive Behavioural Therapy*. London: Sage.

WHO. (2002). *World Health Report (2002): Reducing Risks, Promoting Healthy Life*. Geneva: World Health Organization.

——(2010), *ICD-10 Version: 2010. Mental and Behavioural Disorders F10–F19*. Available at: http://apps.who.int/classifications/icd10/browse/2010 (accessed 23 January 2013).

Williams, E.C., Horton, N.J., Samet, J.H. and Saitz, R. (2007). Do brief measures of readiness to change predict alcohol consumption and consequences in primary care patients with unhealthy alcohol use? *Alcoholism: Clinical and Experimental Research*, 31: 428–435. Available at: www.alcoholandyou.org (accessed 24 January 2013).

Xu, X., and Chaloupka, F.J. (2011). The effects of prices on alcohol use and its consequences. *Alcohol Research and Health*, 34(2).

York Cornwell, E. and Waite, L.J. (2009). Social disconnectedness, perceived isolation and health among older adults. *Journal of Health and Social Behavior*, 50(1): 31–48.

8 Smoking

Learning objectives

At the end of this chapter you will:
- be able to understand the current extent and demographics of tobacco smoking in the UK
- appreciate the health and economic consequences of tobacco smoking
- realise how the Stages of Change model can and has been applied to smoking, and smoking cessation
- understand the approaches to smoking cessation at an individual and community level whilst recognising how health professionals can aid cessation
- be able to apply the motivational interviewing technique to smoking cessation
- understand the development of assessment, action and intervention plans for smoking
- appreciate some of the difficulties faced when attempting to quit smoking and how to cope with them.

Case study

Joe is a 53-year-old window cleaner who is currently working in his own business but is looking forward to retiring shortly. He has worked continuously since he started work when he left school without any qualifications when he was 14 years old. He has few hobbies but loves to play with his grandchildren in the back garden. However, more recently he has found himself getting breathless frequently and thus not able to enjoy playing with them as much as he would like. He does enjoy socialising and likes a couple of pints in the evening with his friends and family at the local working men's club.

Joe has smoked cigarettes since he was a teenager and still smokes some 25–30 per day, with his first cigarette being on waking. He used to smoke more heavily but has recently cut down. Joe has developed frequent chest and breathing problems – he often has bouts of bronchitis and recently suffered four cracked ribs due to prolonged and severe coughing. In addition to his chest problems he also suffers from early peripheral vascular disease and has a mild degree of lower limb neuropathy. Joe knows that he has to stop smoking but he has been doing it for over 40 years and he feels he cannot stop.

He sees you in the clinic and you realise that his health is severely compromised by his behaviour and he must change it or suffer ever more serious consequences. Joe reports that he only 'smokes now and again', although you think it is much more frequent than this. Joe has now noticed that his grandson, JJ, has started acting like him, plays 'smoking cigarettes' and is refusing to eat anything other than chips and bacon butties.

Applying this to Joe

You have to be able to assess Joe's smoking behaviour and work with him to reduce (and stop) his smoking. You also need to ensure that JJ does not start smoking.

Introduction

Surely everyone appreciates the health damage that cigarette smoking causes? It remains the single most avoidable cause of death and disability in the UK and the Western world (Fiore *et al.*, 2008). Some 10 per cent of all deaths in 2020 are predicted to be as a result of smoking (WHO, 2011) and if current trends continue, tobacco will have killed one billion people in the twenty-first century (ASH, 2011), Despite the health effects of smoking being known for over 40 years, and the health impact being publicised considerably, some 12 million individuals in the UK still smoke: 21 per cent of men and 20 per cent of women (ASH, 2012a). However, the number of young people starting to smoke has decreased, with a decline of 26 per cent since 1982 but there is still a core number of individuals that smoke (ASH, 2011a).

Trends in smoking prevalence across the four home countries in the UK

Across the four home countries, prevalence of cigarette smoking in adults aged 16 years and above is lowest in England at 21 per cent. Similar prevalence rates are observed for Scotland, Wales and Northern Ireland across the same time period (25 per cent, 23 per cent and 24 per cent respectively). Smoking rates for men and women followed a similar trend for all home countries in 2010/2011, with smoking prevalence being slightly higher amongst males than females. Again, England demonstrates lower prevalence for smoking in men and women compared to Scotland, Wales and Northern Ireland (see Table 8.1).

The prevalence of smoking is not the same in different groups; about a third of those in the manual groups smoke compared to less than 20 per cent of the professional and managerial groups. Similarly, smoking is highest in the 20–24-year age group (at about 28 per cent) and the lowest in the over-65 years (at about 14 per cent) (The Health and Social Care Information Centre, 2011). Individuals from lower socio-economic backgrounds tend to have different attitudinal beliefs regarding their health than the individuals from higher socio-economic backgrounds. This difference in attitude is thought to contribute to the variance in smoking rates between socio-economic statuses.

Table 8.1 Smoking prevalence for men and women in the UK

Source of data	% of adults who currently smoke	% of men who currently smoke	% of women who currently smoke
Statistics on Smoking: England 2011 (The Health and Social Care Information Centre, 2011)	21%	22%	20%
Health Survey for Scotland 2010 (Bromley and Given, 2011)	25%	26%	25%
Welsh Health Survey 2010 (Welsh Government, 2011)	23%	25%	22%
Health Survey Northern Ireland 2010/2011 (Department of Health, Social Services and Public Safety, 2011)	24%	25%	23%

Applying this to Joe

Joe is in the lower socio-economic class, which has the highest level of smoking in the UK currently. It is likely that many of his family and peers smoke and hence the healthcare professional needs to be aware of his cultural and social baggage.

The UK government (along with most other governments) is determined to reduce smoking across their population through both health promotion and clinical 1:1 interventions. In the UK, the Department of Health's tobacco programme is split into 'strands', each of which, it is hoped, will contribute to an overall reduction in smoking. These strands include:

1. *'Smoke-free' legislation:* From March 2006 in Scotland, April 2007 in Northern Ireland and Wales and from July 2007 in England virtually all enclosed public places and workplaces in England became smoke free, including all pubs, clubs, membership clubs, cafés and restaurants.
2. *Reducing exposure to second-hand smoke:* Legislation such as that introducing smoke-free public buildings and workplaces has reduced the exposure to second-hand smoke.
3. *Tobacco media/education programmes:* A key strand of the government's tobacco control programme is the provision of an on-going media/education campaign.
4. *Reducing availability of tobacco products:* Price increases have been a highly successful way of helping people become non-smokers: UK budget changes to tobacco duty have been directed towards increasing the real cost of cigarettes and thereby increasing economic pressures on smokers.
5. *NHS Stop Smoking Services and NRTs:* the government has set up an NHS Stop Smoking Service. Services are now available across the NHS in the UK, providing counselling and support to smokers wanting to quit, complementing the use of stop-smoking aids such as nicotine replacement therapy (NRT) and bupropion (Zyban).
6. *Reducing tobacco advertising and promotion:* the UK has a comprehensive ban, just like many other countries in Europe and beyond, on tobacco advertising and promotion including displays at the point of sale.
7. *Regulating tobacco products:* This strand of the government's tobacco control programme concerns regulating the contents of tobacco products and the labelling of packaging.

Health consequences of smoking

The link between smoking and cancer has been appreciated since the seminal work of Doll and Hill (1952). This report has been followed by a succession of studies highlighting the strong link between poor health and tobacco smoking. For example, in the UK it is suggested that over 100,000 people die annually as a result of their smoking habit (ASH, 2012b). Every year, tobacco smoking kills around 6 million people worldwide, or about one person every six seconds with the figure expected to rise to 7.5 million in 2020 (WHO, 2011).

Deaths caused by tobacco smoking in the UK are higher than the number of deaths caused by road traffic accidents (3,500), other accidents (8,500), poisoning and overdose (900), alcoholic liver disease (5,000), suicide (4,000) and HIV infection (250). Almost half of all regular smokers will be killed by their habit. A man that smokes cuts short his life by 13.2 years and female smokers lose 14.5 years (ASH, 2009).

In terms of morbidity, more than a quarter of all cancer deaths can be attributed to smoking (ASH, 2012c). It has also been linked to a whole host of diseases and chronic conditions, including heart disease, throat cancer, stomach and bowel cancer, lung cancer, leukaemia, peripheral vascular disease, premature and low weight babies, bronchitis, emphysema, sinusitis, peptic ulcers and dental hygiene problems, and can worsen the effects of asthma and infections (see Table 8.2 and Figure 8.1 for overview).

Applying this to Joe

Joe is currently 53 and, given his current smoking pattern and the considerable ill health he now suffers, he will be unlikely to live until he reaches his retirement at 65 years of age. Joe needs to fully appreciate the consequences of his continued smoking.

Table 8.2 Illness associated with smoking

System	Illness
Cardiovascular	Aneurysm Angina (20 × risk) Beurger's disease (severe circulatory disease) Coronary artery disease Myocardial infarction (2–3 × risk) Peripheral vascular disease Stroke (2–4 × risk)

System	Illness
Musculoskeletal	Back pain
	Ligament injuries
	Muscle injuries
	Neck pain
	Osteoporosis
	Osteoarthritis
	Rheumatoid arthritis
	Tendon injuries
	Low bone density
	Hip fractures
Visual	Cataracts (2 × risk)
	Posterior subcapsular cataract (3 × risk)
	Optic neuropathy (16 × risk)
	Macular degeneration (2 × risk)
	Nystagmus
	Ocular histoplasmosis
	Tobacco amblyopia
Genitourinary	Erectile dysfunction
	Impotence (2 × risk)
	Decreased fertility in women
	Pregnancy complications (e.g. premature rupture of membranes, placenta previa or placental abruption, miscarriage, still birth, low birth weight, reduced lung function in infants)
Digestive, metabolic	Gum disease
	Duodenal ulcer
	Colon polyps
	Crohn's disease
	Diabetes
	Stomach ulcer
	Tooth loss
Respiratory	COPD
Cancers	Lung (90% associated with smoking)
	Mouth and throat (90% associated with smoking)
	Breast (60% increased risk)
	Pancreatic (2 × risk)
	Oesophageal cancer
	Stomach
	Liver
	Bladder (2–5 × risk)
	Kidney
	Cervical cancer
	Myeloid cancer
	Urinary tract cancer

System	Illness
Other conditions	Depression Psoriasis (2 × risk) Hearing loss Sudden Infant Death Syndrome (SIDS) Exacerbates: Asthma Chronic rhinitis Diabetic retinopathy Graves' disease MS Optic neuritis Coughing, sneezing, shortness of breath Common colds, influenza, pneumonia

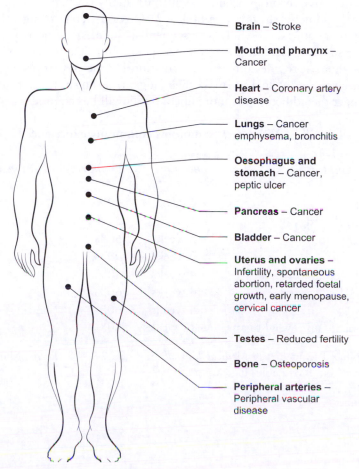

Brain – Stroke

Mouth and pharynx – Cancer

Heart – Coronary artery disease

Lungs – Cancer emphysema, bronchitis

Oesophagus and stomach – Cancer, peptic ulcer

Pancreas – Cancer

Bladder – Cancer

Uterus and ovaries – Infertility, spontaneous abortion, retarded foetal growth, early menopause, cervical cancer

Testes – Reduced fertility

Bone – Osteoporosis

Peripheral arteries – Peripheral vascular disease

Figure 8.1 Health impact of smoking

Those who quit smoking by the age of 40 years retain almost the same life expectancy as lifelong non-smokers. Even those who quit upon diagnosis of early stages of lung cancer are thought to benefit by experiencing an increase in life expectancy (Parsons *et al.*, 2010). Thus, quitting smoking at any age and health status brings with it health benefits.

Assessment of smoking

Smoking behaviour can be best assessed through a subjective recording of cigarettes smoked during a defined period (usually four weeks); however, this can often be an underestimate so this has to be taken into account when making your assessment. However, if an objective measure is required then biochemical assessment of carbon monoxide levels can be assessed (using 10 ppm as a cut-off level) with specialist equipment.

However, aside from whether a confirmed recording of smoking has taken place or whether the subjective record is accurate (which it usually isn't), most important is the need to assess the addiction history (see Table 8.3). Obviously, the stronger the addiction the harder it is to quit successfully. Consequently, there is the need to assess both motivation for smoking (see Table 8.4) and dependency on cigarettes (Table 8.5). These two elements should provide sufficient information for the practitioner to be able to assess adequately the individual and make their judgements on appropriate interventions (e.g. the stronger the addiction the more likely NRTs will be required).

Table 8.3 Withdrawal symptoms commonly experienced

Withdrawal symptom	Duration	Proportion of smokers affected
Light-headedness	< 2 days	10%
Night-time awakenings	< 1 week	25%
Poor concentration	< 2 weeks	60%
Cravings	> 2 weeks	70%
Irritability or aggression	< 4 weeks	50%
Restlessness	< 4 weeks	60%
Depression	< 4 weeks	60%
Increased appetite and weight gain	> 10 weeks	80%

Source: Reproduced from *British Medical Journal*, 328, pp. 277–79 (Jarvis, Martin J. 2004), with permission from BMJ Publishing Group Ltd

Table 8.4 Assessing motivation for smoking

1. What is your reason for smoking?
2. On a scale of 1–10, how much do you enjoy smoking?
      1 – hate, 10 – enjoy very much
3. On a scale of 1–10, how much do you want to stop smoking?
      1 – not at all, 10 – desperately keen
4. What are the negative and positive aspects of smoking for you?
5. How would you benefit from giving up?
6. How do you feel smoking affects your health?
7. How much would you pay/give up if it meant you could stop smoking?

Assess whether – highly motivated
                  – moderately motivated
                  – not motivated

Table 8.5 Fagerstrom Dependence Scale

1. How many cigarettes do you smoke daily?
      10 or fewer (0)
      11–20 (1)
      21–30 (2)
      30+ (3)
2. How soon after waking up do you smoke your first cigarette?
      Less than 6 minutes (3)
      6–30 minutes (2)
      31–60 minutes (1)
      60+ minutes (0)

Scoring

Add up questions 1 and 2

0–1   Low dependence: stopping smoking should be easy.
2   Moderate dependence: guidance and medication to reduce withdrawal symptoms may help.
3   High dependence: guidance and medication may be required.
4–6   Very high dependence: smoking cessation will be difficult and considerable support needed. Medication to reduce withdrawal symptoms will be required.

Source: Adapted from *British Medical Journal*, 328, pp. 338–39 (West, R. 2004), with permission from BMJ Publishing Group Ltd

Joe needs a cigarette when he wakes up in the morning and has been smoking for some considerable time. It is likely that he is heavily addicted. Although his motivation to quit is high, his current surroundings, along with numerous previous failed attempts, count against him. Joe would be classed as in the 'very high dependence' category (Table 8.4) therefore his needs and support when attempting to quit will vary considerably to those smokers classed in the 'low dependence' category. As Joe has a very high dependence, it is important that NRTs are used in conjunction with behavioural therapies in supporting Joe to quit.

Why do people smoke?

Before we explore how to get people to stop smoking, it is first important to see how psychologists have explained why people smoke. People smoke for a variety of reasons and a myriad of explanations have been proposed, from a psychological, social and medical perspective. The psychological explanations have been from both a behavioural and social learning perspective (see Table 8.6 for how elements from the behavioural perspective can help explain why people smoke). The information provided in Table 8.6 goes some way to help us explain why people smoke, and on this basis, how we can help them quit.

Table 8.6 Behavioural explanation of smoking development

Concept	Rules	Example
Classical conditioning	Behaviours acquired through associative learning	Having a cup of coffee and a cigarette equals relaxation
Operant conditioning	Behaviour is likely to increase if it is positively reinforced by the presence of a positive event, or negatively reinforced by the absence or removal of a negative event	Smoking is positively reinforced by social acceptance
Observational learning	Behaviours are learned by observing others	Parents or friends smoking
Cognitive factors	Other factors such as coping mechanisms or self-image may contribute	Belief that smoking looks 'cool'
Social learning perspective	Behaviour is learned by modelling and social reinforcement	Seeing parents and peers smoking – being reinforced as 'part of the gang'

Psychological models of smoking

Several psychological variables have been implicated in the continuance of smoking. Models of health behaviour such as the health belief model, the protection motivation theory, the theory of reasoned action and the health action process approach have been used to examine the cognitive factors that contribute to smoking initiation. Obviously the distinction between these forms of models and the social explanation is somewhat tenuous: there is clear overlap between these factors and attempting to explain smoking (or any) lifestyle behaviour mono-theoretically is a flawed task.

Another approach is based on the theory of planned behaviour (TPB) (Ajzen, 1991) which appears to be one of the most popular and successful models for studying health behaviour (Armitage and Conner, 2001). The TPB has been successful in predicting smoking among adolescents (e.g. Smith *et al.*, 2007). These studies have provided good predictions of intentions and subsequent behaviours.

According to the TPB the proximal determinants of behaviour are the intentions to engage in the behaviour. Intentions reflect an individual's decision to exert effort to perform the behaviour and are assumed to be a function of a number of related factors such as attitudes, subjective norms, perceived behavioural control and self-efficacy. Smoking can be assumed to be different from some of the other behaviours in this book. In particular, smokers might become addicted (whether psychologically or biologically) to cigarettes, but this should not suggest that they have lost control over their behaviour but it is difficult behaviour to change in the sense that their perception of control over the behaviour appears incomplete.

Biological factors associated with smoking

The biological model suggests that smoking is a result of individuals becoming physically dependent on nicotine and the multitude of chemical substances found in cigarettes. The nicotine entering the lungs from a cigarette is transported through the blood supply and to the brain, where it leads to an activation of the autonomic nervous system (ANS). Consequently, there is an increase in heart rate and blood pressure which leads to the body becoming more aroused and alert. Once the person has stopped smoking, the level of nicotine reduces as do the 'positive' effects of smoking. From this, a model of nicotine regulation can be proposed: smokers continue to smoke in order to avoid withdrawal symptoms (Schachter *et al.*, 1977).

However, there are some people who stop smoking for a number of years (and hence all of the nicotine has disappeared from their bodies) but then start smoking again. Furthermore, there are smokers who are known as 'chippers' who smoke a few cigarettes a day for a number of years but do not increase the amount they smoke (hence they do not show tolerance). Because of these issues it is recognised that the biological theories are not the complete picture; there must be other social and psychological factors involved.

Social factors of smoking

The social context in which smoking develops and is maintained is key. The social factors implicated in the initiation of smoking behaviour (e.g. parents, siblings and peers) all have a part to play in the maintenance of this behaviour. Although the relative importance of these various groups has been debated, most research has agreed that they do have a role.

Smoking is a social activity for many but this can differ from individual to individual and from cigarette to cigarette (Perkins *et al.*, 2008). Thus, for somebody at work, smoking a cigarette may provide an opportunity to escape from the drudgery of the workplace and to have a break. In contrast, down the pub, the sharing of a cigarette can be a means of strengthening social bonds with friends. For low-income mothers, smoking is often used as a means of dealing with problems relating to employment and personal relationships (Sperlich *et al.*, 2011). The positive enhancement of image is often cited as a reason for starting smoking amongst young children (Hrubá & Zaloudíková, 2010).

Applying this to Joe

Joe tends to smoke more at the pub (although he now has to go into the pub garden to do so) and when he is around people who are smoking. It is important to appreciate some of the triggers that may be prompting Joe's smoking behaviour such as peer influence.

Interventions to reduce smoking

Evidence suggests that the majority of smokers want to stop smoking (The Health and Social Care Information Centre, 2011), with about a third of smokers attempting to quit each year. Just over a half of smokers do succeed in quitting smoking before they die, although for many it is too late. It can be argued that every healthcare practitioner has a moral duty to try to encourage people to quit smoking. Research suggests that unplanned quit attempts were mostly triggered by advice from a healthcare professional (Murray *et al.*, 2009). However, it is also suggested that such advice is only given if related to the patient's complaints otherwise the patient will not be as compliant (Guassor and Baarts, 2010). There are techniques, both medical and psychological, that can support people in smoking cessation attempts. It is essential that the healthcare professional is aware of the extent of these, and how they can be accessed by clients/patients.

Although it undoubtedly has considerable health benefits, quitting can be fraught with difficulties and many people report getting irritable, depressed, anxious, restless and craving tobacco. There are methods that can help overcome some of these difficulties with a range of pharmacological treatments developed to help relieve them. For example, there are sprays, chewing gum, patches and inhalers – all of which have proven benefits for the smoker (Hung *et al.*, 2011). However, there is always a psychological element to cessation and the healthcare professional is in a prime position to maximise motivation, technique and emotional and cognitive engagement with the cessation programme.

Stopping people smoking

Encouraging and enhancing smoking cessation is now recognised as an important part of public health and a key role of the healthcare practitioner. Mohiuddin *et al.* (2007) reported a reduction in total mortality as a result of an intensive smoking cessation programme when compared to a usual care group. Other studies have also suggested that interventions to improve smoking results in beneficial changes in other health behaviours, such as exercise, which is routinely recommended as an aid to smoking cessation (Ussher *et al*, 2008). Cardiovascular exercise has been shown to reduce the withdrawal symptoms associated with quitting smoking, as well as smoking cravings, but may also reduce weight gain and increase fitness levels. So getting people to stop smoking can have positive consequences on health behaviours other than smoking.

Individual level interventions

Interventions aimed at the individual in relation to smoking cessation can take many forms. In this section, a selection of the individual level approaches, interventions and policies will be discussed. From doing so it will be possible to understand the underlying theory behind them in addition to understanding how psychological principles can be used in addressing smoking cessation. Clinical smoking cessation includes (either alone or in combination) behavioural and pharmaceutical interventions and they range from brief advice and counselling to intensive support, and administration of medications that contribute to reducing or overcoming dependence in individuals and in the population as a whole (Hays *et al.*, 2009).

Clinical interventions

The simplest individual interventions are those brief interventions that most healthcare professionals can engage in without any specific training. The Five As model which is presented in Table 8.7 is one that is promoted for all healthcare professionals. A flow diagram is presented in Figure 8.2 which highlights the process that healthcare professionals should follow whenever they are in a position to offer guidance and advice.

Applying this to Joe

Joe has come to you and asked for support to give up smoking. Arrange to see Joe within seven days of your first appointment. This will enable you to fully assess and provide support and guidance for Joe throughout his lifestyle behaviour change.

Table 8.7 The Five As model for facilitating smoking cessation

Five As	Example	Key points
Ask about tobacco use	Always include questions about tobacco use	Include questions about smoking in all consultations
Advise smokers to quit	Use clear, strong, and personalised language	'Quitting tobacco is the most important thing you can do to protect your health.'
Assess smokers' willingness to quit	Ask every tobacco user if he/she is willing to quit at this time. • If willing to quit, provide resources and assistance • If unwilling to quit at this time, help motivate the patient: – Identify reasons to quit in a supportive manner. – Build patient's confidence about quitting.	'On a scale of 1–10, how ready are you to quit smoking?'
Assist the patient	• Set a quit date, ideally within 2 weeks. • Remove tobacco products from their environment. • Get support from family, friends and co-workers. • Review past quit attempts – what helped, what led to relapse? • Anticipate challenges, particularly during the critical first few weeks, including nicotine withdrawal. • Identify reasons for quitting and benefits of quitting.	Help the patient make a quit plan (see later)

Five As	Example	Key points
	Give advice on successful quitting: • Total abstinence is essential – not even a single puff. • Drinking alcohol is strongly associated with relapse. • Allowing others to smoke in the household hinders successful quitting. Encourage use of medication: • Recommend use of over-the-counter nicotine patch, gum or lozenge; or give prescription for varenicline, bupropion SR nicotine inhaler or nasal spray, unless contraindicated.	
Arrange follow-up	Follow-up should occur.	Arrange for follow-up within a fortnight

Source: Adapted from Okuyemi *et al.*, 2006

Obviously, the 'Assist stage' can vary and these interventions are many and varied, with most (but not all) improving smoking cessation rates efficaciously (e.g. Fiore *et al.*, 2008). For example, these therapies include self-help methods, physician advice, telephone counselling, cognitive behaviour therapy, nicotine replacement therapy (NRT) and non-nicotine medication such as bupropion (Willemsen *et al.*, 2006). These interventions will be explored in more detail later.

But do patients get to know about all (or indeed, any) of these treatment options? Surveys have shown that the majority of smokers (64 per cent in 2010) want to stop smoking (Office for National Statistics, 2012) but the success rate remains low, and in England, although 6 in 10 say they want to stop smoking, less than half make an actual attempt in any given year (Department of Health, 2011). Although a majority (some 60 per cent) of smokers do use methods (Hyland *et al.*, 2004), not all will be efficacious and evidence-based interventions (Willemsen *et al.*, 2006). Many, indeed the majority, of smokers will not seek professional help and consequently the likelihood of success may be low (Chapman and MacKenzie, 2010).

There is also evidence to suggest that many individuals, particularly those in the 'hard to reach groups' (see Chapter 3) where smoking prevalence is often greater, are less likely to have access to cessation programmes and are less likely to receive advice on quitting from primary care providers (Browning *et al*, 2008). Alongside this it is also understood that deprived individuals require a greater level of support when undertaking smoking cessation (Henderson *et al.*, 2011). Hence, all healthcare professionals should be aware of local services and facilitate access to these services.

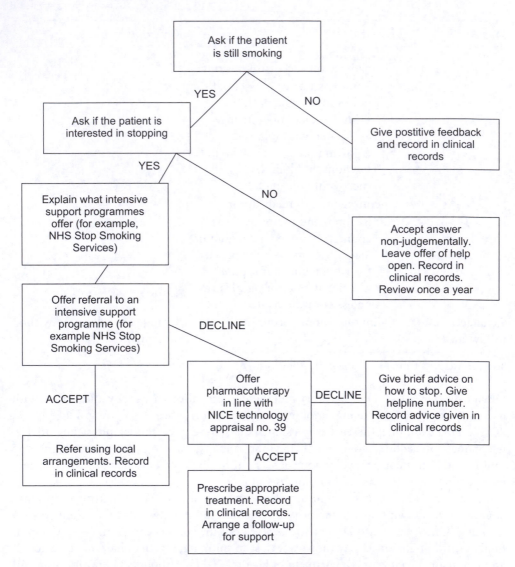

Figure 8.2 Brief intervention for smokers attending the clinic

Source: National Institute for Health and Clinical Excellence (2006). Adapted from *Brief Interventions and Referral for Smoking Cessation in Primary and Other Settings*. London: NICE. Available from www.nice.org.UR/PH001. Reproduced with permission.

Pharmacological treatments

Pharmacological treatments (see Table 8.8) are popular methods for assisting individuals with quitting. These include five forms of nicotine replacement therapy (NRT) (gum, patch, nasal spray, inhaler and lozenge) and bupropion sustained release. In a recent review of 150 trials, Stead *et al.* (2012) surmised that all forms of NRT increase people's

Table 8.8 Pharmacological interventions for smoking cessation

Intervention	Advantage	Disadvantage	Quit rates (%)
Bupropion	Non-nicotine Easy to use Can be used with NRT	Can cause insomnia, dry mouth, headache, tremors, nausea or anxiety	21–30
Nicotine gum • Use 4 mg if smoking 10 cigarettes or more • Use 2 mg if smoking fewer than 10 • Chew each piece slowly for 30 minutes when there is an urge to smoke • Max 15 per day. Reduce slowly over 3 months	Over the counter Flexible Quick delivery Different flavours Low compliance	No food or drink 15 minutes beforehand Frequent use required Jaw pain, mouth soreness, dyspepsia Under-dosing is common	7–10
Nicotine inhaler • 6–12 cartridges daily for 8 weeks • Reduce to half in next 2 weeks • Gradually stop over the next 2 weeks	Flexible dosing Mimics hand-to-mouth action of smoking Few side effects Comes in menthol flavour	Frequent dosing necessary May cause mouth and throat irritation Low compliance Under-dosing is common	23
Nicotine lozenge • 1 or 2 tabs per hour under the tongue • Maximum 40 per day • Continue for at least 3 months and then withdraw slowly until only 1 or 2 tabs needed per day	Over the counter Flexible dosing Quick delivery Oral administration	Frequent dosing necessary May cause mouth soreness or dyspepsia Low compliance Under-dosing is common No food or drink 15 minutes beforehand	24

Intervention	Advantage	Disadvantage	Quit rates (%)
Nicotine patch • 21 mg patch for 6 weeks • 14 mg patch for 2 weeks • 7 mg patch for 2 weeks • If smoking 10 cigarettes or fewer, start with the 14 mg patch and reduce after 6 weeks to the 7 mg patch for the last 2 weeks • Apply in the morning to non-hairy area of skin on trunk or upper arm • Replace in 24 hours • Use for 10 weeks maximum	Over the counter Daily application Overnight use	Less flexible dosing Slow delivery of nicotine May cause skin irritation or sleep problems Not good at treating acute cravings	8–21
Nicotine nasal spray • 1 spray to each nostril as required for 8 weeks • Maximum 1 spray to each nostril twice per hour or 64 sprays per day • Reduce by half over the next 2 weeks • Stop gradually over the last 2 weeks • Maximum treatment is 3 months	Flexible dosing Fastest delivery Reduces craving within minutes	Frequent dosing necessary May cause nose and eye irritation Most addictive of the NRTs	30

chance of quitting by 50 to 70 per cent. NRTs can, in some circumstances, double the rate of abstinence at five months plus.

Even with the pharmacological intervention, it is important to provide psychological support and encouragement for the individual smoker: the psychological factors involved in NRT use are considerable. Without continued motivation the success of NRT would be compromised. Simply focusing on NRTs may be 'doomed to failure' because nicotine is only part of the explanation for smoking behaviour. For example, behavioural techniques or denicotinised cigarettes may be required in order to deal with the sensory-motor activities associated with smoking. A recent review (Stead *et al.*, 2008; Cofta-Woerpel *et al.*, 2007) has suggested that these therapies can be considered an important aspect in a 'vital component' (Stead *et al.*, 2008, p. 47) of smoking cessation programmes and thus should be available to all quitters.

Although NRTs are successful in assisting people to quit smoking, NRTs have not been as influential as would be predicted. It has been suggested that NRTs are less beneficial for individuals who wish to reduce the amount they smoke or partake in temporary abstinence in comparison to individuals who aim to make a permanent change. Smokers wishing to reduce their consumption or partake in temporary abstinence were found to be using NRT in addition to a non-reduction in cigarette smoking (Beard *et al.*, 2011). It could be suggested that individuals who do not aim to fully quit have less motivation and therefore other methods should be suggested.

Consequently, the use of NRTs has not removed the need for psychological input into smoking cessation, rather it has increased it. It is recognised that the most effective cessation technique combines personal support and NRT (Fiore *et al.*, 2008). There are a large number of studies that highlight that some type of personal or telephone support with NRT increases quit rates (Hollis *et al.*, 2007). This support works by increasing motivation for quitting and remaining tobacco-free. However, in England, the majority of individuals who are attempting to quit do not use the National Health Service Stop Smoking Service (NHS-SSS) which is effective, free and combines behavioural and pharmacological approaches (Kotz et al., 2009). When behavioural aspects of quitting are not addressed individuals may not receive the required support and motivation to continue. There are a number of ways of assessing motivation and these will be explored in more detail in a later section. However, three simple questions can be used:

- Do you want to stop smoking for good?
- Are you interested in making a serious attempt to stop in the near future?
- Are you interested in receiving help with your quit attempt?

These provide a qualitative indicator of motivation to stop smoking (West, 2004).

> ## Applying this to Joe
>
> Given Joe's level of smoking and the number of years that he has been smoking, some form of NRT will probably be required. You should explore all the options with Joe to see which one he feels most comfortable with. It is important to discuss options with the client as they need to feel confident and comfortable with any changes they make.

Psychological approaches

Psychological approaches to smoking cessation are important, either alone or in conjunction with pharmacological approaches, and this has been recognised since the 1960s. There are, of course, a number of psychological methods to the interventions and Table 8.9 summarises the effectiveness of particular psychosocial treatment contents (adapted from US Surgeon General, 2008).

> ## Applying this to Joe
>
> Joe would benefit from additional social support: you could arrange for him to contact a Quit-line or the local Stop Smoking clinic. You may also want to discuss with his family so he obtains support from that quarter as well.

Table 8.9 Psychosocial content and abstinence rates

Psychosocial content	Estimated abstinence rate (95% CI)
No counselling (i.e. nothing)	11.2
Relaxation (muscle and imagery relaxation)	10.8 (7.8, 13.8)
Contingency contracting (e.g. 'If you give up smoking I will give you £10')	11.2 (7.8, 14.6)
Cigarette fading (reducing number of cigarettes smoked over specified time period)	11.8 (8.4, 15.3)
Intratreatment social support (support from practitioners during treatment)	14.4 (12.3, 16.5)

Psychosocial content	Estimated abstinence rate (95% CI)
Extratreatment social support (support from practitioners after treatment)	16.2 (11.8, 20.6)
Other aversive smoking (negative consequence associated with smoking cigarette)	17.7 (11.2, 24.9)
Rapid smoking (i.e. smoke one cigarette, followed by another and another until sick)	19.9 (11.2, 29.0)

Source: Adapted from US Surgeon General, 2008

BOX 8.1 Applying research in practice

A randomised controlled trial of an appearance-related smoking intervention (Grogan *et al.*, 2011)

This paper investigated whether exposure to a smoke-related facial age-progression technique impacted on quit smoking cognitions, nicotine dependence and self-reported and objectively assessed smoking in women aged between 18 and 34 years using a randomised control trial.

All the women were randomised to either an appearance related intervention or a control group. Women completed questionnaires assessing attitudes, subjective norms, perceived behavioural control and intention to quit smoking immediately before, immediately after and four weeks after receiving the intervention or usual care.

Findings found that compared to the control group the appearance related intervention group had significantly more positive attitudes, subjective norms, perceived behavioural control and intention to quit smoking immediately after exposure.

It was concluded that an appearance related smoking intervention may be useful with usual care for women smokers.

As we can see from Table 8.9, there are a number of psychological approaches to smoking cessation. One of the earliest and most successful forms of psychological intervention is behavioural in nature. According to behaviourists, all behaviour is learnt from the environment, can be reduced to simple stimulus – response associations – and, regardless of its complexity, can be described and explained without reference to internal states (motivation, emotion etc.) or mental events (i.e. perception, attention, memory, thinking and so on). Thus learning and experience are fundamental to the behaviourist approach.

Behavioural approaches

Behavioural approaches to smoking cessation are many and varied, yet are usually based on the relapse prevention model of Marlatt and Gordon (1985). This model suggests that common events (whether these are cognitive, behavioural or affective) lead to high-risk situations that threaten abstinence, for example an argument with a partner or getting stressed out when driving into work. These situations can be identified with guided support by the individual smoker, although sometimes a table such as that presented in Table 8.10 may be useful to assist the smoker identify any triggers.

Consequently, it is suggested that individuals can prevent relapse by anticipating these events and learning to cope with them. This model has been taken up enthusiastically, however the effectiveness of the method is thought to be questionable (Hajek *et al.*, 2009). At its simplest, any intervention based on the behavioural perspective would explore if there were any triggers for a person smoking and then either eradicate these triggers or teach the individual how to cope with them. For example, if every time a person sat down for a cup of coffee in the morning they had a cigarette, they would be taught to have the coffee in a place where they could not smoke, or to take up some other activity during this time (e.g. reading the newspaper). Obviously it would not be sensible to substitute one unhealthy behaviour for another, so replacing a cigarette with a cream cake would not be a good idea! On the other hand, if the person reached for a cigarette every time they got stressed out with the children and they wanted a 'five-minute break with a fag' then different coping mechanisms for relaxation could be taught.

Table 8.10 Why do you continue to smoke?

Antecedents (before the behaviour)	Behaviour (what did you do?)	Consequences (what happened after this)
• What were you doing? • What were you thinking? • What were you feeling? • Who were you with?	• Smoke!	• What happened after this? • How did you feel?
A	B	C
Example: I was stressed out because of the children	I had a cigarette Or I went and sat down for five minutes to watch TV and relax	I felt guilty Or I felt relaxed and ready to play with the children

Applying this to Joe

Joe has a number of identified triggers – the pub and his friends. He needs to be taught coping mechanisms so he can deal with any potential triggers in these situations.

Another behavioural method much favoured in the past was aversive smoking – for example, rapid smoking and rapid puffing (Danaher, 1977). These methods involve getting the smoker to smoke intensively to the point of discomfort, nausea or vomiting. Evidence indicates that such techniques can be successful and can be used with smokers who have not succeeded with other techniques (Vidrine *et al.*, 2006). However, there are of course associated health risks and consequently aversive smoking interventions should be used with caution (if at all).

Transtheoretical model of change (TTM)/Stages of Change

The most influential psychological model that has been used in smoking cessation has been the 'transtheoretical model of change' or 'Stages of Change' (TTM; DiClemente and Prochaska, 1982). The model suggests that change proceeds through six stages, summarised in Figure 8.3. Importantly, relapse can occur at any stage, and can mean that the individual goes back to the very first stage – it is not a linear model of simple progression from one stage to another. Relapse means that you simply revert to the previous stage: you can revert to *any* previous stage.

The Stages of Change model has been used extensively to promote health and assist individuals in quitting smoking. This model is important because it allows professionals to identify where individuals are in their behaviour and then develop appropriate interventions (whether these be computer or media based, community or individual based, pharmacologically or psychologically based). If, for example, an individual smokes and has no intention of giving up (i.e. in the pre-contemplation stage), the intervention to be developed will be different from that of the individual who is preparing to give up (i.e. in the contemplation stage) or has started the process (i.e. action stage). In the first case, our obligation should be to try to get quitting into the person's thought processes. We want to try to get the individual to consider giving up smoking – we want to shift them from the pre-contemplation stage to the contemplation stage. The most common method in this approach is a simple consciousness-raising exercise: increasing information about the problem and how it can affect the individual concerned. So, at this stage it would simply be a case of getting them to realise that smoking is health damaging, that it can affect them individually, and then spelling out the individual health problems. This example demonstrates that interventions have to be tailored to the individual's position in the cycle.

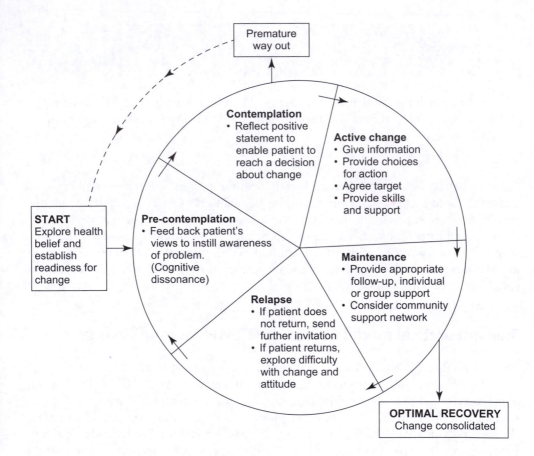

Figure 8.3 Stages of Change model

Source: Adapted from Silverman and Draper, 2005

Interventions based on the stages of changes model usually incorporate two key elements. Firstly, it is necessary to identify accurately an individual's stage of change (or readiness to change), so that an appropriate intervention can be designed and applied. Secondly, the stage of change needs to be reassessed frequently, and the intervention modified in light of this assessment. In this way, stage-based interventions evolve and adapt in response to the individual's movement through the stages. It is suggested that such interventions are better than the 'one size fits all' model and that the intervention will be more efficient and effective than such models.

The first task that we have to do is identify at what stage the individual smoker is. This is not as difficult as it sounds and can be completed using a simple 'readiness ruler' as indicated in Figure 8.4 along with a 'confidence ruler' (see Figure 8.5) which can assist the practitioner in planning the intervention and the support that will be required.

On a scale of 1 to 10, how certain are you that you want to change your smoking behaviour?

1	2	3	4	5	6	7	8	9	10
Not certain at all									Very certain
Pre-contemplation			Contemplation				Action		

Figure 8.4 Readiness ruler for assessing stage of change of smoker

On a scale of 1 to 10, how confident are you that you *want* to change this smoking behaviour?

1	2	3	4	5	6	7	8	9	10
Not confident at all									Very confident

Figure 8.5 Confidence ruler for assessing individual smoker

Applying this to Joe

Joe is in the contemplation stage and you have managed to push him through into the action stage. It is important that the methods you now adopt are appropriate to this stage. Such methods could include providing Joe with information on quitting including preparing him for the physiological and psychological effects this may have. For example, Joe will experience physiological withdrawal symptoms. In addition, it is also now the perfect time to set Joe some targets. Doing all of this will in turn provide Joe with help and support during his attempt to quit.

The TTM has been primarily applied to smoking (West, 2005 reported that a third of all TTM studies dealt with smoking, compared to only 13 per cent for alcohol, cocaine, heroin, opiates and gambling) and has been *the* model for developing interventions. Indeed, surveys have suggested that the Stages of Change model and motivational interviewing were the main topics covered in training courses, as well as the primary theory used to explain behaviour change (West, 2005). The Stages of Change model has been popular with practitioners as a practical intervention guide for clinicians, and as an example of how to apply complex theories of behaviour change in an approachable and understandable form.

Motivational interviewing

The concept of the TTM can be used clinically to work with smokers. Motivational Interviewing (MI), an innovative therapeutic approach for promoting behavioural change, is increasingly being applied to smoking cessation (Hettema and Hendricks, 2010). Motivational interviewing can be defined as 'a directive patient-centred style of counselling, designed to help people to explore and resolve ambivalence about behaviour change' (Lai *et al.*, 2010).

Motivational interviewing (MI) has as its goal the simple expectation that increasing an individual's motivation to consider change rather than showing them how to change should be the key step. If a person is not motivated to change, it is irrelevant whether or not they know how to do it. However, if a person is motivated to change, the interventions aimed at changing behaviour can begin.

Motivational interviewing is a technique based on cognitive behavioural therapy which aims to enhance an individual's motivation to change health behaviour. The whole process aims to help the patient understand their thought processes and to identify how their thought processes help produce the inappropriate behaviour and how their thought processes can be changed to develop alternative, health-promoting, behaviours. Motivational interviewing differs from counselling because it is directive – the healthcare professional elicits and selectively reinforces change talk that resolves ambivalence and moves the smoker towards change.

Motivational strategies include eight components that are designed to increase the person's level of motivation towards changing a specific behaviour. It is important to note that the motivation is specific to one behaviour, so being motivated to quit smoking does not simply transfer to being motivated to reduce alcohol consumption. The eight components are:

- Giving advice (about specific behaviours to be changed);
- Removing barriers (often about access to particular help);
- Providing choice (making it clear that if they choose not to change, that is their right and it is their choice; the therapist is there to encourage change but not insist on change);
- Decreasing desirability (of the ambivalence towards change or the status quo);
- Practising empathy;
- Providing feedback (from a variety of perspectives – family, friends, health professionals – in order to give the patient a full picture of their current situation);
- Clarifying goals (feedback should be compared with a standard (an ideal), and clarification of the ideal can provide the pathway to the goal);
- Active helping (such as expressing caring or facilitating a referral, both of which convey a real interest in helping the person to change).

Motivational interviewing has been considered a successful technique in aiding long-term behaviour change in relation to smoking (Hettema and Hendricks, 2010). Although the method sounds relatively simple and straightforward and, to a certain extent, it is, there are a number of key skills that you need to employ in order to be successful in motivating smokers to quit. Some of these are presented in Table 8.11.

Table 8.11 Key skills for motivational interviewing

Skill	Comment
Express empathy	There should be no criticism or blame as acceptance facilitates change
Develop discrepancy	Change is motivated by a perceived discrepancy between present behaviour and personal goal
Roll with resistance	Avoid arguing for change or providing change – see the smoker as the source of information
Support self-efficacy	The smoker's belief in the possibility of change is an important motivator for change
Use open-ended questions	Encourage the client to do most of the talking: 'What are your concerns about smoking?'
Use reflective listening	Reflect back change talk in a statement: 'I had real cravings this morning' to 'You are a little concerned about the cravings in the morning'
Use affirmation	Use to build rapport: 'You are right to be concerned about smoking in front of the children'
Summarise	Link together and reinforce what has been discussed: 'You are concerned that your smoking may cause lung cancer'
Reframe or agree with a twist	Address resistance by reinterpreting: 'My kids nag me about giving up smoking' to 'It sounds like they really care about your health'
Emphasise personal choice	Reinforce that it is the client's choice to change their behaviour
Evocative questions	
Increasing confidence	Use open questions to evoke confidence talk: 'How might you go about making this change?'
Confidence ruler	Use the ruler to ask 'What would it take to score higher?'
Strengths and successes	Review obstacles and how the client has overcome them
Reframing	'I've tried three times to quit and failed' to 'You have had three good attempts already and are learning new skills'
Prompt coping strategies	Ask for potential obstacles and putative coping strategies

Source: Adapted from Miller and Rollnick, 2002

Applying this to Joe

It is important that Joe also progresses from the action stage and is able to maintain his ability to quit in order for his health to benefit. In continuing to support Joe motivational interviewing could be used and obstacles which impact on his ability to maintain his quitting behaviour can be addressed.

With an estimated 67 per cent of smokers reporting a desire to quit smoking (The Health and Social Care Information Centre, 2011) it is important to highlight some of the specific interventions which are available to all individuals. These interventions have increased in popularity over recent years with government expenditure on NHS Stop Smoking Services exceeding £84 million between 2010 and 2011 (The Health and Social Care Information Centre, 2011). Examples of such programs follow.

The National Health Service Stop Smoking Service

The NHS provides a free stop smoking service across England which is available to anyone who is trying to quit. The service offers a combination of NRTs, counselling and support at either a one-to-one or a group basis. Individuals who wish to quit start their support before any attempt is made to reduce smoking rates. The trained staff offer advice on how to quit alongside recommending the best strategy for that individual. Once the individual decides to quit, carbon monoxide monitors are used to take biochemical measures of the carbon monoxide levels in the breath of the individual. The higher the level of carbon monoxide in the breath, the more the individual is smoking. For example a non-smoker should measure 0–10 on the reader as opposed to a heavy smoker who will show a range of >20. This tool is used to motivate the individual to continue to quit as they will be able to see the benefits of their efforts. A recent evaluation concluded that over 250,000 people had managed to quit smoking through using the service (NHS stop smoking services, 2012).

Quit4life

Provided by the NHS, the service delivers smoking cessation support for individuals across Hampshire. The program adopts a multi-focused approach including psychological and physiological support throughout the quitting process. Similar to the NHS Stop Smoking Service, smoking cessation support is offered in the form of support groups from trained smoking cessation advisers. In addition, the service offers advice on tackling issues related to quitting and NRT. It is suggested that providing individuals with a combination of support mechanisms such as that seen in Quit4life cessation rates can be enhanced (Fiore et al., 2008).

Stoptober

In October 2012, the NHS launched their 'Stoptober' campaign for the first time. Backed by Cancer Research UK and the British Heart Foundation, the campaign encouraged smokers to stop smoking for 28 days, as those who do so are five times more likely to stay smoke free (Department of Health, 2012). Participants could download the Stoptober app or access the Facebook page, where they were provided with tips, advice and encouragement. The results are yet to be seen.

Community level interventions

Having considered individual level interventions, it is also important to consider community based interventions and policies. Such interventions are aimed to promote behaviour change to individuals who would not consider individual level assistance. Tobacco controlling interventions and policies have been found to be successful in reducing smoking prevalence (Wilson *et al.*, 2012). Outlined below are some examples of community level interventions.

Second-hand smoke campaign

We have seen a number of interventions aimed directly at the impact of smoking on the smoker; however, attention also needs to be paid to the effects of cigarette smoke on individuals who don't smoke. A recent national advertising campaign warning of the dangers of second-hand smoke was launched in 2012. This campaign aims to increase smokers' awareness of the dangers of their second-hand smoke. In doing so it aims to increase the number of quit attempts and reduce air pollution for non-smokers. The importance of raising the awareness of second-hand smoke comes from the potentially dangerous chemicals that are thought to be affecting individuals who don't smoke. It is thought that alongside physiological symptoms, individuals such as children can be affected psychologically by second-hand smoke (Bandiera *et al.*, 2011), thus inferring that there are always health implications of second-hand smoke (ASH, 2011b).

Smokefree generation

The Department of Health has launched many advertising campaigns over the years in an attempt to encourage smokers to quit. One recently launched campaign was 'Smokefree Generation'. Re-launched in November 2011, the campaign focused on the children of smokers and emphasised on their worries regarding the parents' smoking habits. This is conveyed through short video clips using real children and their accounts instead of child actors. Within these campaigns the children make stop smoking appeals in an attempt to make the parent realise that their smoking habits affect others around them.

Smoke-free legislation

The smoke-free legislation introduced in 2007 saw enclosed public spaces such as bars and restaurants becoming a smoke-free environment. Since the introduction of this, many benefits have been seen. One benefit includes reduced exposure to second hand smoke for individuals who do not smoke (Sims *et al.*, 2012). More specifically benefits have been seen in the quality of the air in pubs and bars (Brennan *et al.*, 2010). In addition to direct health benefits, it is also thought that the introduction of the smoke-free legislation can impact quit rates and intentions to quit. Research suggests that the perceived unacceptability of smoking due to the smoke-free legislation encouraged quit attempts by smokers (Brown *et al.*, 2009). This highlights the attitudinal changes of individuals in relation to smoking and social norms. This can have future implications in not only quitting but the uptake of the behaviour in the first place. Overall, the legislation has not only been effective at a health and behavioural level but also at an attitudinal level. It is this level that is considered an important factor in successful behaviour change as outlined in health theories and models such as the Theory of Planned Behaviour (Ajzen, 1991; Middlestadt *et al.*, 2012).

Applying this to Joe

Community level campaigns, such as the second-hand smoke campaign, could be shown to Joe as part of educating him about the potential health consequences of smoking. It is important that Joe realises the extent to which his second-hand smoke can affect his grandchild JJ. This factor could then impact upon his motivation to maintain his quitting behaviour.

Working effectively with others

In attempting to reduce smoking rates it is important to provide individuals with the professional advice that they will need. Below are examples of how health professionals can help with smoking cessation and contribute to the successful maintenance of the behaviour to prevent relapse.

Nurses

Nurses have a wide patient base, and as such, provide a good basis for promoting smoking cessation to the general population (Sheffer *et al.*, 2011). This in turn could help with the government's aims to reduce smoking. More specifically, the NHS provides special training and resources to specific healthcare professionals such as midwives. The need to reduce and stop pregnant women smoking is important due to the detrimental health implications for both the mother and the child. Effects of smoking during pregnancy have been well documented. Alongside health implications, foetal development is also seen to be affected (Vardavas *et al.*, 2010). The National Institute for Health and Clinical Excellence (NICE) recognised the importance of midwives in this role and produced an updated outlined guidance on the matter (National Institute for Health and Clinical Excellence, 2010). Recommendations for midwives include making the mother aware of the risks of smoking, providing support for partners who also smoke and referring them to a stop smoking service.

GPs

In addition to nurses having a good access to the general population, GPs also have a wide client base and provide a means of advice for smoking cessation. However, it has been noted that many individuals who talk to their GP regarding smoking cessation are advised to stop but not offered any support (National Institute for Health and Clinical Excellence, 2010). When support and advice was offered by the GP, positive associations were noted in attempted quit rates (National Institute for Health and Clinical Excellence, 2010). This highlights the importance of the GP in promoting smoking cessation to their patients and providing a first point of call for them.

When looking to permanently change behaviour it is important that once the smoker is ready to quit, a plan for change is developed. This can be used alongside any other methods when attempting to quit and comes from the smoker, although it is a process best shared with a healthcare professional. This plan involves setting goals, considering change options, arriving at a plan and eliciting commitment (see Table 8.12). It can be helpful for smokers to complete a physical plan as this will provide reinforcement and something concrete to explore when predicaments occur.

Maintaining the quit behaviour

Once the initial behaviour change is undertaken, it is important to work on maintaining it. The majority of quit attempts fail within the first week and hence it is important to follow up the individual on a frequent and regular basis – probably after the first one, two and three weeks. It may also be useful to have follow-up text messages or phone calls during the first 10 days.

Following withdrawal of nicotine, there may be unpleasant symptoms of nicotine withdrawal (see Table 8.13). These physical and mental symptoms occur because of adaptation of the brain to long-term administration of nicotine. Withdrawal symptoms are normally temporary but for the first few weeks can be very distressing and may lead to relapse. It takes considerable will-power and support to deal with the withdrawal symptoms and the cravings often prompt people to go straight back to the cigarettes. There is a necessity to provide appropriate psychological support during this time, and this is where NRTs can be particularly effective (see previous discussion).

Relapse

Cigarette smoking is a behaviour that is relatively difficult to change. Despite the health risks associated with smoking, relatively few smokers succeed in their quit attempts (Piasecki, 2006). Even with successful treatment relapse can occur quickly – with many smokers not even attaining 24 hours of continuous abstinence (Piasecki, 2006) and the majority abandoning their quit attempts within 5–10 days. In order to explore relapse, researchers have explored psychological processes such as withdrawal, urge and craving, and negative affect.

Table 8.12 Developing a change plan

Aspect of change	Comment	Questions to ask
Setting goals	The smoker's goals are the ones that matter most	What do you want to achieve?
Considering change options	Useful to provide range of optional strategies	What do you think will work for you?
Arrive at a plan	Summarise the smoker's plan	How will you go about it?
Elicit commitment	Useful to agree some immediate steps to implement the plan	What date are you going to quit?

Table 8.13 Withdrawal symptoms commonly experienced

Withdrawal symptom	Duration	Proportion of smokers affected
Light-headedness	< 2 days	10%
Night-time awakenings	< 1 week	25%
Poor concentration	< 2 weeks	60%
Cravings	> 2 weeks	70%
Irritability or aggression	< 4 weeks	50%
Restlessness	< 4 weeks	60%
Depression	< 4 weeks	60%
Increased appetite and weight gain	> 10 weeks	80%

Source: Reproduced from *British Medical Journal*, 328, pp. 277–79 (Jarvis, Martin J. 2004), with permission from BMJ Publishing Group Ltd

Applying this to Joe

It is essential and important to maintain contact during the first four weeks to provide support for Joe through the initial changes that he will experience as a result of quitting. After the initial four weeks, it is still important to monitor Joe but this can be less frequent.

Factors associated with successful cessation

Although the majority of smokers want to stop smoking and some 26 per cent of current smokers have tried to quit in the previous 12 months, the success rate is low with 71 per cent of individuals only giving up for six months or less (Lader, 2009). A number of studies have been undertaken exploring factors associated with successful quitting and these were often interrelated. For example, Zhou *et al.* (2009) found that individuals who experienced sleep disturbance, anxiety and depression were more likely to be unsuccessful in their quit attempt. Furthermore, the environment was also found to be important – being in daily contact with other smokers, for example, is associated with less success, whether this is in the workplace or at home (see Table 8.14).

As an individual's confidence grows, a number of problem situations may arise with which he or she must cope. It is in these situations that the healthcare professional may have a key role in assisting the smoker review the problem situations and suggesting potential coping strategies (see Table 8.15).

Table 8.14 Factors associated with successful smoking cessation

Positive	Negative
Smoke-free home	Multiple previous attempts
No-smoking policy at work	Switching to low-tar products
Aged 35+	
Having university education	
Being married/cohabiting	
One previous attempt at quitting	
Social support	

Table 8.15 Potential coping strategies

Situation	Potential coping strategy
When stuck in the car in a traffic jam	Chew NRT gum or have a lozenge
In the pub	Let the smokers go outside by themselves Stop going to the pub!
After a meal	Move on to something else – cleaning table etc. – rather than mulling over a cigarette
On waking	Use patch or gum, or clean teeth/shower immediately
When stressed	Relaxation techniques, exercise
When bored	Displacement
When anxious	Relaxation techniques
When relaxed	Displacement or avoidance
When angry	Relaxation techniques
Cravings	NRT Use support – either personal or professional Have a healthy snack (fruit, vegetables) Keep hands occupied Think positively about reasons for quitting

Applying this to Joe

You need to ensure that the positive factors associated with quitting are in place in Joe's life such as social support from his friends and family and ensuring his home is smoke free so behavioural triggers are reduced.

Many smokers who are willing and ready to quit struggle and often lapse at moments where some form of support would have seen them succeed. Support can make all the difference – whether this comes from the family, friends, some healthcare professional (e.g. nurse, health trainer), a support group or a helpline.

Conclusion

Smoking results in significant health problems, including an abbreviated life expectancy. Consequently, it is important for all healthcare professionals to explore with their clients and patients how they can assist them in stopping smoking. In those groups at risk for starting to smoke (e.g. adolescents or those with a family history of smoking), appropriate messages about the harm caused by smoking should be provided.

In order to assist those smokers, there are a number of resources and pharmacological and psychological methods that can be used to support smoking cessation. The Stages of Change model and motivational interviewing are key methods that can be employed by the healthcare professional.

Key points

- Cigarette smoking remains the single most avoidable cause of death and disability in the UK and the Western world.
- There are differences in prevalence rates of smoking in England, Wales, Scotland and Northern Ireland.
- The number of people smoking, including the young and older generations, has decreased considerably. Smoking has been linked to a whole host of diseases and chronic conditions, including heart disease, cancer, peripheral vascular disease, premature and low weight babies, bronchitis, emphysema, sinusitis, peptic ulcers and dental hygiene problems, and can worsen the effects of asthma and infections.
- Despite knowledge of the health risks associated with smoking, people continue to smoke and to display unrealistic optimism regarding the impact of their smoking behaviour.
- The most influential model used in smoking cessation is the transtheoretical or Stages of Change model. This suggests that people move between different stages of 'readiness' for change. People can move forwards or backwards and relapse can occur at any time. However, there is limited evidence that smoking cessation programmes based on the TTM are effective.
- Motivational interviewing can be used to attempt to increase a smoker's motivation to quit.
- Individual level smoking cessation interventions include (either alone or in combination) behavioural and pharmaceutical interventions ranging from brief advice and counselling to intensive support and administration of medications that contribute to reducing or overcoming dependence.
- Community level interventions and legislations have been useful in raising awareness of the health consequences of smoking alongside impacting upon attitude change towards the behaviour.
- It is important that society as a whole continues to work together in the attempt to impact smoking rates. Working effectively with others and having a multi-angled approach is key in implementing behaviour change.
- Lapse and relapse rates are high in smokers attempting to quit. Contact with other smokers, age, gender and previous quit attempts can all impact on the likelihood that a quit attempt will be successful.

Points for discussion

- Critically discuss the importance of attitudes in relation to smoking cessation.
- Consider the current and future implications of smoke free legislation from a psychological stance.
- Evaluate the importance of social support in quit attempts.

Further resources

Coleman, T. (2004a) Cessation interventions in routine health care. *British Medical Journal,* 328: 631–3.
Wilson, A., Agarwal, S., Bonas, S., Murtagh, G., Coleman, T., Taub, N. andChernova, J. (2010). Management of smokers motivated to quit: a qualitative study of smokers and GPs. *Family Practice*, 27(4): 404–409. DOI:10.1093/fampra/cmq027

Useful web links

British Heart Foundation 0800 169 1900 www.bhf.org.uk
NHS Stop smoking quitline 0800 169 0169 www.givingupsmoking.co.uk
Quitline 0800 002 200 www.quit.org.uk
Ash 0207 739 5902 www.ash.org.uk
Smokefree – help to quit website http://smokefree.nhs.uk/ways-to-quit/local-nhs-stop-smoking-service/
Smokefree helpline 08000224332
Quitting during pregnancy helpline 08001699169
Quit4life website http://www.quit4life.nhs.uk/about_quit4life.html

References

Ajzen, I. (1991). The theory of planned behavior. *Organizational Behavior & Human Decision Processes*, 50(2): 179.
Armitage, C. J & Conner, M. (2001). Efficacy of the theory of planned behaviour: ameta-analytic review. *British Journal of Social Psychology* 40(4): 471–499.
ASH (2009). *Essential Information: Who Smokes and How Much*. London: ASH.
——(2011a). *Smoking Statistics: Young People and Smoking*. London: ASH.
——(2011b). *Research Report: Second-hand Smoke*. London: ASH.
——(2012a). *Smoking statistics: Who Smokes and How Much*. London: ASH.
——(2012b). *Facts at a Glance: Smoking Statistics*. Available at http://www.ash.org.uk/files/documents/ASH_93.pdf (accessed 28 December 2012).
——(2012c). *Facts at a Glance: Smoking and Disease*. Available at http://www.ash.org.uk/files/documents/ASH_94.pdf (accessed 28 December 2012).
Bandiera, F., Richardson, A., Lee, D., He, J. and Merikangas, K. (2011). Second-hand smoke exposure and mental health among children and adolescents. *Archives of Paediatrics & Adolescent Medicine*, 165(4): 332–338.

Beard, E.E., McNeill, A.A., Aveyard, P.P., Fidler, J.J., Michie, S.S. and West, R.R. (2011). Use of nicotine replacement therapy for smoking reduction and during enforced temporary abstinence: a national survey of English smokers. *Addiction*, 106(1): 197–204.

Brennan, E., Cameron, M., Warne, C., Durkin, S., Borland, R., Travers, M.J., Wakefield, M. A. *et al.* (2010). Second-hand smoke drift: Examining the influence of indoor smoking bans on indoor and outdoor air quality at pubs and bars. *Nicotine & Tobacco Research*, 12(3): 271–277.

Bromley, C. and Given, L. (2011). *The Scottish Health Survey 2010, Volume 1: Main Report*. Edinburgh: The Scottish Government. Available at: http://www.scotland.gov.uk/Publications/2011/09/27084018/91 (accessed 10 January 2013).

Brown, A., Moodie, C. and Hastings, G. (2009). A longitudinal study of policy effect (smoke-free legislation) on smoking norms: ITC Scotland/United Kingdom. *Nicotine & Tobacco Research*, 11(8): 924–932.

Browning, K.K., Ferketich, A.K., Salsberry, P.J. and Wewers, M.E. (2008). Socioeconomic disparity in provider-delivered assistance to quit smoking. *Nicotine & Tobacco Research: Official Journal of the Society for Research on Nicotine and Tobacco*, 10(1): 55–61.

Chapman, S. and MacKenzie, R. (2010). The global research neglect of unassisted smoking cessation: causes and consequences. *PLOS Medicine*, 7(2): e1000216

Cofta-Woerpel, L., Wright, K.L. and Wetter, D.W. (2007). Smoking cessation 3: multicomponent interventions. *Behavioural Medicine*, 32: 135–149.

Danaher, B.G. (1977). Rapid smoking and self control in the modification of smoking behaviour. *Journal of Consulting and Clinical Psychology*, 45(6): 1068–1074.

Department of Health (2011). *Healthy Lives, Healthy People: A Tobacco Control Plan for England*. London: Department of Health.

——(2012). *Stoptober Campaign Will Encourage Smokers to Quit for 28 Days*. Available at: http://www.dh.gov.uk/health/2012/09/stoptober/ (accessed 28 December. 2012).

Department of Health, Social Services and Public Safety. (2011). *Health Survey Northern Ireland: First results from the 2010/11 Survey*. Belfast. Available at: http://www.dhsspsni.gov.uk/index/stats_research/stats-public-health.htm (accessed 10 June 2012).

DiClemente, C.C. and Prochaska, J.O. (1982). Self-change and therapy change of smoking behaviour: a comparison of processes of change in cessation and maintenance, *Addictive Behaviours*, 7: 133–142.

Doll, R. and Hill, A.B. (1952). A study of the aetiology of carcinoma of the lung. *British Medical Journal*, ii: 1271–1286.

Fiore, M.C., Jaén, C.R., Baker, T.B. *et al.* (2008) *Treating Tobacco Use and Dependence: 2008 Update. Clinical Practice Guideline*. Rockville, MD: U.S. Department of Health and Human Services. Public Health Service.

Grogan, S., Flett, K., Clark-Carter, D., Conner, M., Davey, R., Richardson, D. and Rajaratnam, G. (2011). A randomized controlled trial of an appearance-related smoking intervention. *Health Psychology*, 30(6): 805.

Guassora, A. and Baarts, C. (2010). Smoking cessation advice in consultations with health problems not related to smoking? Relevance criteria in Danish general practice consultations. *Scandinavian Journal of Primary Health Care*, 28(4): 221–228.

Hajek, P., Stead, L.F., West, R., Jarvis, M. and Lancaster, T. (2009). Relapse prevention interventions for smoking cessation. *Cochrane Database of Systematic Reviews*, Issue 1. Art. No.: CD003999. DOI: 10.1002/14651858.CD003999.pub3.

Hays, J., Ebbert, J. and Sood, A. (2009). Treating tobacco dependence in light of the 2008 US Department of Health and Human Services Clinical Practice Guideline. *Mayo Clinic Proceedings*, 84(8): 730–736. DOI: 10.4065/84.8.730.

Henderson, H., Memon, A., Lawson, K., Jacobs, B. and Koutsogeorgou, E. (2011). What factors are important in smoking cessation amongst deprived communities: a qualitative study. *Health Education Journal*, 70(1): 84–91.

Hettema, J.E. and Hendricks, P.S. (2010). Motivational interviewing for smoking cessation: a meta-analytic review. *Journal of Consulting And Clinical Psychology*, 78(6): 868–884. DOI: 10.1037/a0021498.

Hollis, J. F., McAfee, T. A., Fellows, J. L., Zbikowski, S. M., Stark, M. and Riedlinger, K. (2007). The effectiveness and cost effectiveness of telephone counselling and the nicotine patch in a state tobacco quitline. *Tobacco Control*: 16i53–i59. DOI: 10.1136/tc.2006.019794.

Hrubá, D. and Zaloudíková, I. (2010). Why to smoke? Why not to smoke? Major reasons for children's decisions on whether or not to smoke. *Central European Journal of Public Health*, 18(4): 202.

Hung, W.T., Dunlop, S.M., Perez, D. and Cotter, T. (2011). Use and perceived helpfulness of smoking cessation methods: results from a population survey of recent quitters. *BMC Public Health*: 11592.

Hyland, A., Li, Q., Bauer, J.E., Steger, C. and Cummings, K.M. (2004). Predictors of cessation in a cohort of current and former smokers followed over 13 years. *Nicotine and Tobacco Research* 6(S3): S363–S369.

Jarvis, M.K. (2004). Why people smoke. *British Medical Journal*, 328, 277–279.

Kotz, D., Fidler, J. and West, R. (2009). Factors associated with the use of aids to cessation in English smokers. *Addiction*, 104(8): 1403–1410.

Lader, D. (2009). *Smoking-Related Behaviour and Attitudes 2008/09*. London: ONS.

Lai, D.T., Cahill, K., Qin, Y. and Tang, J. (2010). Motivational interviewing for smoking cessation. *Cochrane Database of Systematic Reviews*. Available at http://www.thecochranelibrary.com/userfiles/ccoch/file/World per cent20No per cent20Tobacco per cent20Day/CD006936.pdf (accessed 28 December 2012).

Marlatt, G.A. and Gordon, G. (eds) (1985). *Relapse Prevention: Maintenance Strategies in Addictive Behavior Change*. New York: Guilford Press.

Middlestadt, S.E., Seo, D., Kolbe, L.J. and Jay, S.J. (2012). Applying the theory of planned behavior to explore the relation between smoke-free air laws and quitting intentions. *Health Education & Behavior*, 39(1): 27–34.

Miller, W.R. and Rollnick, S. (2002). *Motivational Interviewing: Preparing People for Change*, 2nd edn. New York: Guilford Press.

Mohiuddin, S., Mooss, A., Hunter, C., Grollmes, T., Cloutier, D. and Hilleman, D. (2007). Intensive smoking cessation intervention reduces mortality in high-risk smokers with cardiovascular disease. *Chest*, 131(2): 446–452.

Murray, R.L., Lewis, S.A., Coleman, T., Britton, J. and McNeill, A. (2009). Unplanned attempts to quit smoking: missed opportunities for health promotion. *Addiction*, 104(11): 1901–1909.

National Institute for Health and Clinical Excellence (NICE). (2006). *Brief Interventions and Referral for Smoking Cessation in Primary Care and Other Settings*. London: Nice. Available at: www.nice.org.uk/PH001 (accessed 4 July 2012).

——(2010). *Public Health Guidance 26, Quitting Smoking in Pregnancy and Following Childbirth*. Available at http://www.nice.org.uk/nicemedia/live/13023/49345/49345.pdf (accessed 30 June 2012).

Office for National Statistics (2012). *General Lifestyle Survey Overview, a Report on the 2010 General Lifestyle Survey*. Available from www.ons.gov.uk (accessed 28 December 2012).

Okuyemi, K.S., Nollen, N.L. and Ahluwalia, J.S. (2006). Interventions to facilitate smoking cessation. *American Family Physician*, 74: 262–271.

Parsons, A., Daley, A., Begh, R. and Aveyard, P. (2010). Influence of smoking cessation after diagnosis of early stage lung cancer on prognosis: systematic review of observational studies with meta-analysis. *BMJ (Clinical Research Ed.)*: 340b5569. DOI:10.1136/bmj.b5569

Perkins, K.A., Conklin, C.A. and Levine, M.D. (2008). *Cognitive-Behavioural Therapy for Smoking Cessation*. New York: Routledge.

Silverman, J. and Draper, J. (2005). *Skills for Communicating with Patients*, 2nd edn. Oxford: Radcliffe Publishing.

Sims, M., Mindell, J.S., Jarvis, M.J., Feyerabend, C., Wardle, H. and Gilmore, A. (2012). Did smokefree legislation in England reduce exposure to second-hand smoke among nonsmoking adults? Cotinine analysis from the Health Survey for England. *Environmental Health Perspectives*, 120(3): 425–430.

Smith, B., Bean, M., Mitchell, K., Speizer, I. and Fries, E. (2007). Psychosocial factors associated with non-smoking adolescents' intentions to smoke. *Health Education Research*, 22(2): 238–247.

Sperlich, S., Illiger, K. and Geyer, S. (2011). [Why do mothers smoke? Analysing the influence of living circumstances and psychological factors on tobacco consumption among mothers with minor children]. *Bundesgesundheitsblatt, Gesundheitsforschung, Gesundheitsschutz*, 54(11): 1211–1220.

Stead, L.F., Perera, R., Bullen, C., Mant, D. and Lancaster, T. (2008). Nicotine replacement therapy for smoking cessation. *Cochrane Database of Systematic Reviews*, Issue 1. Art. No.: CD000146. DOI: 10.1002/14651858.CD000146.pub3.

Stead, L. F., Perera, R., Bullen, C., Mant, D., Hartmann-Boyce, J., Cahill, K. and Lancaster, T. (2012). Nicotine replacement therapy for smoking cessation. *Cochrane Database of Systematic Reviews*. Available at http://onlinelibrary.wiley.com/doi/10.1002/14651858.CD000146.pub4/abstract (accessed 28 December 2012).

The Health and Social Care Information Centre. Statistics on Smoking: England, 2011. Available online at: https://catalogue.ic.nhs.uk/publications/public-health/smoking/smok-eng-2011/smok-eng-2011-rep.pdf (accessed 5 July 2012).

Ussher, M.H., Taylor, A. and Faulkner, G. (2008). Exercise interventions for smoking cessation. *Cochrane Database Syst Rev*, 1.

US Surgeon General (2008). *Treating Tobacco Use And Dependence. 2008 Update*. Atlanta, GA.: Dept. of Health and Human Services, Centers for Disease Control and Prevention, National Center for Chronic Disease Prevention and Health Promotion, Office on Smoking and Health; Washington, DC.

Vardavas, C.I., Chatzi, L., Patelarou, E., Plana, E., Sarri, K., Kafatos, A. and Kogevinas, M. *et al.* (2010). Smoking and smoking cessation during early pregnancy and its effect on adverse pregnancy outcomes and foetal growth. *European Journal Of Pediatrics*, 169(6): 741–748. DOI: 10.1007/s00431-009-1107-9.

Vidrine, J.L., Cofta-Woerpel, L., Daza, P., Wright, K.L. and Wetter, D.W. (2006). Smoking cessation 2: behavioural treatments. *Behavioural Medicine*, 32(3): 99–109.

Welsh Government (2011). *Welsh Health Survey 2010*. Available at: http://www.wales.gov.uk/statistics (accessed 10 January 2013).

West, R. (2004). ABC of smoking cessation: assessment of dependence and motivation to stop smoking. *British Medical Journal*, 328: 338–339.

——(2005). Time for a change: putting the Transtheoretical (Stages of Change) Model to rest. *Addiction*, 100(8): 1036–1039.

WHO (2011). *Global Status Report on Noncommunicable Diseases 2010*. Available at http://whqlibdoc.who.int/publications/2011/9789240686458_eng.pdf (accessed 28 December 2012).

Willemsen, M.C., Wiebing, M., van Emst, A. and Zeeman, G. (2006). Helping smokers to decide on the use of efficacious smoking cessation methods: a randomized controlled trial of a decision aid. *Addiction*, 101(3): 441–449.

Wilson, L., Avila Tang, E., Chandler, G., Hutton, H., Odelola, O., Elf, J. and Apelberg, B. *et al.* (2012). Impact of tobacco control interventions on smoking initiation, cessation, and prevalence: a systematic review. *Journal of Environmental and Public Health*: 2012961724.

Zhou, X., Nonnemaker, J., Sherrill, B., Gilsenan, A., Coste, F. and West, R. (2009). Attempts to quit smoking and relapse: factors associated with success or failure from the ATTEMPT cohort study. *Addictive Behaviors*, 34(4): 365–373.

9 Sexual activity

Learning objectives

At the end of this chapter you will:
- appreciate how 'sex', 'safe sex' and 'safer sex' have been defined by professionals and the lay public alike
- understand the nature of sexually transmitted diseases and their health consequences
- be able to evaluate the psychological determinants of sexual behaviour and safe sex practices
- recognise and be able to review how psychological interventions can assist in promoting safer sex
- understand how the transtheoretical model (TTM) can be used to develop interventions to promote safer sex.

Case study

Gary is an 18-year-old car mechanic who is enjoying life to the full. He works hard in a local garage and earns a steady income. He has recently moved out of his parents' house to set up home with his fiancée, Debbie, in a rented flat. They have an on-off relationship but have been engaged steadily for three months now. Gary has a varied sexual history and has boasted about having more than 15 sexual partners since his introduction to sex in his early teens. Indeed, despite his determination to remain with Debbie, Gary is having occasional 'flings' with girls he meets at the local pub or night club (although he never has 'full sex' – sexual intercourse). Debbie is 17 years of age and has had a 'few' sexual partners (although the last time she counted, this number was over 10) but is currently monogamous with Gary. She does not want to get pregnant since she wants to complete her training as a hairdresser and is hence using the contraceptive pill. Initially when they got together Gary and Debbie did use condoms but Gary felt it reduced sensation and so Debbie was convinced to go on the pill despite her misgivings. Gary has recently experienced some pain 'down below' and has come to a GUM clinic to get it checked out. He feels that he may have contracted an STI from a recent 'fling' that went too far on a recent night out. You have recognised that Gary may be at risk from a sexually transmitted disease and have to try to promote safer sex for both Gary and Debbie.

Applying this to Gary and Debbie

Consider the potential difficulties Debbie and Gary may face in their relationship and how their lifestyle may compromise their health. Deliberate the ways in which Gary could reduce and change his inappropriate behaviour.

Introduction

The first question we must ask, of course, is what is sexual behaviour? Although most people would not struggle when asked this question, further thought suggests that there are difficulties and this may have implications for assessment by the healthcare professional and any planned intervention. A simplistic, biological definition of 'sexual behaviour' could refer to all actions and responses that make fertilisation possible. In order to effect a fertilisation, a male and female have to perform a specific series of actions and physiological responses. This may be a little restrictive, however, and sexual behaviour is more than vaginal intercourse between a male and a female. A more pragmatic definition refers to any behaviour that involves a 'sexual response' of the body. In this way the physical actions associated with sexual behaviour do not have to result in fertilisation. The definition covers all types of human sexual activity (e.g. sexual self-stimulation, heterosexual and homosexual intercourse), but it does not imply any hierarchical order among them. Moreover, it leaves each of these activities open to interpretation. In short, the above definition does not equate sex with reproduction or any other particular purpose. It merely calls attention to a certain physical response common to a variety of activities.

A final definition includes all actions and responses related to pleasure seeking. This is a modern, very wide definition which can be traced to Sigmund Freud and his psychoanalytic theory. Thus, in this view 'the sex drive' came to stand for man's pursuit of pleasure in all its forms. 'Sex' was the underlying motive of every life-enhancing activity. As we can see, when used in this fashion, the term 'sexual behaviour' becomes quite inclusive. The only question in all of these cases is one of motivation. If the behaviour is somehow motivated by the wish for pleasure, if it is prompted by an individual's inner need for self-fulfilment, if it satisfies or gives the individual comfort, if it heightens the sense of being alive – then it is clearly sexual.

Most sexual researchers use the second of these definitions. The definition does not equate sex with reproduction or any other particular purpose. It merely calls attention to a certain physical response common to a variety of activities. Obviously this definition is important for health researchers. When asking members of the population if they engage in 'sex', 'dangerous sexual behaviour' or 'safe sexual behaviour' it is important to define clearly what this covers.

Applying this to Gary

Sex can be defined as physical actions between two individuals that produces a physiological sexual response which may or may not result in fertilisation. Gary would define sex as a pleasure seeking act.

The majority of UK adults obtain their sexual health information from media such as television, newspapers and magazines (ONS, 2009). This means that individuals may not be defining sexual behaviour in the way that professionals define it. Hence, when asking 'Have you engaged in sex?' or 'When was the last time you had sexual behaviour?' you may not get a consistent response. For example, a study (Byers et al., 2009) of university students' views on what activities count as 'having sex' suggested that a small proportion (1.4 per cent) regarded tongue kissing as having sex, 8 per cent regarded touching of genitals without orgasm, 20 per cent regarded oral sex without orgasm, 25 per cent regarded oral sex with orgasm, as having sex. Over 70 per cent thought that vaginal intercourse was sex, whereas around 80 per cent thought that anal intercourse was sex. This suggests that non-coital sex may not be defined as sex by certain key groups, particularly the younger respondents. Accordingly, the definitions of 'sex', 'sexual activity' and 'risky sexual behaviour' need to be extended and clearly defined, for both the healthcare professional and the individual.

In another study of undergraduate students by Hans et al. (2010) only around 20 per cent of respondents regarded oral sex as 'sex'. This may be a result of some considering safe sex to be that form of sexual intercourse that does not result in pregnancy. There has been seen to be a difference of opinion between undergraduate students and sexual healthcare professionals regarding whether oral sex maintains virginity: 90.4 per cent and 79.3 per cent respectively (Hans and Kimberly, 2011). Supporting this, research has also found that 16.1 per cent of adolescents believe that participating in anal sex also maintains their virginity (Bersamin et al., 2007). It is possible that individuals who engage in oral sex, but do not consider it as 'sex', may not associate the acts with the potential health risks they can bring (Chambers, 2007). In fact, evidence suggests that oral sex can contribute to the development of several sexually transmitted infections (STIs) such as HIV, herpes, syphilis, gonorrhoea, and hepatitis (Saini *et al.*, 2010) and the human papillomavirus virus (HPV) which is linked to various cancers (D'Souza *et al.*, 2009). It is by acknowledging this evidence that sexual health interventions should be implicated.

Having sex (however this may be defined) with more than one partner in a lifetime may be a common experience. This means, of course, that calling on people to refrain from having sex does not work from a public health point of view. If we look at potential chains of sexual networking, as described in Figure 9.1, we can see that from apparently being monogamous the number of potential partners from which STIs could have been contracted expands considerably. For example, in Figure 9.1 the male has had previous sexual contact with three women, who have each had three previous male partners. So, the first male has to consider the consequences not just of having sex with an individual woman but also her partners. Hence, the female in the apparently monogamous relationship would have to deal with the consequences of 13 separate sexual couplings.

Applying this to Gary

Gary has had 15 previous sexual partners and each of those women have had 2 other previous sexual partners. This means that Debbie is being exposed to 45 separate couplings.

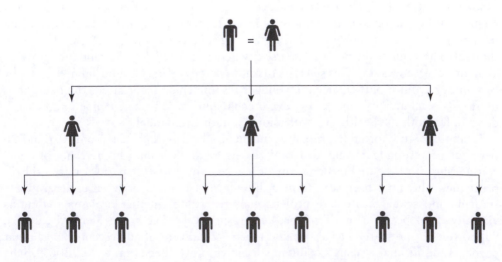

Figure 9.1 An example of a chain of sexual networking

Government recommendations

The UK government has spent millions of pounds on promoting 'safe sex' and has promoted the use of condoms as preventing sexually transmitted infections. The concept of safe sex was derived in response to the HIV/AIDS epidemic and consequently it originally focused on male homosexuals, the community where the outbreak originated, with the earliest reference to this professional term being in 1984 (Morin *et al.*, 1984). A government definition of 'safe sex' involves taking precautions during sex that can keep you from getting a sexually transmitted disease (STD), or from giving an STD to your partner. In 1985, the Coalition for Sexual Responsibility drafted safe sex guidelines to promote the distribution and use of condoms 'to eliminate the exchange of body fluids during anal intercourse or oral sex' (Lindsey, 1985). Subsequently, health promotion officials extended the definition to heterosexual adolescents: 'judicious selection of sexual partners, the use of mechanical and chemical barriers during intercourse, and avoidance of sex practices such as those in which bodily fluids are exchanged' (Slevin and Marvin, 1987).

Applying this to Gary

Gary thinks he is practising safe sex as he is not having 'full sex' with the women that he has occasional flings with.

Recently, and mostly within Canada and the US, the use of the term *safer sex* rather than *safe sex* has gained greater use by health workers, with the realisation that risk of transmission of sexually transmitted infections in various sexual activities is a continuum rather than a simple dichotomy between risky and safe. However, in most other countries, including the UK and Australia, the term *safe sex* is still mainly used by sex educators.

Sexually transmitted infections can be prevented by condom use, but a 2009 survey indicated that individuals are less likely to use condoms for this preventative purpose, with 90 per cent of men and 89 per cent of women citing prevention of pregnancy as their reason for using condoms, and only 45 per cent citing prevention of infection, most of whom cited pregnancy infection as well (NSOS, 2009). Interestingly, the percentage of men who used condoms to prevent infection declined with age: 50 per cent among men aged 25–34 to 33 per cent among men aged 45 and over, perhaps indicating an opinion that STDs only occur amongst the younger generations, which is worrying considering there has been a rise in STDs amongst over 50s in recent years. In 2006, for example, 10 per cent of newly diagnosed HIV cases in the US were amongst the over 50s (Minichiello *et al.*, 2011). The potential for sexually transmitted diseases arising from this lack of knowledge and appropriate usage has to be stressed. For example, the use of condoms during oral sex rather than vaginal or anal intercourse is relatively low and below 20 per cent (Stone *et al.*, 2006) despite the fact that oral sex is a transmission route for many STIs.

The majority of adults (over 50 per cent) report making no changes to their behaviour as a result of what they hear regarding sexual health (NSOS, 2009). It is clear that information and awareness campaigns are ineffective in achieving their goal and other strategies must be implemented.

There is clear evidence to suggest a reduction in STI transmission when consistent and correct use of condoms is employed (McKay, 2007). For example, a Cochrane review found that the consistent use of condoms reduces the risk of contracting HIV by 80 per cent (Weller and Davis-Beaty, 2002). Similarly, Wald *et al.* (2005) found that participants reporting more frequent use of condoms were at a lower risk for acquiring Herpes Simplex Virus-2 than participants who used condoms less frequently.

Abstinence is an absolute answer to preventing STDs. However, abstinence is not always a practical or desirable option. Research has indicated that the individual's underlying attitudes in relation to abstinence and sex are driving forces for the uptake of sexual intercourse in the teenage population (Masters *et al.*, 2008). Therefore attitudes need to be addressed for abstinence to be more popular in the teenage years. Studies have found that a more comprehensive approach to educating adolescents about safe sex, including dispensing contraceptives and condoms, reduces risky sexual behaviour more than abstinence-only education (Underhill *et al.*, 2008). Next to abstinence, the least risky approach is to have a monogamous sexual relationship with someone that you know is free of any STI. Condoms can be used to avoid contact with semen, vaginal fluids or blood. Both male and female condoms dramatically reduce the chance that individuals will get or spread an STI (McKay, 2007). The World Health Organization (WHO) cite the male condom as the single, most efficient, available technology to reduce the sexual transmission of diseases (WHO, 2007). The female condom, though effective and safe, has not achieved its national potential due to its high costs, but both should be readily and consistently available to reduce the spread of STDs.

However, although the 'official' and 'educational' definitions of 'sex' and 'safe sex' are well known and agreed, there is a paucity of literature on how the general public (and those at risk in particular) define 'safe sex' (Moskowitz *et al.*, 2006). A Californian study reported that most defined safe sex in terms of condom use (with 26.3 per cent suggesting that this alone was 'safe sex'). Condom use, in conjunction with other common methods (e.g. abstinence, safe partner or monogamy), was mentioned by two-thirds of respondents. Definitions of safe sex varied across sociodemographic groups. For example, males were more likely to mention monogamy and less likely to mention abstinence. Condom use was mentioned most often by adults aged 18–24 years and tended to decrease with age. Adults aged 25–64 years were most likely to mention monogamy, and those aged 45–64 years were most likely to mention safe partner (Moskowitz *et al.*, 2006). In the study by Bourne and Robson (2009), participants offered an alternative view to 'safe sex' health promotion campaigns, and thought that sex could be safe in a loving relationship, in which partners trusted each other, whether condoms were used or not.

Applying this to Gary and Debbie

Debbie's definition of safe sex would be to take the pill so she doesn't get pregnant.

The NHS Choices website, Livewell – Sexual Health provides a wealth of information on various STDs and their symptoms, how they can be caught, including oral sex and the use of sex toys and 15 different forms of contraception and their availability (NHS Choices, no date). It is an interactive, easy to navigate website that may allow people to gain information without the embarrassment of visiting their clinician.

The National Survey of Sexual Attitudes and Lifestyles (Wellings *et al.*, 1994) examined the sexual behaviour of over 18,000 men and women across Britain and produced considerable data on factors such as age of first intercourse, sexual behaviour and contraception use. The report indicates that for men and women aged 16–24 the most popular form of contraception was condom use (see Figure 9.2). It was rather worrying, however, that many young adults in this age group reported using either no contraception at all, or potentially unreliable methods such as withdrawal or the 'safe period'. In terms of safe sex, healthcare professionals should try to encourage condom use to prevent STDs along with potentially unwanted pregnancies. The third NATSAL began in 2010 and its results will be published in 2013.

Other reports have investigated the views of both men and women. In general, men tend to report a number of negative attitudes towards condom use, including reduction in spontaneity of behaviour and reduced sexual pleasure. It has been found those men's perceptions of comfort while using a condom were a predictor of actual behaviour. The males who perceived condoms as being uncomfortable were less likely to use them for the duration of intercourse (Hensel *et al.*, 2011). Surveys of young women suggest that they also hold these negative attitudes. They also tend to hold unrealistic perceptions of contracting a STI which is seen to differ between men and women especially when considering temporary partners (Leval *et al.*, 2011).

Applying this to Gary and Debbie

Youngsters such as Gary and Debbie tend to underestimate their personal risk of sexually transmitted infections.

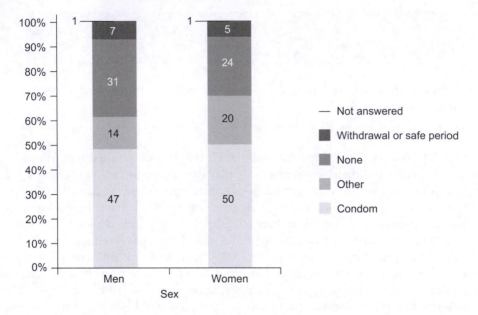

Figure 9.2 Forms of contraception used by both men and women

Source: From Wellings *et al.*, 1994

There are also a number of other negative attitudes held by women that can potentially hinder condom use, including:

*   Anticipated male objection to a female suggesting condom use (denial of their pleasure);
*   Difficulty/embarrassment in raising the issue of condom use with a male partner;
*   Worry that suggesting use to a potential partner implies that either they or their partner is HIV + or has another STI;
*   Lack of self-efficacy or mastery in condom use.

As we will see subsequently, these negative attitudes or misconceptions have to be addressed by the healthcare practitioner in order to promote condom use.

Applying this to Gary and Debbie

Gary holds a view that wearing a condom reduces his sensation. Debbie has not been able to discuss the use of condoms with Gary and has taken the simple route of 'going on the pill'.

Box 9.1 Applying research in practice

Associations between sexually experienced adolescents' sources of information about sex and sexual risk outcomes (Secor-Turner *et al.*, 2011)

This study examined prevalent informal sources of information about sex and examined associations between informal sources of information about sex and sexual risk outcomes among sexually experienced adolescents. The sample included 22,828 sexually experienced adolescents aged between 13 and 20 years.

Findings revealed that peers and siblings were the most commonly reported informal, proximal source of information about sex. It was also reported that parents or parents plus peers and siblings as a source of information lead to significantly lower odds of having multiple sex partners in the past year. Furthermore informal sources of information about sex had significantly lower odds of lifetime pregnancy involvement.

It was concluded that information about sex from adolescents' everyday lives has the potential to diminish the likelihood of involvement in sexual risk behaviours. Therefore formal sex education programmes should engage informal sources of information about sex to adolescents as having these informal, familiar sources of information about sex appears to serve as a protective factor against sexual risk outcomes, especially among younger adolescents.

Consequences of unsafe sex

Sex is, for the main part, a pleasurable activity and one that has to be promoted for the sake of humanity. Sexual pleasure is both physical and psychological in nature and can result from a range of erotic interactions. However, it also comes with potential to do harm – sexually transmitted diseases. Unprotected sex and having multiple sexual partners can lead to unwanted pregnancies and STDs, including human immuno-deficiency virus (HIV). At the end of 2011 there were approximately 34 million people living with HIV worldwide (UNAIDS, 2012). In the UK in the same year, an estimated 96,000 people were living with HIV, a quarter of whom were, worryingly, unaware of their infection (HPA, 2012b). However, STIs are not simply confined to HIV and AIDS; there are a host of other diseases that can result from unsafe sex (see Table 9.1). One common STI which can be contracted as a result of unprotected sex is chlamydia. Over 2 million chlamydia tests were conducted on individuals aged 15 to 24 in 2011; this resulted in over 140,000 new diagnoses being made (HPA, 2012a). Chlamydia and gonorrhoea are the two most common STIs and both are the key cause of preventable infertility amongst women, and along with other STIs make the acquisition and transmission of HIV more likely (Ward and Rönn, 2010) although there is some debate as to whether this is causal.

Table 9.1 Symptoms of sexually transmitted diseases

STI	Comment
Chlamydia trachomatis	Can be transmitted in vaginal or seminal fluids. Although chlamydia is most often asymptomatic, untreated infections can progress to pelvic inflammatory disease, and approximately 40% of women later have decreased fertility
Gonorrhoea	Transmitted via seminal and vaginal fluids and easily transmitted through sexual activity. Gonococcal urethritis causes painful urination and discharge, although approximately 25% of men have no symptoms. Among women, gonorrhoea can cause cervicitis, with vaginal discharge, pain with intercourse, or painful urination; however, approximately half of infected women are asymptomatic
Nongo-nococcal urethritis (NGU)	NGU is the most common clinical sexually transmitted syndrome among men and is characterised by painful urination with or without discharge
Syphilis	Clinical manifestations of syphilis are varied, and its natural history is complex. It can be transmitted through sexual intercourse or direct contact with syphilitic sores or rash
Herpes	Genital herpes is the most common ulcerative STI in the UK, with diagnosis rates showing an increasing trend (HPA, 2011). There is no cure, and as with other STIs transmission of herpes simplex virus (HSV) can occur with unprotected sex or direct contact with genital ulcers. There is an especially high risk of transmission when those infected have an active genital sore or an active oral cold sore
Hepatitis B virus (HBV)	Can be passed via seminal and vaginal fluids and is approximately 100 times more transmissible than HIV. About a fifth of all new HBV infections occur among men having sex with men (MSM) and people are often unaware of their status. Vaccination is the most effective strategy against HBV (HPA, 2009)
Hepatitis C virus	The virus can be transmitted through seminal and vaginal fluids; however, the risk of sexual transmission is low. It is likely that if condoms are used consistently then sexual transmission of hepatitis C will be avoided
Human papilloma-virus (HPV)	In total, 40 types of HPV can infect the genital tract. HPV-16 or -18 causes over 70% of cervical cancers worldwide, whereas HPV-6 or -11 causes over 90% of genital warts. HPV infection is extremely common. At least 50% of sexually active men and women acquire genital HPV infection at some point in their lives and may develop warts. The disease can be transmitted through unprotected sex or direct contact with genital warts

STI	Comment
Human immuno-deficiency virus (HIV)	An uninfected individual is most at risk of acquiring HIV from receptive anal or vaginal sex. Infection is initially asymptomatic. Signs of primary HIV include: fever, swollen glands, sore throat, rash on the body or face, painful muscles or joints, headache, feeling sick and vomiting, ulcers on the mouth, genitals and oesophagus. After the early symptoms, HIV may remain undetected for a number of years until the body's ability to fight infections is reduced. This leaves the body vulnerable to infections. If a person develops certain life-threatening illnesses it is known as AIDS.

In the UK, the number of reported cases of STIs has risen considerably, particularly amongst young people (see Table 9.2). For instance, between 1995 and 2003, diagnoses of new episodes of gonorrhoea and chlamydia increased by 197 per cent and 409 per cent respectively among men aged 16–19 years (HPA, 2008). From Table 9.3 (adapted from HPA, 2011) the increases are truly massive – a 135 per cent increase in chlamydia, for example. Given the increase in STIs and unwanted pregnancies in adolescence, it is hard to disagree with the contention that the sexual health of England and Wales is in crisis and the worst in Europe (Evans and Tripp, 2006) The UK has the highest rates of teenage pregnancy in Western Europe (WHO, 2011) and Scotland have recently introduced a new sexual health and blood borne virus policy to tackle the level of STIs in the country, drawing parallels with other policy areas such as drugs and alcohol misuse (The Scottish Government, 2011). Obviously, from this perspective, sexual behaviour moves from the pleasurable to the irresponsible and dangerous. However, not surprisingly, most people who engage in sexual activity are thinking of pleasure rather than any concerns over sexually transmitted diseases (Philpott et al., 2006). Thus, the healthcare professional has to deal with a tricky dilemma – the promotion of safe sex without denying the pursuit of pleasure. Indeed, some have argued that denying the possibility of pleasure in sexual relations has a negative impact on their active negotiation of safer sex especially within adolescents (Brown et al., 2008).

Table 9.2 Rates per 100,000 of population of STI diagnoses by country (2011)

	Gonorrhoea	Syphilis	Chlamydia	Genital warts	Genital herpes
England	30.8	4.8	359.4	141.7	55.6
Wales	16	1.1	126	125	22
Northern Ireland	11	1.7	115	125	22
Scotland	17	3.7	170	135	27
UK	32	4.6	189	139	36

Table 9.3 New STI diagnoses at GUM (genitourinary medicine) clinics
in England: 2002–2011

Year	Syphilis	Gonorrhoea	Chlamydia	Herpes	Genital warts	All new diagnoses
2002	1,560	24,123	79,271	17,259	62,982	285,870
2003	2,005	23,346	86,595	16,903	64,319	305,297
2004	2,626	20,669	94,216	16,694	67,251	319,602
2005	3,186	17,632	97,291	17,379	67,852	322,110
2006	3,116	17,191	100,377	19,254	69,700	327,263
2007	3,207	17,119	108,507	23,487	75,272	347,341
2008	2,874	14,985	176,941	26,094	78,156	415,837
2009	2,851	16,144	189,356	27,536	77,845	426,735
2010	2,650	16,835	189,314	29,794	75,451	419,773
2011	2,915	20,965	186,196	31,154	76,071	426,867
% change	87%	-13%	135%	81%	21%	49%

Source: Adapted from HPA, 2011

Applying this to Gary and Debbie

Gary and Debbie are both exposing themselves to a number of possible sexually transmitted diseases. As Gary is already experiencing pain 'down below' he could have contracted gonorrhoea.

Why do people have safe/unsafe sex?

To combat the spread of STDs the government's message is to use a condom. Research evidence has supported the contention that consistent condom use is associated with reduced risk of STDs (e.g. Gallo et al., 2007) and use of condoms during each risky sexual encounter is the only efficient way to prevent the spread of most STDs (Carey et al., 1992). In one US study some 82 per cent of individuals attending a follow-up study conducted in a STD clinic reported using a condom at least once in the last year. However, 94 per cent of individuals reported that they had participated in sex and not used a condom. In addition, it is also concluded that only 5 per cent of this high risk population reported using condoms consistently over the year of the study (Peterman et al., 2009). Not only does the condom have to be used, but it has to be used effectively (i.e. properly). Hatherall et al. (2007) report that a sizeable minority (between 12 per cent and 40 per cent) applied a condom imperfectly. Given that imperfect use of condoms fails to maximise their effectiveness as a method of STI prevention, it is obviously important to address this through appropriate public health messages.

So, why do couples not use a condom? And if they do, why don't they use them correctly? Why is it that, despite the risks, individuals still take the risk and have unsafe sex? There are, of course, a number of possible reasons why this might be, and many of these are psychological in nature.

There may be some external factors to consider as well. For example, young people's sexual encounters are often unplanned, sporadic and sometimes the result of social pressure, coercion or alcohol. It is estimated that 11 per cent of teenagers regret a sexual encounter that they had while being under the influence of alcohol (Hibell et al., 2007). One American study amongst close to 1,000 college students found that around 25 per cent had encountered one or more alcohol-related regretted sex occurrences in the past month; a very short space of time (Orchowski et al., 2012). Early sexual activity is strongly associated with alcohol use and both may be in relation to poor wellbeing at school (Philips-Howard et al., 2010). It is possible that the two decisions (young age of first sex and non-use of condom) are related and it may be that younger teens are less able to negotiate condom use or that younger age at first sex is a marker for other underlying risk-taking propensities. However, it is clear that alcohol plays a significant role in sexual behaviour for adolescents. For example, in one study (Phillips-Howard et al., 2010) reported that alcohol increased the chances of children (11–14 year olds) partaking in sexual activity and intercourse. The chances of individuals experiencing some sort of sexual behaviour increased by up to twelvefold when the individual drank alcohol at least once a week, therefore inferring that alcohol had contributed to them doing 'more' sexually than they would when sober.

Buhi and Goodson (2007) reviewed the predictors of risky sexual behaviour in adolescents and classified these factors under common themes (see Table 9.4).

There are a number of psychological variables that may be important when discussing sexual behaviour. Potentially one of the most important of these is self-efficacy. Studies (e.g. Buhi and Goodson, 2007) have indicated a protective effect of self-efficacy. For example, intention was found to be a predictive factor towards adolescents' sexual behaviour, alongside perceived norms and time spent at home while being alone (Buhi and Goodson, 2007).

A different approach was adopted by Reissing et al. (2012) who reported the experiences of an individual's first sexual experience in relation to future sexual attitudes. It is suggested that an individual's first sexual experience can influence psychological factors in several ways. For example, it was concluded that women who were older at the time of their first sexual experience had less sexual self-efficacy. This again highlights the importance of psychology and attitudes in relation to sexual behaviour.

Table 9.4 Summary of predictors of sexual behaviour

Theme	Element
Intention to have sex	• Initiation of sexual behaviour (+);
Environmental constraints	• Greater parental involvement (+/0); • High quality of relationship with parents (+/0); • Fewer rules/boundaries (–/0); • Increased parental support (+/0/–); • Greater parental monitoring/supervision (+/0); • Increased peer support (0); • Increased time home alone (without a parent) (–);
Norms	• Perceptions of peer sex behaviours (believing most peers have had sex) (–/0); • Perception of peer disapproval of sex or negative attitudes towards sex (+/0); • Perceived parental disapproval of engaging in sexual intercourse (+); • Self-efficacy (+/0); • Pro abstinence self-standards (+); • Negative emotions regarding sex/positive emotions towards sexual abstinence (+/0); • Positive attitudes toward abstinence/fewer sexually permissive attitudes (+/0);

Note: (–) indicates that this element is a risk factor, (+) indicates a protective factor, (0) indicates a non-statistically significant finding.

Source: Buhi and Goodson, 2007

Applying this to Gary

Gary is not as likely to practise safe sex as he reports of sensation loss when using a condom.

In relation to the impact of psychological variables on safe sex, it is thought that moral norms impact upon condom use and safe sex practices (Sarkar, 2008). This variable represents a measure of personal feelings of moral obligation or responsibility for adopting a given behaviour. This is perceived as a variable of growing importance in the health-related domain and has implications for the development of appropriate interventions and media campaigns.

Other reasons why unprotected sex may occur is that there may be other goals besides health. For example, sharing intimacy, experiencing belongingness and increasing one's own self-esteem are some of the goals which may override thoughts of health in an immediate situation (e.g. Gebhardt *et al.*, 2006). These psychological functions served by sexual behaviour may impact on safe sex behaviour. For example, heterosexual men's accounts of sexual pleasure while using a condom can be found to correlate with negative perceptions of psychological factors such as perceived penis size (Hensel *et al.*, 2012). Investigations into condom use and sexual pleasure concluded that sexual pleasure and age were correlated, the older age the male is, the higher the sexual pleasure that is experienced whilst using a condom (Hensel *et al.*, 2012). In particular men who believe condoms reduce sexual pleasure are less likely to engage in safe sex and use condoms (Randolph *et al.*, 2007)

Finally, psychological research on the determinants of unsafe sexual practice has usually employed the social cognition models outlined in Chapter 3, including theories such as the Health Belief Model (Rosenstock, 1990), the Protection Motivation Theory (Rogers, 1975), the Theory of Reasoned Action (Fishbein and Ajzen, 1975) and the Theory of Planned Behaviour (Ajzen, 1985). Within this type of conceptualisation, it is assumed that individuals are motivated to use a condom if the benefits of doing so outweigh the costs, and that they are able to perform the behaviour.

All of these factors have to be used by the healthcare professional when attempting to devise intervention strategies.

Applying this to Gary

Environmental factors should be considered when designing an intervention to assist Gary and Debbie due to Gary's 'flings' with women in pubs and nightclubs.

Interventions to promote safer sex

Individual level interventions

Shrier *et al.* (2001) explored whether an individual intervention based on various psychological models, including the Stages of Change (SoC) (Prochaska and DiClemente, 2002), and implemented through motivational interviewing (Miller and Rollnick, 2002) could improve condom use. The intervention they suggested began with a seven-minute video in which popular entertainers and sports figures discussed and dramatised condom names, buying condoms and negotiating condom use, and two female adolescents demonstrated condom use to their peers. Condom use was portrayed as normative behaviour.

In addition to this, a series of female health educators were employed and trained in various theories and were taught to use a standardised intervention manual that outlined key points to cover, activities to perform and the motivation strategies to employ. At the outset, participants were asked about how much they needed and wanted to change their sexual risk behaviour (on a so-called 'wheel of change'). The intervention ensured that the same information was provided to all participants but the educator tried to individualise the session based on the stage of change. On the basis of this intervention, there was an improvement in condom use in that more of the participants used condoms during sex than previously. However, this is one specific example and there are many others which are based on the Stages of Change model.

Support for the use of the SoC model has also been seen from a recent meta-analysis (Noar *et al.*, 2009) which considered 12 randomised control trials of computer based HIV prevention interventions. Interventions that adopted the SoC model were found to be more effective. This is thought to be due to the tailoring of the intervention to the individual and using a personalized approach.

Applying this to Gary and Debbie

Healthcare professionals could work with Gary and Debbie to encourage Gary to use a condom. The Stages of Change model could be considered as a starting point as this will allow the health professional to tailor the intervention specifically to Gary and Debbie. They will be able to identify the stage of change that they are currently at and gradually move them forward through activities and strategies such as motivational interviewing. This will allow both Gary and Debbie to explore the underlying reasons of Gary's negative views of condoms and endeavour to change his condom use behaviour in the long term.

There are other psychological models that can contribute to the promotion of safer sex and can be incorporated into any intervention based on the SoC model. One example would be from the Theory of Planned Behaviour (Fishbein and Ajzen, 1975), which suggests that subjective norms, including peer norms, are important factors related to stage of change. For example, adolescents who perceive a greater support for safer sex are more likely to improve and maintain their own sexual behaviour (e.g. Sieving *et al.*, 2006).

The Stages of Change model has been described extensively elsewhere in this book, for example how it can be applied to smoking cessation in Chapter 8. However, it serves as a useful model for developing and implementing intervention strategies for a range of lifestyle behaviours and safe sex is one of them. The Stages of Change model (Prochaska and DiClemente, 1983) has been used as a foundation for intervention design and its benefit is that it allows an intervention to be tailored to an individual's needs and their specific stage. A further strength of the model is that the individual's current stage can be used as an indicator of success. If we look at the Stages of Change model when applied to condom use we can explore how we can place individuals within each of the stages (see Figure 9.3).

In this model, women who reported using condoms consistently (i.e. every time they had sex) for at least six months with their main partners were in 'maintenance', those using condoms consistently but for less than six months were in 'action', those who intended to use condoms consistently in the next month were in 'preparation', those who intended to use condoms consistently sometime within the next six months were in 'contemplation', and those who did not intend to use condoms consistently were in 'pre-contemplation'.

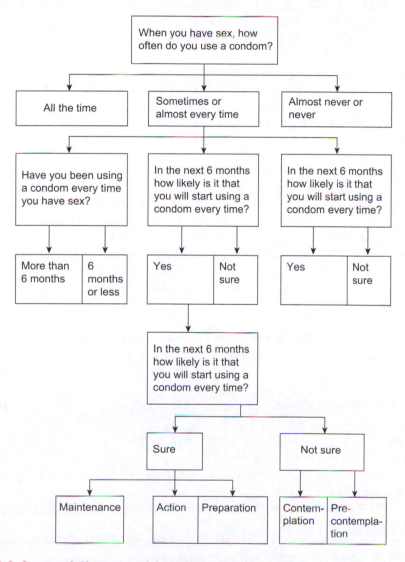

Figure 9.3 Stages of Change model applied to condom use

Source: Adapted from Gielen *et al.*, 2001

Gary is in the pre-contemplation stage of change when considering condom use.

This is one simple way of classifying individuals into stage of change and basing interventions on this assessment. However, there are other, more sophisticated models. Level of motivation to practise safer sex can be reported in a number of ways. For example, asking individuals a set of questions allows them to be categorised into each of the stages (see Table 9.5).

Alternatively (in a less formal manner), the healthcare professional could simply ask the individual what their sexual behaviour was and whether they intended to change it.

According to the SoC model, there are two important factors for predicting movement towards adoption of safer behaviour: self-efficacy and decisional balance. An individual's self-efficacy for performing the behaviour has been shown to have a linear relationship with more movement to safer behaviour. As individuals progress towards maintenance of positive health behaviour, their confidence in their ability to carry out the behaviour increases (see Chapter 4 for fuller discussion on self-efficacy). Decisional balance is simply weighting the perceived pros and cons of behaviour change and how these cognitions about health behaviour relate to stage of change. Typically, people in the pre-contemplation stage identify more cons associated with the behaviour, whereas those in the action or maintenance stages perceive greater pros of engaging in the behaviour. Some of the pros and cons of condom use most frequently reported are presented in Table 9.6.

Table 9.5 Allocating individuals to stage of change

Question	Stage of change
Are you basically satisfied with your sexual behaviours and don't want to change them?	Pre-contemplators
Are you thinking about making changes to your sexual behaviour soon (i.e. in the next month)?	Contemplators
Are you going to make changes to your sexual behaviour in the next month?	Preparation
Have you made changes to your sexual behaviour in the past six months?	Action
Have you made changes to your sexual behaviour in the past six months and not returned to the previous pattern?	Maintenance

Applying this to Gary and Debbie

Presented in Table 9.6 are the pros and cons of condom use. Another way of looking at this is the pros and cons of unprotected sex. In relation to Gary, a con of Gary having unprotected sex is the possibility that he may have contracted an STI. A pro of this behaviour (according to Gary) is that sensation during sexual activity is increased.

Studies have indicated that, not surprisingly, the pros and cons of condom use are consistently the best predictor of progression to and maintenance of consistent condom use. Hence, the message for the healthcare professional is clear: deal with the pros and cons of condom use at the outset. One of the major tasks may be dealing with the negative aspects of condom wear and correcting misconceptions.

Community level interventions

Within the UK, the Department of Health suggested that there were a number of actions that needed to be put in place. The first of these was to develop a national campaign aimed at younger men and women to ensure that they understand the real risk of unprotected sex and persuade them of the benefits of using condoms to avoid the risk of STIs or unplanned pregnancies (see, for example, www.nhs.uk/Livewell). Furthermore, there was a longer-term strategy to ensure that children and young people were on the right path towards improving their sexual health by reducing teenage pregnancy and consumption of alcohol and illicit drugs. Developments of new resources for the health service (e.g. confidential email service, websites such as www. teenagehealthfreak.org and www.nhs.uk/Livewell/Sexandyoungpeople/Pages/Sex-and-young-people-hub.aspx) are all part of this approach.

Table 9.6 Pros and cons of condom use

Pros	Cons
Protects from STIs	Sensation reduced
Prevents unwanted pregnancy	Interrupts the moment
Reduces mess	Added expense/inconvenience to obtain
Increases female pleasure	Embarrassment when communicating with partner
Lengthens time for intercourse	

Such interventional programmes aimed at promoting condom use have used a range of strategies and media, including, amongst others, lectures, leaflets, interactive games and websites, films, role-modelling and posters. Public health campaigns have employed poster campaigns, TV, newspaper and cinema advertising, interactive computer and web programs and health promotion leaflets (for example, www.nhs.uk/Livewell/Sexandyoungpeople/Pages/Sex-and-young-people-hub.aspx and www.wheredidyouwearit.com).

The theoretically derived interventions have concentrated on the social cognition models approach to safer sexual behaviour. These models have suggested that knowledge about STDs and beliefs about infection, risk and symptom severity are weaker predictors of condom use than action-specific cognitions, such as attitudes towards condom use, perceived self-efficacy in relation to condom use, the social acceptability of condom use and condom use intentions. The Theory of Planned Behaviour (TPB) has been widely used as a basis for both understanding condom use behaviour in addition to being utilised as a basis for developing interventions. In addition, it has been shown to be a useful model for varying sub-samples of the population including drug addicts in relation to safe sex practices (Mausbach *et al.*, 2009).

Recent research by Abraham *et al.* (2011) investigated the predictive ability of the TPB on condom use while accounting for social structure. It was recognised that accounting for social structure whilst using this theory enabled the theory to be a more reliable predictor of condom use behaviour. The study identified key messages and recommendations in relation to the application of cognitive theory and condom use. Some of these are:

- Cognition models do not successfully account for social structure such as socio-economic status (SES) on behaviour.
- Mother's SES status accounted for 5 per cent of the variance.
- Condom use was correlated with condom use cognitions.
- Individuals from areas with greater levels of deprivation reported using a condom less frequently.
- Positive attitudes towards condom use were associated with greater educational aspirations, lower parental aspirations and being female.
- College aspirations explained 4 per cent of the variance in consistent condom use, thus highlighting the importance of social structure in predicting behaviour.

Overall it was suggested that more research should be conducted into the effects of the social structure including SES, aspirations, gender and deprivation alongside cognitions when considering teenagers' behaviours in relation to condoms. In addition, the research highlighted the potential underlying factors that influence condom related behaviour in this sample of teenagers. It can be suggested that by considering social structural factors health behaviour in relation to condoms could be better understood. Other such research has demonstrated similar conclusions with acknowledging the need for the TPB to be used in conjunction with other variables in a better attempt to predict condom use (Turchik and Gidycz, 2012).

Investigations into the effectiveness of leaflet based interventions derived from the TPB highlight interesting findings and implications for the use of this model in health promotion relating to condom use. Krahé *et al.* (2005) considered an experimental condition into the effectiveness of a leaflet promotion aimed to impact upon safe sex practices. The leaflet was developed based on research into cognitive correlates in relation to condom use (Sheeran *et al.*, 1999). However, mixed results into the effectiveness of the leaflet alone were seen. In the experimental conditions tested by this research, it was considered that the leaflet alone provided similar results to the no leaflet condition. The research highlighted the importance of motivation with regards to getting the individual to spend time and read the leaflet. Thus, the experimental group that were given an intrinsic reward for reading and processing the leaflet produced lasting effects on the behaviour at one month follow-up. Consequently, it is important to note that the specifically tailored interventions for individuals have to attempt to overcome this deficit and develop appropriate materials.

Research has shown that abstinence programs can be successful in preventing adolescent sexual involvement (Jemmott III *et al.*, 2010). There is a growth of such a movement within the US (e.g. The Silver Ring Thing: http://www.silverringthing.com/) but similar trends have not been seen in the UK. It may be because health educators fear that their audience will be unwilling to contemplate delaying sexual intercourse. The other problem with this approach, as discussed above, is: what is abstinence? Does it mean only 'not having sexual intercourse'? Or does it mean not kissing or touching as well? Furthermore, all adolescents experience some form of sexual desire. As Berer (2006) suggests, 'The prescription of abstinence is a potential death sentence for anyone who wants to have sex if the means to make it safe, at whatever age, are withheld' (p. 7).

A potential strategy to attempt to change individual behaviour in relation to condom use is to attempt to reinterpret the use of condoms; for example, moving from the condom as 'safety wear' to condoms as 'pleasure promoters' or eroticising the condom. One project, the Pleasure Project (Philpott *et al.*, 2006), aims to promote condoms as sexy and pleasurable and lists a number of 'quick and dirty ways' to illustrate the benefits of condoms. So, for example, opening a male condom packet can be a sign that a person is ready for sex. Carrying condoms in a pocket or handbag when going out, and showing them to a potential partner, can illustrate how interested the person is in sex, while also encouraging condom use (Philpott *et al.*, 2006, p. 25). A Turkish condom company saw a considerable boost in sales through the use of social networking sites by reinventing the condom, using slogans like 'safe and fun sex is your right', and aimed to market condoms as playful and fun through colourful packaging and a range of flavours, shapes and textures (Purdy, 2011). For example, Table 9.7 outlines the previously highlighted negatives associated with condom wear and suggests how these can be corrected or addressed.

A second key element derived from the studies exploring the SoC is that interventions need to be tailored to the stage of change. The model suggests that different processes in behaviour change, such as raising consciousness and self-reinforcement, are necessary at different stages. Thus, interventions focusing on cognitive and emotional factors will be the most influential in early stages, whereas action-orientated approaches are effective in later stages.

Table 9.7 Misconceptions around condom wear

Cons	How
Sensation reduced	Add additional lube which can enhance the experience for both partners
Interrupts the moment	Can add to the moment, as it can signify to the partner that they are ready for sex
Added expense/inconvenience to obtain	Can be obtained free from a number of sources
Embarrassment when communicating with partner	Should be able to embrace the moment and actually can add to the pleasure for both parties

For example, for inconsistent condom users, interventions should first target increasing the advantages of using condoms (e.g. lengthen duration of sexual intercourse, decrease messiness, increase female pleasure) and then promote and model skills for communication with partners about condoms. Maintaining consistent condom use is a challenge and interventions will need to focus on novel ways to sustain interest in the effectiveness and positive aspects of condoms. For individuals who use condoms consistently, interventions might adhere to relapse prevention models whereby the goals are to preserve the positive attitude towards condoms, maintain consistent communication with partners about condoms and reinforce perceptions of vulnerability to STIs.

There is a difference between some of the other behaviours discussed in this book and safer sex: for example, with smoking, diet and exercise, behaviour change is largely an individual choice. The adoption of condom use, however, is a behaviour that often demands communication and agreement between partners. It may necessitate an assessment of one's own risk, and also the risk of one's partner(s). Therefore, communication with partners about condom use and perceived personal vulnerability to STIs and HIV must be taken into account. Furthermore, we must return to our original point: sex is a pleasurable activity and this has to be encouraged with partners and individuals. The fear message will not work.

Applying this to Gary

It is important for Gary and Debbie to talk about using condoms within their relationship, reconcile their differences regarding the use of them and in turn for them to use contraception that they are both 100 per cent happy with.

Working effectively with others

Given that attempting to provide safer sex education can be problematic, it is essential that some broad-based messages are promoted and these are provided in Table 9.8. As can be noted, the emphasis is on pleasure rather than fear. It is about promoting the activity in a safe way rather than attempting to scare people into changing.

Table 9.8 Tips for sexual health educators

Tip	Comment
Have a realistic attitude	Appreciate that different sexual practices and attitudes are evident
Get advice from the target audience	Pleasure and sexiness are often culturally specific, so tailor the message appropriately
Remain comfortable about talking about sex and pleasure	Trainers and health educators need to be able to talk about sex and pleasure seeking in appropriate language
Focus on pleasure and sex rather than disease	It is important to strike a balance between promoting pleasure and promoting health
Promote positive messages rather than messages of fear or shame	If people are fearful or shamed then they are less likely to request assistance
Focus on the individual issues	Ensure that any counselling/intervention is tailored to deal with the individual concerns and not a predetermined agenda
Be realistic in an assessment of risk	Ensure the individual client assesses their own risks and acceptable measures of risk reduction
Support positive changes	Small steps are positive, and moving from one stage to another can be seen as positive
Clarify misconceptions	Clarify rather than deal with general discussions
Use appropriate language	Ensure that over-technical language is avoided and that the individual feels comfortable when discussing sex

School nurses and sexual education

School nurses provide students with a wide variety of services during school hours, one of which is free confidential advice on sexual health and contraception. The use of school nurses to provide this service enables the young population to gain accurate advice and information relating to sexual health. Although the use of school nurses could potentially positively impact on teenagers' sexual health, it is suggested that such staff are not used to their full advantage when considering sexual health (Westwood and Mullan, 2009).

Research into the experiences of sex education by children in schools has provided some insightful findings. Children were found to want the most advice on STIs and wide variation between preferred delivery method was seen throughout the sample (Newby *et al.*, 2012). This provides challenges for schools when trying to make messages in the sex education sessions effective for all especially when society is becoming increasingly diverse. Therefore better thought-out recourses should be put in place; this will not only address the worries regarding the transmission of STIs but also intend to impact upon the teenage pregnancy concerns. Working together with the school nurse, schools could potentially develop a more successful sex education programme.

Sexual health and family planning clinics

Sexual health clinics or genitourinary medicine (GUM) clinics provide a vast range of services available to the general population. The services available include treatment for STIs, contraception advice, sexual health advice, free condoms and counselling services for individuals who have suffered sexual attacks or been diagnosed with an STI. Trained health professionals from a variety of backgrounds such as doctors, nurses and counsellors are all available to offer free, confidential advice which is offered in a non-judgmental way. The non-judgmental attitude of staff is a crucial element of the service and younger people especially consider the attitudes of the staff to be important in reducing barriers to sexual health advice (Baxter *et al.*, 2011).

In addition, research has identified that using psychological behaviour change techniques within this setting and family planning clinics can have positive effects on emergency contraception consultation rates (Martin *et al.*, 2011). It is suggested that by using techniques which specifically outline behaviours such as the 'if-then' technique, implications can be seen in relation to effective contraception behaviour. Again in turn this technique could be applicable in aiming to reduce STIs and unwanted pregnancy rates.

Applying this to Gary

Gary and Debbie could both visit their local sexual health clinic to get tested for STIs. In addition, they could also get some advice on safe sex and using condoms correctly so they don't 'reduce sensation' for Gary.

Conclusion

Sexual behaviour is a natural behaviour that has, at its root, a fundamental physiological purpose. However, it serves a range of other cultural, emotional, psychological and social purposes which have to be considered when attempting to promote safe sexual behaviour. The promotion of a safe sex message is important given the rise in sexually transmitted diseases both nationally and worldwide. Psychological factors contribute to whether people engage in safe sex or not, and social cognitive models have proved successful in predicting condom use. There are a number of key elements from the Stages of Change model that can be used in promoting safe sex.

Key points

- Researchers generally define sexual behaviour as any behaviour that involves a sexual response of the body; however, individuals (particularly adolescents) will define it differently.
- Safe sex is hard to define but involves taking steps to reduce the chance of contracting or transmitting STIs. Most people associate this with condom use and/ or monogamy.
- The UK has seen the largest rise in the number of HIV cases since 2000 and cases of other STIs, such as chlamydia and herpes, are also increasing.
- Evidence suggests that consistent and correct condom use is associated with reduced STI transmission. Despite this, many people in the UK are not consistently practising safe sex.
- Alcohol is associated with risky sexual behaviours.
- Social cognition models have been shown to predict some safe sex practices.
- Self-efficacy is a key variable in promoting safe sex.
- Interventions to reduce unsafe sex include providing sex education in schools and mass media campaigns.
- Interventions have been shown to be more effective when they are targeted to specific audiences and are based on psychological theory.
- Individuals can be classified according to their stage of change and this information used to promote condom use.
- Misconceptions about condom use must be addressed and these can be redefined positively.
- Sexual behaviour change is more effective if promoted within a positive pleasure framework.

Points for discussion

- Consider how attitudes towards condom use have changed through the decades and discuss the potential reasons underlying the attitude change. In doing so identify any sub-groups in the population where attitudes are less positive.

- Critically evaluate psychological theory in relation to the promotion of safe sex.
- Consider Gary and Debbie:
  - What sort of problems are Debbie and Gary potentially facing?
- Develop an action plan for Gary (and discuss how to involve Debbie).

Further resources

Condom essential wear http://www.condomessentialwear.co.uk/
Teenage Health Freak www.teenagehealthfreak.org
NHS – sexual health www.nhs.uk/Livewell
Brook – Free and confidential information for under 25s – Ask Brook 0808 802 1234
or http://www.brook.org.uk/

References

Abraham, C., Sheeran, P. and Henderson, M. (2011). Extending social cognition models of health behaviour. *Health Education Research*, 26(4): 624–637.

Ajzen, I. (1985). From intention to actions: a theory of planned behaviour. In J. Kuhl and J. Beckman (eds) *Action-Control: From Cognition to Behaviour*. Available at: http://www.people.umass.edu/aizen/publications.html (accessed 20 December 2007).

Baxter, S., Blank, L., Guillaume, L., Squires, H. and Payne, N. (2011). Views of contraceptive service delivery to young people in the UK: a systematic review and thematic synthesis. *Journal of Family Planning & Reproductive Health Care*, 37(2): 71–84.

Berer, M. (2006). Editorial: Condoms, yes! Abstinence, no. *Reproductive Health Matters*, 14(28): 6–16.

Bersamin, M., Fisher, D., Walker, S., Hill, D. and Grube, J. (2007). Defining virginity and abstinence: adolescents' interpretations of sexual behaviors. *Journal of Adolescent Health*, 41(2): 182–188.

Brown, L., DiClemente, R., Crosby, R., Fernandez, M., Pugatch, D., Cohn, S. and Schlenger, W. *et al.* (2008). Condom use among high-risk adolescents: anticipation of partner disapproval and less pleasure associated with not using condoms. *Public Health Reports*, 123(5): 601–607.

Bourne, A. H. and Robson, M. A. (2009). Perceiving risk and (re)constructing safety: the lived experience of having 'safe' sex. *Health, Risk & Society*, 11(3): 283–295.

Buhi, E.R. and Goodson, P. (2007). Predictors of adolescent and sexual behaviour and intention: a theory-guided systematic review. *Journal of Adolescent Health*, 40(1): 4–21.

Byers, E., Henderson, J. and Hobson, K. M. (2009). University students' definitions of sexual abstinence and having sex. *Archives of Sexual Behaviour*, 38(5): 665–674.

Carey, R.F., Herman, W.A., Retta, S.M., Rinaldi, J.E.R., German, B.A. and Athey, T.W. (1992). Effectiveness of latex condoms as a barrier to human immunodeficiency virus-sized particles under conditions of simulated use. *Sexually Transmitted Disease*, 19: 230–234.

Chambers, W.C. (2007). Oral sex: varied behaviours and perceptions in a college population. *Journal of Sex Research*, 44(1): 28–42.

D'Souza, G., Agrawal, Y., Halpern, J., Bodison, S. and Gillison, M. (2009). Oral sexual behaviors associated with prevalent oral human papillomavirus infection. *Journal of Infectious Diseases*, 199(9): 1263–1269. .

Evans, D.L. and Tripp, J.H. (2006). Sex education: the case for primary prevention and peer education. *Current Paediatrics*, 16: 95–99.

Fishbein, M. and Ajzen, I. (1975). *Belief, Attitude, Intention and Behaviour: An Introduction to Theory and Research*. London: Addison-Wesley.

Gallo, M.F., Steiner, M.J., Warner, L., Hylton-Kong, T., Figueroa, J.P., Hobbs, M.M. and Behets, F.M. (2007). Self-reported condom use is associated with reduced risk of chlamydia, gonorrhoea, and trichomoniasis. *Sexually Transmitted Diseases*, 34(10): 829–833.

Gebhardt, W.A., Kuyper, L. and Dusseldorp, E. (2006). Condom use at first intercourse with a new partner in female adolescents and young adults: the role of cognitive planning and motives for having sex. *Archives of Sexual Behaviour*, 35(2): 217–223.

Gielen, A.C., Fogarty, L.A., Armstrong, K., Green, B.M., Cabral, R., Milstein, B., Galavotti, C. and Heilig, C.M. (2001). Promoting condom use with main partners: a behavioural intervention trail for women. *AIDS and Behaviour*, 5: 193–204.

Hans, J. D. and Kimberly, C. (2011). Abstinence, sex, and virginity: do they mean what we think they mean? *American Journal of Sexuality Education*, 6(4): 329–342.

Hans, J. D., Gillen, M. and Akande, K. (2010). Sex redefined: the reclassification of oral-genital contact. *Perspectives on Sexual and Reproductive Health*, 42(2): 74–78.

Hatherall, B., Ingham, R., Stone, N. and McEachran, J. (2007). How, not just if, condoms are used: the timing of condom application and removal during vaginal sex among young people in England. *Sexually Transmitted Infections*, 83: 68–70.

Hensel, D.J., Stupiansky, N.W., Herbenick, D., Dodge, B. and Reece, M. (2011). When condom use is not condom use: an event-level analysis of condom use behaviors during vaginal intercourse. *Journal of Sexual Medicine*, 8(1): 28–34. DOI: 10.1111/j.1743-6109.2010.02031.x.

——(2012). Sexual pleasure during condom-protected vaginal sex among heterosexual men. *Journal of Sexual Medicine*, 9(5): 1272–1276. DOI: 10.1111/j.1743-6109.2012.02700.x.

Hibell, B., Balakireva, O., Bjarnason , T., Kokkevi, A. and Kraus, L. (2007) *European School Survey Project on Alcohol and Other Drugs (ESPAD)*. CAN, Sweden.

Health Protection Agency. (HPA). (2008). *All New Episodes Seen at GUM Clinics: 1998–2007. United Kingdom and Country Specific Tables*. London: Health Protection Agency.

——(2009). *Hepatitis B – General Information*. Available at http://www.hpa.org.uk/Topics/InfectiousDiseases/InfectionsAZ/HepatitisB/GeneralInformationHepatitisB/hepbGeneralInfo/(accessed 16 July 2012).

——(2011) *Number and Rates of new STI Diagnoses in England, 2002 – 2011*. Available at http://www.hpa.org.uk/webc/HPAwebFile/HPAweb_C/1215589015024 (accessed 7 January 2013).

——(2012a). *HIV/Sexually Transmitted Infections (STIs): Health Protection Report*. London: Health Protection Services, Colindale. Available at http://www.hpa.org.uk/hpr/archives/2012/hpr2212.pdf (accessed 13 July 2012).

——(2012b). *HIV in the United Kingdom: 2012 Report*. Available at http://www.hpa.org.uk/webc/HPAwebFile/HPAweb_C/1317137200016 (accessed 19 December 2012).

Jemmott III, J.B., Jemmott, L.S. and Fong, G.T. (2010). Efficacy of a theory-based abstinence-only intervention over 24 months: a randomized controlled trial with young adolescents. *Archives of Paediatrics & Adolescent Medicine*, 164(2): 152.

Krahé, B., Abraham, C. and Scheinberger-Olwig, R. (2005). Can safer-sex promotion leaflets change cognitive antecedents of condom use? An experimental evaluation. *British Journal of Health Psychology*, 10(2), 203–220.

Leval, A., Sundström, K., Ploner, A., Dahlström, L., Widmark, C. and Sparén, P. (2011). Assessing perceived risk and STI prevention behaviour: a national population-based study with special reference to HPV. *PLOS ONE*, 6(6), 1–10.

Lindsey, R. (1985). Bathhouse curbs called help in coast AIDS fight. *New York Times*, 24 October, p. A19.

Martin, J., Slade, P., Sheeran, P., Wright, A. and Dibble, T. (2011). 'If-then' planning in one-to-one behaviour change counselling is effective in promoting contraceptive adherence in teenagers. *Journal of Family Planning & Reproductive Health Care*, 37(2): 85–88.

Masters, N., Beadnell, B., Morrison, D., Hoppe, M. and Gillmore, M. (2008). The opposite of sex? Adolescents' thoughts about abstinence and sex, and their sexual behaviour. *Perspectives on Sexual & Reproductive Health*, 40(2): 87–93.

Mausbach, B., Semple, S., Strathdee, S. and Patterson, T. (2009). Predictors of safer sex intentions and protected sex among heterosexual HIV-negative methamphetamine users: an expanded model of the Theory of Planned Behaviour. *AIDS Care*, 21(1): 17–24.

McKay, A. (2007). The effectiveness of latex condoms for prevention of STI/HIV. *Canadian Journal of Human Sexuality*, 16(1–2): 57–61.

Minichiello, V., Hawkes, G. and Pitts, M. (2011). HIV, sexually transmitted infections, and sexuality in later life. *Current Infectious Disease Reports*, 13(2): 182–187.

Miller, W.R. and Rollnick, S. (2002). *Motivational Interviewing: Preparing People for Change*, 2nd edn. New York: Guilford Press.

Morin, S.F., Charles, K.A. and Malyon, A.K. (1984). The psychological impact of AIDS on gay men. *American Psychologist*, 39: 1288–1293.

Moskowitz, J.M., Assunta Ritieni, A., Tholandi, M. and Xia, M. (2006). How do Californians define safe sex? *Californian Journal of Health Promotion*, 4(1): 109–118.

Newby, K., Wallace, L. M., Dunn, O. and Brown, K. E. (2012). A survey of English teenagers' sexual experience and preferences for school-based sex education. *Sex Education*, 12(2): 231–251.

NHS Choices (No date). Available at: www.nhs.uk/Livewell/STIs (accessed 19 December 2012).

Noar, S.M., Black, H.G. and Pierce, L.B. (2009). Efficacy of computer technology-based HIV prevention interventions: a meta-analysis. *Aids*, 23(1): 107–115.

ONS (2009). Opinions Survey Report No. 41 Contraception and Sexual Heath, 2008/09. Available at: http://www.ons.gov.uk/ons/rel/lifestyles/contraception-and-sexual-health/2008-09/2008-09.pdf (accessed 23 September 2013).

Orchowski, L. M., Mastroleo, N. R. and Borsari, B. (2012). Correlates of alcohol-related regretted sex among college students. *Psychology of Addictive Behaviors*, 26(4): 782–790.

Peterman, T., Tian, L., Warner, L., Satterwhite, C., Metcalf, C., Malotte, K., Douglas, J. *et al.* (2009). Condom use in the year following a sexually transmitted disease clinic visit. *International Journal of STD & AIDS*, 20(1): 9–13. DOI: 10.1258/ijsa.2008.008177.

Phillips-Howard, P., Bellis, M., Briant, L., Jones, H., Downing, J., Kelly, I.,Cook, P. *et al.* (2010). Wellbeing, alcohol use and sexual activity in young teenagers: findings from a cross-sectional survey in school children in North West England. *Substance Abuse Treatment, Prevention, And Policy*, 527.

Philpott, A., Knerr, W. and Boydell, V. (2006). Pleasure and prevention: when good sex is safer sex. *Reproductive Health Matters*, 14: 23–31.

Prochaska, J.O. and DiClemente, C.C. (1983). Stages and processes of self-change of smoking: toward an integrative model of change. *Journal of Consulting and Clinical Psychology*, 51: 390–395.

——(2002). Transtheoretical therapy: toward a more integrative model of change. *Psychotherapy: Theory, Research and Practice*, 19: 276–288.

Purdy, C. H. (2011). Using the Internet and social media to promote condom use in Turkey. *Reproductive Health Matters*, 19(37): 157–165.

Randolph, M.E., Pinkerton, S.D., Bogart, L.M., Cecil, H. and Abramson, P.R. (2007). Sexual pleasure and condom use. *Archives of Sexual Behaviour*, 36(6): 844–848. DOI: 10.1007/s10508-007-9213-0.

Reissing, E.D., Andruff, H.L. and Wentland, J.J. (2012). Looking back: the experience of first sexual intercourse and current sexual adjustment in young heterosexual adults. *Journal of Sex Research*, 49(1): 27–35.

Rogers, R.W. (1975). A protection motivation theory of fear appeals and attitude change. *Journal of Psychology*, 91: 93–114.

Rosenstock, I. (1990). The Health Belief Model: explaining health behaviour through expectancies. In K. Glanz, F.M. Lewis and B.K. Rimmer (eds). *Health Behaviour and Health Education: Theory, Research and Practice*. San Francisco: Jossey-Bass.

Saini, R., Saini, S. and Sharma, S. (2010). Oral sex, oral health and orogenital infections. *Journal of Global Infectious Diseases*, 2(1): 57–62

Sarkar, N.N. (2008). Barriers to condom use. *European Journal of Contraception & Reproductive Health Care*, 13(2): 114–122.

Secor-Turner, M., Sieving, R.E., Eisenberg, M.E. and Skay, C. (2011). Associations between sexually experienced adolescents' sources of information about sex and sexual risk outcomes. *Sex Education*, 11(4): 489–500.

Sheeran, P., Abraham, C. and Orvell, S. (1999). Psychosocial correlates of heterosexual condom use: a meta-analysis. *Psychological Bulletin*, 125: 90–132.

Shrier, L.A., Ancheta, R., Goodman, E., Chiou, V.M., Lyden, M.R. and Emans, S.J. (2001). Randomized controlled trials of safer sex intervention for high-risk adolescent girls. *Archives of Paediatrics and Adolescent Medicine*, 155: 73–79.

Sieving, R., Eisenberg, M., Pettingell, S. and Skay, C. (2006). Friends' influence on adolescents' first sexual intercourse. *Perspectives on Sexual and Reproductive Health*, 38: 13–19.

Slevin, A.P. and Marvin, C.L. (1987). Safe sex and pregnancy prevention: a guide for health practitioners working with adolescents. *Journal of Community Health Nursing*, 4: 235–241.

Stone, N., Hatherall, B., Ingham, R. and McEachran, J. (2006). Oral sex and condom use among young people in the United Kingdom. *Perspectives on Sexual and Reproductive Health*, 38: 6–12.

The Scottish Government (2011). *The Sexual Health and Blood Borne Virus Framework 2011–15*. Available at http://www.scotland.gov.uk/Resource/Doc/356286/0120395.pdf (accessed 7 January 2013)

Turchik, J.A. and Gidycz, C.A. (2012). Prediction of sexual risk behaviors in college students using the theory of planned behaviour: a prospective analysis. *Journal of Social & Clinical Psychology*, 31(1): 1–27.

UNAIDS (2010). *UNAIDS/WHO Report on the Global AIDS epidemic 2010*. Available at: http://www.unaids.org/globalreport/global_report.htm (accessed July 2012).

——(2012). UNAIDS Report on the Global AIDS epidemic 2012. Available at: http://www.unaids.org/en/media/unaids/contentassets/documents/epidemiology/2012/gr2012/20121120_UNAIDS_Global_Report_2012_en.pdf (accessed 19 December 2012.)

Underhill, K., Montgomery, P. and Operario, D. (2008). Abstinence-plus programs for HIV infection prevention in high-income countries. *Cochrane Database of Systematic Reviews (Online)*, (1): CD007006.

Wald, A., Langenberg, A.G.M., Krantz, E., Douglas, J.M., Handsfield, H.H., DiCarlo, R.P., Adimora, A.A., Izu, A.E., Morrow, R.A. and Corey, C. (2005). The relationship between condom use and herpes simplex virus acquisition. *Annals of Internal Medicine,* 143: 707–713.

Ward, H. and Rönn, M. (2010). The contribution of STIs to the sexual transmission of HIV. *Current Opinion in HIV and AIDS,* 5(4): 305–310.

Weller, S.C. and Davis-Beaty, K. (2002). Condom effectiveness in reducing heterosexual HIV transmission. *Cochrane Database of Systematic Reviews,* Issue 1. Art. No.: CD003255. DOI: 10.1002/14651858.CD003255/

Wellings, K., Field, J., Johnson, A.M. and Wadsworth, J. (1994). *Sexual Behaviour in Britain: The National Survey of Sexual Attitudes and Lifestyles.* Harmondsworth: Penguin.

Westwood, J. and Mullan, B. (2009). Teachers' and pupils' perceptions of the school nurse in relation to sexual health education. *Sex Education,* 9(3): 293–306.

World Health Organization (WHO) (2007). *Global Strategy for the Prevention and control of Sexually Transmitted Infections: 2006–2015.* Available at: http://whqlibdoc.who.int/publications/2007/9789241563475_eng.pdf (accessed 19 December 2012).

——(2011). Sexual health: a public health challenge in Europe. *Entre Nous, The European Magazine for Sexual and Reproductive Health.* Available at http://www.euro.who.int/__data/assets/pdf_file/0019/142570/en72.pdf (accessed 7 December 2013).

10 Specific conditions

Learning objectives

At the end of this chapter you will:
- appreciate the impact that lifestyle can have on the onset and progression of specific diseases
- understand the importance of health promotion in their management
- have explored available interventions to promote the health of people with specific disorders
- understand how psychology can influence behaviour change in different client groups
- identify the role that health and allied professionals play in promoting health for each condition.

Introduction

The burden of lifestyle-related ill health in the UK cannot be ignored. Modifiable risk factors such as physical inactivity, diet-related factors, smoking and alcohol use have been closely linked to the rising prevalence of many common chronic diseases, including coronary heart disease (CHD), type 2 diabetes, obesity and chronic obstructive pulmonary disease (COPD). Unhealthy behaviours not only increase a person's risk of developing health problems over time but they can also hasten disease progression and contribute to greater morbidity and early mortality for those already diagnosed with a condition (Buck and Frosini, 2012). Clearly, there is a differential influence of these lifestyle behaviours on the course and development of specific conditions. It is well known that smoking cessation significantly improves outcomes for people with COPD and the influence of increased physical activity in the prevention and management of type 2 diabetes is well recognised. Understanding the impact of these behaviours on health and well-being for different medical conditions is therefore essential.

Behaviour change has a critical role to play in reducing and managing the burden of preventable and treatable diseases (Department of Health, 2011). Consequently, the need for effective lifestyle interventions and improved management of these conditions through behaviour change is essential. However, changing lifestyle behaviour is challenging and requires time, effort and motivation from both health professional and client (Noordman *et al.,* 2012). Insight into effective behaviour change techniques can facilitate health care providers to better understand and support clients to adapt their lifestyle to manage their condition/s more effectively.

Health consequences of behaviour

Having a chronic condition is often the consequence of an unhealthy lifestyle and this is particularly true for multi-factorial disorders such as type 2 diabetes, CHD, common mental health problems and COPD. Lifestyle factors play an important role not only in the onset but also in the progression of these conditions so an important aspect of their management is the promotion of healthful behaviours and the modification of risky behaviours.

Type 2 diabetes

Case study

Janet is a 48-year-old woman who works as an accounts clerk. Following the birth of her second daughter 10 years ago Janet's weight has steadily increased and she is now overweight for her height. Over the past six months Janet has often complained of feeling tired and has less energy to do everyday activities which she has put down to 'her age'. Compensating for this tiredness, Janet has resorted to snacking frequently between meals for an energy boost.

Recent symptoms of increased thirst during the day and at night have prompted Janet to see her GP because her nights are becoming increasingly disturbed as she will get up at least twice to pass water. Following tests, Janet has been diagnosed with type 2 diabetes. She is not entirely shocked by the diagnosis because her father similarly has type 2 diabetes and has lived with the condition since his 50s. Having been told by her GP that type 2 diabetes can 'run in the family' Janet is unsure how changes in her current lifestyle will help to control and manage the progression of the condition. Although Janet had previously enjoyed attending aerobics classes in her early 20s, she believes her increasing family and work commitments have prevented her from sustaining a physically active lifestyle.

Introduction

Type 2 diabetes is a chronic and progressive disorder which, owing to its rapidly increasing prevalence, has reached epidemic proportions both nationally and on a global scale. Currently there are 2.6 million people who have been diagnosed with diabetes in the UK. This figure is expected to almost double by 2025 if the national prevalence of diabetes continues its upward trend (Diabetes UK, 2010). Characterised by defects in both insulin secretion and insulin action, type 2 diabetes accounts for around 90 per cent of all diagnosed cases of diabetes (Nolan et al., 2011). It is the leading cause of kidney failure, blindness in adults and amputation in the UK and is an independent risk factor for heart disease and stroke, reducing life expectancy on average by 10 years (Diabetes UK, 2010). The macro-vascular and micro-vascular complications and associated organ damage resulting from poorly managed diabetes represent an enormous cost, both economically in terms of the financial cost to diabetes care and in terms of its impact on quality of life for the individual (Nolan et al., 2011). Although there is a genetic component to its aetiology, the environment also plays an important role in the onset of type 2 diabetes (Scheumer et al., 2008). With levels of obesity rising and Western lifestyles accepting sedentary behaviour as the norm, the climbing prevalence of this condition is only set to continue (Jarvis et al., 2010).

Type 2 diabetes is a complex condition to manage. Careful regulation of blood glucose means that a person living with type 2 diabetes must often manage their own condition outside of the clinical setting. Daily choices about diet, physical activity, taking medication and blood glucose monitoring are made by individuals with a diagnosis of diabetes and the consequences of these choices can affect health and progression of the disease (Jarvis et al., 2010). Monitoring and regulating blood glucose levels requires considerable effort on the part of the individual and these activities may be particularly onerous if the individual generally feels well and the complications of the condition have yet to manifest (Department of Health, 2001a). There is however promising evidence that behavioural interventions can improve diabetes control and health outcomes for people diagnosed with type 2 diabetes.

Interventions to promote the health of people with type 2 diabetes

Given its multi-factorial aetiology, people's lifestyle choices clearly play an important role in the onset and progression of type 2 diabetes. Traditional approaches to its treatment have focused on drug interventions to stabilise blood glucose levels and manage cardiovascular risk factors. However, long-term data from the UK Prospective Diabetes Study has shown that despite initial improvements, drug therapy was not effective in maintaining blood glucose control over time (UKPDS, 1998). These findings raise questions about the effectiveness of drug interventions alone for the long-term management of type 2 diabetes (Jarvis et al., 2010).

It is important to recognise that effective diabetes management lies mainly in the hands of the person with the condition (Department of Health, 2001a). It is not surprising therefore that current evidence indicates that self-management skills are required for people to manage their diabetes successfully and this is best delivered through structured educational courses (Steinsbekk *et al.*, 2012). Unlike patient education within the medical model, where health professionals are considered to be the experts and patients the recipients of care (Brennan, 1996), structured educational programmes are patient-centred and aim to empower patients to become active self-managers of their condition.

Individual level interventions

Structured patient education

Structured educational programmes are a relatively new approach to diabetes education within the UK. Based on theories of patient empowerment (Anderson and Funnell, 2000) and problem-based learning (Barrows, 1996), these programmes aim to provide individuals with the confidence, tools and techniques that will enable them to manage their condition more effectively (Loveman *et al.*, 2008). The diabetes education and self-management for ongoing and newly diagnosed (DESMOND) intervention (Davies *et al.*, 2008) and the Diabetes X-PERT programme (Deakin *et al.*, 2006) are two examples of structured education programmes that are available nationally for people with type 2 diabetes. In particular the X-PERT programme, which runs over six weeks, has been shown to be particularly effective in improving clinical, lifestyle and psychosocial indicators in people with newly diagnosed and existing type 2 diabetes (Deakin, 2012).

Course contents for the X-PERT diabetes programme:
*   What is diabetes?
*   The eatwell plate and energy balance
*   Carbohydrate awareness and glycaemic index
*   The benefits of physical activity
*   Supermarket tour and understanding food labels
*   Possible complications of diabetes and their prevention
*   Lifestyle experiment
*   Are you an X-PERT? game
*   Care Planning: the lifestyle experiment
            www.expertpatients.co.uk/course-participants/courses/x-pert-diabetes

Structured educational programmes utilise behavioural strategies such as problem solving, goal setting and social support to facilitate dietary and physical activity behaviour change and self-monitoring among people with type 2 diabetes. Self-directed behavioural goal setting is a strategy often used in structured programmes to increase self-efficacy and empowerment. It refers to the process of creating an action plan whereby individuals can accomplish behaviours necessary for the self-management of their condition. This process allows the individual to develop concrete, usually short-term goals to facilitate lifestyle change (Funnell, 2010). Behavioural goals to improve diabetes self-management may include:

- Avoidance of foods with high sugar content in order to regulate blood glucose levels
- Reduction of daily calorie intake to achieve weight loss and reduce BMI
- Avoidance of foods high in fat to achieve weight loss and reduce BMI
- Increasing daily physical activity levels.

Diabetes self-management education can be delivered in many forms. A systematic review by Steinsbekk *et al.* (2012) concluded that group based training for diabetes self-management improves diabetes control and knowledge of the condition in the short and longer term. The Diabetes X-PERT programme, which is a group-based intervention, has proven to be particularly effective in improving blood glucose control up to 14 months after the intervention. By contrast to structured education delivered in a group, the efficacy of one-to-one patient education to improve clinical outcomes has not been demonstrated. Careful consideration of the delivery mode for diabetes education is therefore essential (Duke *et al.*, 2009).

Opportunities clearly exist for individuals to establish social support when structured education is delivered within a group setting. As discussed in Chapter 4 of this book, specific social support can work at the individual level by providing positive feedback about successful behaviour change thereby improving self-efficacy (Gruber, 2008). It can also provide instrumental and emotional support whereby members can draw on and learn from the experiences of others in the group (Jarvis *et al.*, 2010). Designed to run over a six-week period, the X-PERT programme (Deakin *et al.*, 2006) may provide individuals with the necessary social support for diabetes self-management and lifestyle change unlike the DESMOND programme which is delivered over one day or two half day equivalents (Davies *et al.*, 2008).

Applying this to Janet

Referring Janet to the X-PERT programme will enable her to develop knowledge and self-management skills to optimise her diabetes management. Janet's self-efficacy for dietary and physical activity behaviour change may be enhanced through the setting of individualised self-directed goals. The social support she receives from group membership may facilitate her to adapt to her condition and make the necessary lifestyle changes to control its progression.

Promoting health through physical activity

Low cardio-respiratory fitness, an independent marker of long-term mortality in individuals with diabetes, is a modifiable risk factor that can lead to poor health outcomes for people with type 2 diabetes (Wei *et al.*, 2000). Physical activity is the only intervention that directly influences cardio-respiratory fitness and is essential to the management of the condition (Kavookjian *et al.*, 2007). Frequently described as the cornerstone of type 2 diabetes management (Chudyk and Petrella, 2011; Kirk *et al.*, 2009; Yates *et al.*, 2009), regular physical activity has a positive effect on glycaemic control and has been associated with decreases in cardiovascular risk by lowering blood pressure, BMI and improving lipid profiles (Marwick *et al.*, 2009). Despite its many health benefits, physical activity is underutilised by people with the condition who, according to Morrato *et al.* (2007), are less likely to meet physical activity guidelines compared to the general population. Challenges clearly exist for the successful promotion of physical activity in individuals with type 2 diabetes.

Structured exercise programmes

Simply advising people to become more physically active is generally ineffective when promoting lifestyle change (Upton and Thirlaway, 2010). A recent systematic review and meta-analysis of randomised controlled clinical trials supports this view by concluding that physical activity advice alone for people with diabetes was ineffective in reducing blood glucose concentrations over time (Umpierre *et al.*, 2011). By contrast, structured exercise training that consisted of aerobic exercise, resistance training or a combination of the two was associated with reductions in blood glucose levels, the effects of which were similar across the three exercise modalities. This effect was greater again for people who engaged in structured exercise of moderate intensity for at least 150 minutes per week (Chudyk and Petrella, 2011; Umpierre *et al.*, 2011), giving support to the positive effect of current physical activity guidelines on health (Department of Health, 2011).

Despite structured exercise regimes of moderate intensity exhibiting a more significant impact on diabetes-related outcomes (Umpierre *et al.*, 2011; Chudyk and Petrella, 2011), it is important to appreciate that higher intensity exercise may not be tolerated or may even be hazardous for individuals who have previously been sedentary and/or present with co-existing complications. It is generally accepted that physical activity at any level is better than no exercise at all (Kavookjian *et al.*, 2007), and emerging evidence also suggests that breaks in sedentary behaviour, such as non-exercise standing activity, and light intensity exercise are independently associated with improved blood glucose regulation for people with type 2 diabetes (Healy *et al.*, 2008; Healy *et al*, 2008; Department of Health, 2011). For individuals who are already exercising at a moderate level of intensity, health professionals may wish to consider encouraging exercise of a higher intensity and sustained duration because of the potential additional benefits on metabolic regulation and cardio-respiratory fitness (Kavookjian *et al.*, 2007). It is vital therefore that interventions promoting physical activity for people with type 2 diabetes are tailored to the specific health needs of the individual. An assessment of previous activity levels, cardiovascular risk factors and co-existing complications is therefore essential.

Applying this to Janet

An assessment of Janet's current health status, to include baseline measures of blood pressure, pulse, weight, BMI and current activity level, is required before she decides which form of physical activity is acceptable and appropriate for the management of her diabetes.

Her previous enjoyment of aerobics classes may allow Janet to consider improving her cardio-respiratory fitness through this more structured form of exercise.

Exercise referral schemes

Exercise referral schemes have been discussed in detail in Chapter 6. It is worth mentioning that these schemes are available through the NHS to patients with type 2 diabetes; however their efficacy in promoting sustained behaviour change has not been demonstrated.

Box 10.1 Applying research in practice

Type 2 diabetes and dog walking: patients' longitudinal perspectives about implementing and sustaining physical activity (Peel *et al.*, 2010)

This study explores the ways in which people with type 2 diabetes talk about implementing and sustaining physical activity in their everyday lives.

Interviews were conducted with 40 patients newly diagnosed with type 2 diabetes living in the Lothian region of Scotland. Participants were interviewed at baseline, 6 and 12 months. Twenty-one of the original sample not lost to follow-up were interviewed again after four years.

Regular physical activity was considered unsustainable by most participants and information and guidance about physical activity from health professionals was considered to be vague and non-specific. Walking, especially with a dog, was considered an achievable and sustainable form of exercise for people with type 2 diabetes. Participants' accounts revealed how dog walking provided regular routine activity for the self-management of type 2 diabetes which was maintained over the four-year study period.

In conclusion, ascertaining patients' preferences and constraints on physical activity would facilitate the setting of individualised achievable goals. The potential for physical activity maintenance through dog walking is noteworthy in this client group.

Community level interventions

Many of the community level interventions promoting physical activity and healthy eating can be easily applied to people with type 2 diabetes. The influence of obesity, overweight and physical inactivity in the onset and progression of type 2 diabetes is well documented (Diabetes UK, 2010), so community-wide promotional activities that target important modifiable risk factors such as diet and exercise could greatly help the treatment of this condition (Bailey, 2011). One such example is the Change4Life campaign which has been described at length in Chapter 2 (Department of Health, 2009). Although this intervention aims to tackle obesity in people of all ages through changes in dietary and exercise habits, these lifestyle measures are equally important for the management of type 2 diabetes. Similarly, the Traffic Light System devised by the Food Standards Agency facilitates people to make healthy dietary choices by indicating the nutritional values in food. This informational intervention is particularly relevant to people with type 2 diabetes because they are required to closely monitor and regulate their daily sugar intake in order to stabilise their blood glucose levels.

Public health campaigns addressing physical activity are equally as important for people with type 2 diabetes. Active Transport schemes, which promote cycling and walking, and green activities such as allotment gardening as part of a community group, have the potential to increase daily activity levels in people with diabetes. These community approaches may be particularly effective in promoting an active lifestyle because they enable people with the condition to incorporate physical activity into their daily lives more flexibly (these interventions are discussed in detail in Chapter 4).

Applying this to Janet

Janet could use the Traffic Light system on food packaging to ensure that she successfully regulates her blood sugar by avoiding foods with high sugar content. This labelling system could also enable Janet to monitor her dietary fat intake in an attempt to reduce her weight and BMI.

Environmental schemes encouraging active transport could enable Janet to schedule physical activity into her otherwise busy work and home life. This could be achieved through either walking or cycling to work.

Working effectively with others

Multi-disciplinary team support is available to all people with type 2 diabetes from diagnosis. GPs, practice nurses, dieticians, podiatrists and other allied health professionals all have an important role to play in the provision of diabetes care. Traditionally, diabetes education was delivered in a didactic setting whereby health professionals were assumed to be the experts. However, the emphasis is shifting and patients are now encouraged to have autonomy by working in alliance with professionals to identify successful strategies for diabetes self-management (Deakin *et al.*, 2006).

Peer support

Peer support is a promising approach for diabetes care. It harnesses the ability and experience of patients with diabetes to support others with the condition (World Health Organisation, 2008). It is usually provided within a volunteering framework and can be delivered in many ways, including group or individual support (Smith *et al.*, 2011). In the UK, the Expert Patient Programme (Department of Health, 2001b) advocates the development of peer educators. However, the efficacy of these peer-led interventions is mixed with some studies indicating that 'expert' patients are as effective as specialist health professionals in imparting diabetes self-management knowledge (Baksi *et al.*, 2008) and others saying there is no effect of group-based peer support interventions on diabetes control or psychosocial measures (Cade *et al.*, 2009; Smith *et al.*, 2011). Perhaps more promisingly, a study investigating the effect of peer-led self-management coaching for type 2 diabetes demonstrated improvements in self-efficacy for a subgroup of patients who were experiencing low self-efficacy shortly after diagnosis (van der Wulp *et al.*, 2012). Although the effectiveness of peer support has not been consistently demonstrated, as an adjunct to other diabetes self-management programmes, peer support may offer the kind of emotional, social and practical support that is necessary to achieve and sustain complex behaviour change necessary for the self-management of diabetes (Boothroyd and Fisher, 2010).

Applying this to Janet

Janet will work closely with members of the primary care team in order to establish self-directed goals to manage her diabetes autonomously.

Joining a peer support group would enable Janet to meet and gain support from other people with type 2 diabetes.

Coronary Heart Disease (CHD)

Case study

Graham has recently been discharged from hospital following a sudden heart attack at the age of 52. He had collapsed early one morning with crushing chest pain whilst collecting papers for his newsagency business which he has run for the past 30 years. Living in a rural location, Graham relies on his car to deliver papers to his clients. Starting work at 5am most mornings to collect paper deliveries and working through until early evening when the shop closes means that Graham works long, often unsociable hours to meet the needs of the business. Weekends are similarly as busy in the shop and he has limited leisure time activities as a consequence. These demands have taken a toll on Graham's mood and stress levels over the years and he admits that he has used smoking as a coping strategy. Graham and his wife are keen to make changes to his current lifestyle because he is overweight for his height and has been for many years. However, they are fearful that by becoming more physically active he will increase his risk of having another heart attack.

Introduction

Coronary heart disease (CHD) is the term used to describe the build-up of fatty deposits in the coronary arteries and it affects the heart by restricting the flow of blood to the heart muscle. This can lead to a feeling of tightness or pain in the chest, known as angina, or to a myocardial infarction (heart attack). The condition is caused by a combination of genetic factors and unhealthy lifestyle behaviours therefore long-term modification of behavioural-risk factors is key to reducing the risk of future health problems. CHD is a largely preventable disease yet it affects an estimated 2.6 million people in the UK (NACR, 2010) and accounts for approximately 124,000 myocardial infarctions (heart attacks) every year (British Heart Foundation, 2010). Despite decreasing trends in incidence and mortality, CHD continues to be the leading cause of premature death in the UK, accounting for around one in four deaths in men and one in six deaths in women (British Heart Foundation, 2010).

Having an acute cardiac event is a frightening and often life-changing experience (British Heart Foundation, 2007). Indeed, many people with CHD experience reduced quality of life, often suffering from anxiety, depression, and emotional and social disturbances all of which can affect the development and progression of the condition (Goulding *et al.*, 2010). Even if the physical implications of an acute coronary event are minimised by prompt medical interventions such as angioplasty and antithrombotic drugs, many individuals find the long-term modification of lifestyle behaviours daunting and difficult to sustain (British Heart Foundation, 2007). The importance of pharmacological treatments to combat the associated risk factors of CHD is indisputable; however, Mozaffarian *et al.* (2008) suggest that more attention should be focussed on helping individuals to make and sustain positive changes to their lifestyle. Smoking, poor diet and lack of exercise are important modifiable risk factors for CHD and even modest changes in these lifestyle behaviours can substantially improve outcomes for people with the condition (Artinian *et al.*, 2010).

Individual level interventions

Cardiac rehabilitation

Cardiac rehabilitation is a complex intervention that utilises a variety of therapies, including exercise, risk factor education, behaviour change, psychological support, and strategies to manage the clinical risk factors for heart disease (Heran *et al.*, 2011). The National Service Framework for Coronary Heart Disease (Department of Health, 2000) recommends that 85 per cent of post myocardial infarction and re-vascularisation (angioplasty and bypass) patients should be offered cardiac rehabilitation. However, according to the latest figures from the 2011 National Audit for cardiac rehabilitation just 43 per cent of heart patients in England participated in the programme. In Wales, participation rates were 35 per cent and in Northern Ireland the figure was 40 per cent. Opportunities to promote health and reduce cardiac risk factors in the period immediately following a cardiac event are clearly being missed for patients who do not attend CR.

What do patients receive through CR programmes?

Group-based educational classes are the preferred method for delivering behaviour change in Cardiac Rehabilitation at the individual level (British Heart Foundation, 2011). Programmes aim to support patients to become active self-managers in their health (BHF, 2007) through participation in the four phases of Cardiac Rehabilitation:

- **Phase I:** pre-discharge care which includes medical risk factor assessment, education, correction of cardiac misconceptions and reassurance.
- **Phase II:** the immediate post-discharge period which includes home visits, telephone contact and supervised use of the Heart Manual (a self-help programme for patients recovering from a heart attack).
- **Phase III:** a 6- to 14-week multidisciplinary behaviour change and rehabilitation programme, consisting of group sessions once or twice a week
- **Phase IV:** maintenance of lifestyle changes made in the preceding phases, including exercise opportunities accessed through local sports and leisure centres. This phase is not currently part of the NHS pathway.

In order to reduce the risk of a recurrent heart attack, Graham would benefit from Cardiac Rehabilitation. His participation in the four phases of CR is essential to optimise early behaviour change that will support self-management of the condition.

Behaviour change in cardiac rehabilitation

Lifestyle modification is a central feature of cardiac rehabilitation. Patients are encouraged to develop skills in self-management and this often means making positive changes to their lifestyle in order to reduce behavioural-risk factors and promote cardiovascular health. Chow *et al.* (2010) highlight the early benefits of lifestyle modification after acute coronary events. They found that adherence to diet, exercise and smoking recommendations just 30 days following an MI was associated with a substantially lower risk of recurrent cardiovascular events and mortality at six months. Patient collaboration is essential to the behaviour change process, with health professionals taking on a facilitative role by assisting patients to identify patterns of helpful and unhelpful health behaviour in order to self-generate solutions for behaviour change. This partnership allows the patient to decide which health behaviour, if any, he/she would like or is ready to change (Tierney *et al.*, 2011). NICE (2007a) have developed guidelines relating to behaviour change in the healthcare context and these guidelines can be used by health professionals to facilitate patients receiving CR to effectively change their health behaviour (Table 10.1).

Table 10.1 NICE guidelines: generic principles for effective health behaviour change at the individual level

Select interventions that motivate and support people to:
- Understand the short-, medium- and long-term consequences of their health-related behaviours, for themselves and others
- Feel positive about the benefits of health-enhancing behaviours and changing their behaviour
- Plan their changes in terms of easy steps over time
- Recognise how their social contexts and relationships may affect their behaviour, and identify and plan situations that might undermine the changes they are trying to make
- Plan explicit 'if-then' coping strategies to prevent relapse
- Make a personal commitment to adopt health-enhancing behaviours by setting (and recording) goals to undertake clearly defined behaviours, in particular context, over a specified time
- Share their behaviour with others

Source: National Institute for Health and Clinical Excellence, 2007a

Strategies supporting behaviour change in cardiac rehabilitation

Cognitive-behavioural strategies are an integral component of any behaviour change intervention (Artinian *et al.*, 2010). Chapter 4 provides a detailed discussion of the psychological interventions that are available to help people make changes to their lifestyle; these include CBT, goal setting and motivational interviewing. In terms of cardiac rehabilitation, these strategies enable individuals with CHD to:

1. Modify their lifestyle
2. Develop adaptive coping strategies
3. Change maladaptive illness beliefs
4. Improve physical and psychosocial outcomes.

In their review, Janssen *et al.* (2012) found that lifestyle interventions that incorporated four self-regulation strategies: goal-setting, self-monitoring, planning and feedback resulted in greater improvements in dietary and exercise behaviour for patients with CHD than interventions that included none of these techniques.

Goal setting

Goal setting is an effective technique to achieve desired behaviour change within clinical groups. This technique is generally more successful when goals are specific in outcome, short term and realistic in terms of the patients' current capabilities and health status (Artinian *et al.*, 2010). Behavioural goals to facilitate CHD self-management may include:

- Avoidance of foods high in saturated fats in order to improve cholesterol levels
- Reduction of daily calorie intake to achieve weight loss and reduce BMI
- Reduction of daily/weekly alcohol consumption in line with current government guidelines
- Increasing physical activity levels to improve cardiovascular fitness
- Smoking cessation/reduction of tobacco use,

Self-monitoring

Self-monitoring is an important self-regulatory strategy and refers to the process of observing one's behaviour and evaluating it in relation to identified goals. Simple diaries can be used for self-monitoring of behaviours; individuals can chart their physical activity/dietary intake by logging number of steps taken, distance walked, calories consumed or amount of weight lost (Burke *et al.*, 2008). This strategy provides the individual with direct feedback on progress thus enhancing self-efficacy for behaviour change and facilitating the adoption of self-management behaviours for CHD management.

Planning

Action planning has been described as a simple yet promising strategy to increase the uptake of phase IV CR (Sniehotta *et al.*, 2010). As previously outlined, phase IV cardiac rehabilitation groups are usually community-based and provide patients with the opportunity to make sustained lifestyle changes generally through participation in physical activity programmes (British Heart Foundation, 2011). A recent study by Sniehotta *et al.* (2010) demonstrated that among participants who planned where and when to attend phase IV CR in the third phase of this programme, 65.9 per cent subsequently went on to attend a phase IV program compared to 18.5 per cent of those who did not make a plan. These findings suggest that both intention and action planning are good predictors of phase IV CR attendance and give support to the utility of an extended Theory of Planned Behaviour to explain cardiac rehabilitation behaviour.

Feedback

Feedback is frequently included in successful behaviour change interventions and, when delivered by a health professional, it can act as a gauge upon which the individual can assess their progress (Artinian *et al.*, 2010). Feedback about behavioural performance can motivate an individual to sustain changes made to their lifestyle, or it can facilitate them to make adjustments to their behaviour in order to reach their goal/s for CR self-management.

Social support

Phase III of CR is particularly well placed to provide individuals with the necessary social support for an adaptive psychological coping response following an acute cardiac event (Barth *et al.*, 2010). This group-based approach incorporates scheduled follow-up sessions for ongoing contact with multi-disciplinary team members and social support from the peer group. The frequency and duration of this group-based intervention may have the advantage of enhancing perceived social support for lifestyle change among patients referred to CR. In their review, Barth *et al.* (2010) distinguish between different dimensions of social support and their impact on CHD prognosis. They concluded that functional social support (e.g. perceived social support) was more important than structural support (e.g. living alone) for reducing cardiac mortality. Social support through group participation is an important intervention strategy that may improve risk factors and related health behaviours for individuals with CHD.

Applying this to Graham

Encouraging Graham to attend the group-based CR programmes will provide him with the necessary social support to make changes to his current lifestyle and reduce the risk factors associated with poor cardiovascular outcomes.

The role of physical activity in cardiac rehabilitation

Despite overwhelming evidence promoting an active lifestyle, the majority of people in the UK fail to meet government guidelines for being active (Department of Health, 2011). This is clearly problematic because cardio respiratory fitness is closely associated with overall risk of CHD (Lavie *et al.*, 2009). The beneficial effects of increased physical activity in people with CHD is well documented (Artinian *et al.*, 2010; Held *et al.*, 2012) and when delivered as a component part of Cardiac Rehabilitation favourable cardiovascular and psychosocial outcomes are observed (Lavie *et al.*, 2009; Heran *et al.*, 2011). Held *et al.* (2012) importantly identify that even minimal amounts of either mild or moderate intensity physical activity (e.g. from 0 to 30 minutes/week) can have a protective effect on the heart and this effect is greater when physical activity is performed during leisure time rather than at work. However, clinical guidelines regarding myocardial infarction secondary prevention suggest that any increased physical activity may be enhanced by 'tailored advice from a suitably qualified professional' (p. 9, NICE, 2007b) and clearly 'some form of pre-exercise assessment is essential' (p. 20, Department of Health, 2001) in order to establish the individual's specific health needs.

A common misconception for people with heart disease is the belief that physical activity may further damage their heart or indeed increase their risk of sustaining another heart attack (Riegel, 1993). Evidence suggests that faulty illness beliefs in people with CHD can lead to maladaptive health behaviours such as abstaining from even low levels of physical activity. This inappropriate behavioural response can lead to low cardio-respiratory fitness, exacerbating the symptoms of CHD and making recurrence of an acute event more likely. In their review, Goulding *et al.* (2010) suggest that health professionals should endeavour to correct maladaptive illness beliefs in order to encourage positive coping strategies and adaptive health behaviours. They conclude that cognitive behavioural interventions are particularly effective in both challenging cardiac misconceptions and creating positive belief change in people with CHD.

A substantial body of evidence demonstrates a strong link between depression and CHD (Goldston and Baillie, 2008; Wellenius *et al.*, 2008; Whooley, 2006). Interventions promoting physical activity have a clear role to play in the management of these co-existing conditions because physical exercise is known to improve both depressive symptoms and markers of cardiovascular risk (Blumenthal *et al.*, 2007). The association between depression and cardiovascular events is, according to Whooley *et al.* (2008), largely explained by health behaviours, most notably physical inactivity. It is therefore crucial that patients with CHD who are also depressed are encouraged to increase their physical activity levels to concurrently reduce their risk of any further adverse coronary events and manage their symptoms of depression (Lett *et al.*, 2004).

Applying this to Graham

Tailoring physical activity advice to Graham's specific health needs will require a pre-exercise assessment by a health professional or exercise specialist. This will establish how exercise can be incorporated into Graham's daily life to ensure that he achieves improvements in cardio-respiratory fitness.

Correcting Graham's and his wife's faulty illness beliefs that exercise could further damage his heart is essential if he is to make an adaptive response to engage in physical activity for cardiac rehabilitation.

Engaging in physical activity could have the added benefit of improving Graham's overall mood.

Community level interventions

Many of the community level interventions that target specific lifestyle behaviours such as smoking, eating healthily and being physically active are important to people with CHD because these health behaviours are also important modifiable risk factors for the development and progression of the disease. Public health smoking campaigns are particularly relevant to people with CHD who smoke because smoking cessation or any reduction in cigarette use can have considerable benefits for coronary health. The Smokefree legislation introduced by the Department of Health in 2007 has been particularly successful in changing attitudes to smoking in public places, making this behaviour less socially acceptable. Smoke free policies seek to encourage smoke free environments to benefit the health of smokers and non-smokers alike, therefore this intervention can both directly and indirectly influence the health of people with CHD.

Public health campaigns to improve dietary habits and increase physical activity are equally important to people with CHD. The Change4Life intervention (Department of Health, 2009) is one such example that targets these important risk factors for heart disease and aims to encourage a healthier lifestyle to reduce obesity. Similarly, the Traffic Light System can assist individuals with heart disease to make healthier food choices. The colour coded labelling system can guide people to select foods that are low in saturated fats, salt and sugar in order to facilitate weight loss and/or lower dietary fat intake to improve cholesterol levels.

A number of community interventions aim to increase physical activity and there has been much debate around the obesogenic environment. Active transport has emerged as an important intervention that could yield many benefits including improvements of public health by increasing physical activity and reducing air pollution and traffic congestion (Jarrett *et al.*, 2012). Increased walking and cycling and reduced use of private cars all have a positive effect on many health outcomes, and environments that support these activities are particularly important for coronary health.

Applying this to Graham

The opportunity for Graham to smoke in public places will be restricted by the enforcement of smoke free policies. These smoke free campaigns may alter Graham's attitude towards smoking through the alteration of social norms which makes smoking less socially acceptable.

Graham could use the Traffic Light System on food packaging to ensure that he reduces his intake of foods which are high in saturated fats. This food labelling system would enable him to make healthier food choices and monitor his overall calorie intake in order to reduce his weight and BMI.

Active transport is a strategy that Graham could use to increase his physical activity levels, either to get back and forth to work or to make deliveries to clients who are within easy reach of the business. Reducing his reliance on the car will ensure that he reduces time spent in sedentary activities.

Working effectively with others

Clinical guidelines emphasise the importance of a multi-disciplinary approach to CR (BHF, 2011). Nurses, physiotherapists, dieticians, exercise specialists, occupational therapists and psychologists all have a role to play in supporting individuals with CHD to become active self-managers in the control of their condition. Since 2007 there has been a significant increase in the number of exercise specialists available through CR programmes (BHF, 2011). The beneficial influence of physical activity on clinical and psychosocial outcomes is indisputable therefore any investment to promote this behaviour in people with CHD is clearly warranted. However, by contrast there has been a worrying decline in access to psychology time through CR. Between 2007 and 2010 the proportion of people receiving relaxation training through CR programmes fell from 44 per cent to 29 per cent. During this same time period the number of patients receiving psychology talks similarly fell from 32 per cent to 19 per cent (BHF, 2011).

Psychologists importantly address the psychological aspects of CHD management. Cognitive-behavioural therapy (CBT) is one such approach that clinical psychologists may use to enable patients to change any negative patterns of thinking or behaviour that may be impacting on their ability to manage their condition. A recent randomised controlled trial that compared cognitive behavioural therapy based on stress management and standard treatment for people with CHD found that group-based CBT delivered over a year was significantly more effective in lowering the rate of fatal and non-fatal recurrent coronary events (Gulliksson et al., 2011). Similarly, Olivio et al. (2009) demonstrated the efficacy of a mindfulness-based stress management programme for patients with CHD. Significant reductions in depression and perceived stress were observed for patients participating in a 4-week programme that encouraged awareness of day-to-day experiences such as breathing, walking, working, listening and talking through mindfulness meditation. Having access to these psychological therapies is clearly fundamental because psychosocial factors such as work-related stress, depression, anxiety and hostility have been shown to account for approximately 30 per cent of the attributable risk of acute heart attacks (Yusuf et al., 2004)

Applying this to Graham

In order to manage his current stress and low mood, Graham would benefit from cognitive behavioural therapy focussed on stress management. Attending a group-based stress management intervention run by a psychologist as part of a cardiac rehabilitation programme would enable Graham to garner emotional social support from peers to enable him to manage his responses to stress more adaptively.

Mental health

Case study

Emily is a 22-year-old undergraduate student in the final year of her sociology degree. The past six months have been particularly difficult for Emily because she has been feeling very low and has been unable to get any enjoyment out of life. Emily has actively avoided any social activities at college and when asked how she is feeling she will often become tearful and upset. Emily is particularly concerned because her sleep pattern has changed and she is constantly over-tired because she wakes very early most mornings and is unable to get back to sleep. Her college work is suffering as a consequence and this is adding to

Emily's feelings of hopelessness. Her recent weight loss due to her decreased appetite prompted Emily to visit her GP and having discussed her symptoms, Emily has been diagnosed with depression. Although Emily has been prescribed anti-depressant medication she is also keen to understand how changes to her lifestyle may help her to cope with her symptoms of depression.

Common mental health disorders

One in four people in the UK will experience some form of mental health problem in the course of a year, with mixed anxiety and depression being the most common mental health disorder (Mental Health Foundation, 2012). Common mental health disorders, which comprise of different types of anxiety and depression, cause emotional distress for the individual and interfere with physical and social functioning if left untreated (Adult Psychiatric Morbidity Survey [AMPS], 2009). Based on AMPS data, Table 10.2 shows that overall prevalence of common mental health problems in the UK has gradually increased between 1993 and 2007. With the exception of obsessive compulsive disorder, all other mental health conditions have risen to some degree within this time period (Table 10.2). Data from the 2007 AMPS also indicates that prevalence of common mental disorders is higher for women than men: overall, 1 in 5 women had a common mental health disorder compared to 1 in 8 men. Indeed, the impact of gender on mental health outcomes is well established, although many other biopsychosocial factors are also thought to influence a person's vulnerability to depressive and/or anxiety disorders.

Table 10.2 Prevalence of common mental health problems

	Mixed anxiety and depression	Generalised anxiety disorder	Depressive episode	Phobias	Obsessive compulsive disorder	Panic disorder	Any common mental health condition
1993 survey	7.5	4.4	2.2	2.2	1.4	1	15.5
2000 survey	9.4	4.7	2.8	2.8	1.2	0.7	17.5
2007 survey	9.7	4.7	2.6	2.6	1.3	1.2	17.6

Source: Adapted from The Health & Social Care Information Centre 2009, http://www.mind. org.uk/help/research_and_policy/statistics_1_how_common_is_mental_distress#common

Depression

Depression refers to a range of mental health problems that are typically characterised by low mood, loss of interest and enjoyment in everyday experiences and other behavioural, emotional and physical symptoms (NICE, 2009). The ICD-10 uses a list of ten depressive symptoms to categories depression according to its severity (WHO, 2010). In terms of treatment and management, the common form of major depressive episode is divided into four distinct groups based on the number of depressive symptoms experienced within the list.

ICD-10 diagnostic criteria for depression: an agreed list of ten depressive symptoms

Key symptoms:

1. persistent sadness or low mood; and/or
2. loss of interests or pleasure
3. fatigue or low energy
4. disturbed sleep
5. poor concentration or indecisiveness
6. low self-confidence
7. poor or increased appetite
8. suicidal thoughts or acts
9. agitation or slowing of movements
10. guilt or self-blame.

The 10 symptoms then define the degree of depression, and management is based on the particular degree:

* **not depressed** (fewer than four symptoms)
* **mild depression** (four symptoms)
* **moderate depression** (five to six symptoms)
* **severe depression** (seven or more symptoms, with or without psychotic symptoms).

Symptoms should be present for a month or more and every symptom should be present for most of every day (WHO, 2010, cited in National Institute for Health and Clinical Excellence, 2004).

Commonly, people with depression remain low throughout the course of the day, although for some, mood may gradually improve during the day only to return to low mood upon waking (NICE, 2004). The symptoms of depression are often extremely distressing for the affected individual and for those close to them (Adult Psychiatric Household Survey, 2009). Apart from the personal suffering experienced by individuals who are depressed, the impact of the condition on social and occupational functioning, physical health and mortality is substantial (NICE, 2004). This has been demonstrated by the World Health Organisation (2005) who have calculated that 31.7 per cent of all years lived with disability are due to mental health disorders, with depression making the greatest contribution.

Interventions to improve the health of people with common mental health disorders

Mental health disorders increase the risk of communicable and non-communicable diseases, and strong associations between depression and coronary heart disease have been found (Tylee *et al.*, 2012). Treatment is therefore essential in order that the physical and psychosocial consequences of common mental health disorders are minimised. Traditionally, depression and anxiety have been treated with medication and psychological interventions, however, lifestyle interventions also have an important role to play in the treatment of these conditions (Forsyth *et al.*, 2009). Smoking, physical inactivity, poor diet and obesity have all been associated with poor mental health and these lifestyle behaviours are also risk factors for the development of depression and anxiety (Prince *et al.*, 2007). Physical activity is probably the one lifestyle behaviour that is most closely associated with improved outcomes for people with depression and/or anxiety. The recurrent nature of these disorders suggests that interventions promoting sustained lifestyle changes are necessary for both symptom control and/or relapse prevention.

Individual level interventions

Physical activity in the treatment of depression and anxiety

There is a general belief that physical activity and exercise have positive effects on mood and anxiety. Indeed, the effect of exercise on depression has been scrutinised over many years and some have advocated its use as an adjunct or alternative treatment for the condition. The National Institute for Health and Clinical Excellence (NICE) guideline for depression recommends structured, supervised exercise programmes 2–3 times a week, for 45 minutes to one hour, over 10 to 14 weeks for the treatment of mild to moderate depression (NICE, 2009). Across the UK, exercise referral schemes are also available for people with depression through primary care (Department of Health, 2001). However, this scheme's effectiveness has not been demonstrated over a sustained period so its utility for the management of long-term mental health problems is questionable.

Although it is reasonable to recommend exercise to people with depression, a recent systematic review of randomised controlled trials found that exercise has but a moderate effect on reducing depressive symptoms for people with major depression (Rimer *et al.*, 2012). This outcome is in contrast to a previous review which concluded that exercise is highly effective as a treatment intervention in depression (Mead *et al.*, 2009). In their review, Rimer *et al.* (2012) importantly state that it is not possible to give people accurate information about how effective exercise might be in the treatment of their depression, nor can they determine the optimum dose necessary for anti-depressant effects (Rimer *et al.*, 2012). These findings perhaps explain why the clinical use of exercise as an alternative to other established treatment approaches like psychotherapy or anti-depressant medication is still in its infancy (Ströhle, 2009).

Nevertheless, research in the field has attempted to establish the optimal dose (frequency, duration and intensity) of physical activity necessary to improve mental health outcomes for people with depression and anxiety. A review by Teychenne *et al*, (2008) found that the greatest benefits of physical activity on mental health were achieved when higher doses of activity were achieved. This higher dose was comparable to current public health guidelines of 150 minutes of moderate-intensity physical activity over a week (Department of Health, 2011). However, support was also obtained for much lower doses of physical activity with evidence suggesting that as little as 20–60 minutes of exercise per week can be protective against depression. It has also been suggested that it is the practice of regular physical activity that is associated with improvements in mental health (Azevedo Da Silva *et al.*, 2012). It is therefore important to initially reinforce frequency so that physical activity becomes habitual. The duration and intensity of the exercise can then gradually build up over time (Otto *et al.*, 2007).

Generally, people with depression and anxiety are at greater risk of being physically inactive than non-depressed individuals (Roshanaei-Moghaddam *et al.*, 2009). The relationship between physical activity and depression/anxiety is likely to be bidirectional: regular physical activity improves symptoms for individuals with these conditions, although having symptoms of depression/anxiety increases the probability of not meeting recommended levels of activity (Azevedo Da Silva *et al.*, 2012). Cognitive-behavioural strategies such as goal-setting, self-monitoring, activity assignments and supportive follow-up are effective techniques that may help depressed individuals to adopt and maintain a more physically active lifestyle. Activity diaries are a particularly useful self-monitoring tool that may promote physical activity in people with common mental health conditions. Diaries that include measures for mood or anxiety can provide individuals with direct feedback of the effect of exercise on subjective well-being. Focusing on short-term mood changes associated with physical activity has been found to be more motivating and tangible to patients than changes in physical fitness because the results are more immediate (Forsyth *et al.*, 2009).

Applying this to Emily

To enhance her mood, Emily would benefit from regular physical activity. Assessing her current activity level and supporting Emily to set realistic yet progressive goals would enable her to gradually increase her exercise to meet the recommended guideline of 150 minutes a week. An activity diary would reinforce the mood enhancing effects of exercise for behaviour change.

Diet in the treatment of depression

Dietary habits have only recently been recognised as having an impact on mental health and a growing body of epidemiological studies has demonstrated an association between depression and unhealthy eating patterns and poor food choices (Jacka and Berk, 2012). It is generally accepted that overall dietary pattern may be more important for the prevention and management of depression than the effect of any single nutrient. A seminal study by Sánchez-Villegas *et al.* (2009) reported that individuals adhering to the Mediterranean style diet reduced their risk of developing depression over time. The Mediterranean dietary pattern includes foods which may be protective against depressive symptoms, for example:

*   high ratio of monounsaturated fats to saturated fats
*   high intake of vegetables
*   high intake of fruit and nuts
*   moderate alcohol intake
*   low intake of meat or meat products
*   high intake of cereal
*   high fish intake.

By contrast, a Westernised dietary pattern, which is typically characterised by the consumption of calorie-dense foods which are high in saturated fats and sugars and low in essential micro-nutrients, has been linked to poorer mental health measures in adolescents and to increased anxiety in men and women (Oddy *et al.*, 2009; Jacka *et al.*, 2011). Indeed, depression itself can have an effect on appetite (decreased or increased) and this may also result in the decline of essential nutrients for physical and mental health (Mikolajczyk *et al.*, 2009). Adherence to national dietary guidelines is an important recommendation for people with depression, particularly when studies examining dietary improvements as a treatment strategy in depression are lacking (Jacka and Berk, 2012).

A number of cognitive-behavioural techniques may be used to strengthen healthy eating patterns in individuals with depression. Forsyth *et al.* (2009) found that a goal-based approach to lifestyle change was well received by patients with depression and/or anxiety in a primary care setting. A key feature of this approach was the inclusion of homework at the end of each session in order that patients could record and monitor their progress towards dietary and exercise goals. Homework activities have been used increasingly in the treatment of mental health conditions (Kazantzis *et al.*, 2000), and a recent meta-analysis has found that daily activity scheduling is effective in the treatment of depression in adults (Cuijpers *et al.*, 2007). Activity scheduling is a behavioural treatment which enables individuals with depression to monitor their mood in response to daily activities in order to establish connections between the two. The Food and Mood Diary (Mental Health Foundation) is a resource that may facilitate people with depression to self-regulate their mood in response to the foods they eat (Figure 10.1). This diary enables people to simply log their dietary intake across the week and record their mood accordingly. Completing the diary allows individuals to recognise how eating patterns and the consumption of particular foods can influence their mood. Dietary behaviour can then be modified to improve mood and reduce depressive symptoms.

Food & Mood Diary

This diary will help you understand how the way you feel is affected by what you drink and eat.

Write down what you have at each meal and for snacks in the table below and circle one of the faces to record how it made you feel in the 1-2 hours afterwards.

You should start to recognise which foods put you in a good mood and which do not. The next page shows you which foods might help improve the way you feel.

Week commencing: _____

	Eg.	Monday	Tuesday	Wednesday	Thursday	Friday	Saturday	Sunday
Breakfast		No breakfast						
Lunch		Tuna sandwich						
Dinner		Lasagne & vegetables						
Snacks		Apple, yoghurt						
Notes								

Visit our website for more on diet and mental health: www.mentalhealth.org.uk/food

mental
health
foundation

Nutritional Info

Eating foods rich in vitamins and minerals can affect the way you feel. This page shows which foods can improve the way you feel, and is taken from our Feeding Minds report.

	Can help with:	Foods that include magnesium:
Magnesium	Anxiety, depression, stress, irritability and insomnia	Spinach, watercress, avacados, peppers, broccoli, brussel sprouts, green cabbage, almonds, brazil nuts, cashews, peanuts, macadamias, pistachios, walnuts, pecans, pumpkin seeds, sunflower seeds, poppy seeds, oats, bran, long grain rice, buckwheat, barley, quinoa, plain yoghurt, baked beans, bananas, kiwi fruit, blackberries, strawberries, oranges, raisins, chocolate

	Can help with:	Foods that include vitamin B3:
Vitamin B3	Stress, depression	Brown rice, rice bran, wheatgerm, broccoli, mushrooms, cabbage, brussel sprouts, courgette, squash, peanuts, beef liver, beef kidney, pork, turkey, chicken, tuna, salmon, sunflower seeds

	Can help with:	Foods that include tryptophan:
Tryptophan	Depression, sleep problems	Skinless turkey, skinless chicken, plain yoghurt, milk, eggs, cheddar, gruyere, swiss cheese, cottage cheese, almonds, pistachios, pecan, hazelnuts, peanuts, soy nuts, poppy seeds, pumpkin seeds, sesame seeds, lentils, chickpeas, kidney beans, lima beans, soya, spinach, watercress, cabbage

	Can help with:	Foods that include zinc:
Zinc	Lack of motivation, poor appetite and depression	Oysters, mussels, shrimp, fortified breakfast cereal, cashews, walnuts, almonds, mozzarella, swiss cheese, cheddar chese, low fat yoghurt, chickpeas, kidney beans, baked beans, lima beans, lentils, miso, chicken (dark meat), turkey, lamb, pork, minced beef, pumpkin seeds, sesame seeds, spinach, mushrooms, squash, asparagus, broccoli, blackberries, kiwi fruit

mental health foundation

Visit our website for more on diet and mental health: www.mentalhealth.org.uk/food

Figure 10.1 Food and mood diary

Source: Available at: www.mentalhealth.org.uk/food

Applying this to Emily

Encouraging Emily to complete a Food and Mood Diary over the course of a week will enable her to recognise which foods improve her mood and which foods are to be avoided to reduce depressive symptoms. Emily can then modify her diet in response to her mood record.

Maintaining a balanced diet through the increased consumption of fruit and vegetables and the avoidance of high fat and sugary foods is a simple yet effective strategy to regulate Emily's mood.

Community level interventions

Interventions targeting physical activity in the community

Being physically active has clear benefits for people with common mental health disorders and community level interventions promoting an active lifestyle are particularly important for these individuals. Active transport is one such strategy that promotes active living at the community level, however, a recent meta-analysis by Barton and Pretty (2010) has also explored the impact of green exercise on mental health outcomes with promising results. They concluded that green space provides communities with a unique opportunity to improve mental health because physical activity in the presence of nature is associated with improvements in self-esteem and mood. Even short duration and light intensity physical activity in green space, such as walking in parks, resulted in immediate mental health benefits. The potential for green exercise as a therapeutic intervention for people with a mental health problem is great; however access to green space, particularly within urban settings, requires planning and investment at a strategic level.

Applying this to Emily

Regular physical activity in green space has important mood enhancing benefits that may improve Emily's depression. Emily could learn to self-regulate her mood by simply walking, jogging or cycling in local parks.

Interventions targeting smoking cessation in the community

Smoking is a known risk factor for depression and some anxiety disorders and smokers who are nicotine dependent tend to have poorer mental health outcomes than non-dependent smokers (Pedersen and von Soest, 2009). Policies promoting smoking cessation have a clear role to play in the physical and mental health of people who smoke. Smoke-free legislation in particular has the potential to reduce smoking prevalence at a population level by limiting people's opportunities to smoke in public places. The added advantage of this approach is that people's exposure to second-hand smoke is also reduced. The effects of this legislation are therefore two-fold because any reduction in smoke-exposure, either directly through smoking behaviour or indirectly through second-hand smoke, has the potential to improve mental health outcomes.

Working effectively with others

People with common mental health problems are usually treated within primary care (NICE, 2009) with GPs playing a pivotal role because they are usually the first person that patients see regarding their symptoms. This puts them in an ideal position to identify unhealthy lifestyle behaviours that may be impacting on patients' mental health. A multi-disciplinary approach to mental health care means that the skill and expertise of health and other allied professionals is often called upon to support and treat people with mental health disorders in primary care. Community mental health nurses, dieticians, psychologists and exercise specialists may all be involved in the care of people with a mental health diagnosis, and the reinforcement of national guidelines for diet and physical activity should be standard practice for all patients with depression and anxiety.

Befriending services for people with depression

Befriending is an intervention that aims to provide individuals with additional social support to be able to deal with the challenges of living with depression or other emotional distresses. In the UK there are over 500 charities and voluntary sector organisations currently offering befriending services. A recent systematic review and meta-analysis demonstrated that befriending interventions have a modest but significant effect on reducing depressive symptoms (Mead *et al.*, 2010). Although these results are promising, the current effectiveness evidence for befriending does not meet the National Institute for Health and Clinical Excellence guidelines for its adoption as a treatment option for depression (Mead *et al.*, 2010). Despite this, befriending is a relatively low cost supportive intervention that utilises the help of volunteers and lay people to support and help others to cope with the emotional distress arising from a mental health condition.

Applying this to Emily

The social support received through a befriending service at the university may help Emily to cope more effectively with her depression and adapt to the lifestyle changes necessary for its management.

Chronic Obstructive Pulmonary Disease: COPD

Case study

Malcolm is 58 and has smoked for most of his life, having started as a young teenager. His early retirement from the steelworks six months ago was inevitable because Malcolm has been suffering with breathing problems which are steadily worsening over time. Having suffered from a persistent productive cough and breathlessness on exertion for the past year, Malcolm reluctantly visited his GP for help. Tests have revealed that Malcolm has moderate COPD. His family are particularly concerned because Malcolm has also lost a significant amount of weight and his breathing problems are beginning to limit his daily activities. Malcolm and his family are keen to make changes to his lifestyle in order to improve his breathing and overall health.

Introduction

Chronic Obstructive Pulmonary Disease (COPD) is a long-term irreversible disease of the lungs in which the flow of air into the lungs is restricted by inflammation and damage to the lung tissue (NICE, 2010). Characteristic symptoms of COPD include a cough, sputum production and breathlessness on exertion and a diagnosis is made when airflow obstruction is detected on spirometry (Gruffydd-Jones and Loveridge, 2011). Bronchitis and emphysema are the two main types of COPD and the important causative factor for their development is smoking. It is estimated that 30–40 per cent of smokers who have smoked for over 25 years will develop COPD (Løkke et al, 2006). Other risk factors for the disease do exist however and these may include workplace exposure to fumes and chemicals, general environmental pollution, genetic disposition and socio-economic status. The condition is described as being progressive because it gradually gets worse over time, and this deterioration is often associated with poorly managed exacerbations. Exacerbations are particularly debilitating for individuals because they accelerate loss of lung function and reduce physical activity in daily life (Bourbeau, 2009). This downward spiral can lead to physical de-conditioning and ultimately death (Figure 10.2). Early treatment is essential to manage acute exacerbations and slow any decline in lung function in order to lengthen the time in which the individual can maintain an active life (Department of Health, 2011).

In the UK annual deaths from COPD have been fairly consistent over the past 25 years, ranging between 25,000 and 30,000 deaths each year (Health and Safety Executive, 2012). It is the fifth biggest killer nationally, with death rates much higher in the 75+ age range for both men and women (this group accounts for two thirds of all deaths from the disease). Accurately estimating prevalence rates for the disease is fraught with difficulties because levels of under-diagnosis and misdiagnosis in the early

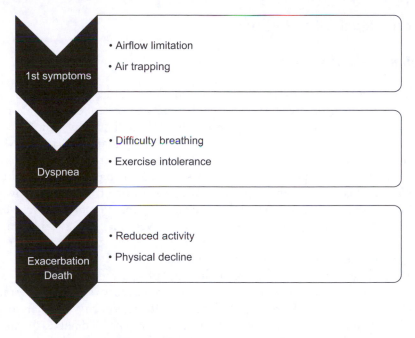

Figure 10.2 Disease course of chronic obstructive pulmonary disease
Source: Adapted from Fromer, 2011

stages are high (Department of Health, 2011). However, any delay in diagnosis can result in patients needlessly suffering symptoms and limitations that could otherwise be alleviated by appropriate management (Price *et al.*, 2011). According to the National Institute for Health and Clinical Excellence, the mean delay from onset to diagnosis is 20 years (NICE, 2010). Opportunities to prevent its progression in the early stages are therefore being missed.

Interventions to improve the health of people with COPD

Although not curable, COPD can be treated at any stage of the disease: mild, moderate or severe (O'Donnell *et al.*, 2008). Key to the successful management of the disease is the need for people to modify or change their health behaviour/s in order to preserve lung function and optimise their general health. In its early stages opportunities exist to prevent disease progression through lifestyle modification. Smoking cessation and physical activity are the two important lifestyle behaviours that impact on the health of people living with COPD (NICE, 2010).

Individual level interventions

Pulmonary rehabilitation

Available through the NHS for patients with a confirmed diagnosis of COPD, pulmonary rehabilitation seeks to restore individuals to the fullest possible physical, social and mental health. This is achieved through individually tailored physical exercise training, self-management advice and multi-disciplinary education (IMPRESS, 2008). Fundamentally, the programme aims to improve patients' exercise tolerance in order to support a more physically active lifestyle. This is particularly important for people with COPD because the negative consequences of prolonged inactivity have far-reaching consequences, with research demonstrating that impaired exercise capacity is a significant determinant of disease burden (van Wetering *et al.*, 2008). Improving exercise tolerance to support an active lifestyle is therefore an important treatment goal for people attending pulmonary rehabilitation.

The effectiveness of pulmonary rehabilitation programmes to improve exercise tolerance, dyspnoea (breathlessness) and health-related quality of life is well established (Maltais *et al.*, 2008; van Wetering *et al.*, 2010). Its approach is similar to that of Cardiac Rehabilitation and Structured Education for type 2 diabetes because it is underpinned by training in self-management and empowerment for behaviour change. Exercise training is a central focus of the programme and a combination of aerobic and strength training is advocated to concurrently increase exercise tolerance and improve muscle function. Indeed, low muscle mass due to skeletal muscle dysfunction is a strong predictor of mortality in COPD (Man *et al.*, 2009). In contrast to the irreversible abnormalities of the lungs, the skeletal muscle abnormalities in COPD can be improved or reversed by exercise training. In turn, exercise training through Pulmonary Rehabilitation can restore the patient to the highest level of functional capacity possible relative to their breathing impairment (Rochester, 2003).

Pulmonary rehabilitation typically consists of twice-weekly supervised sessions for a minimum of six weeks. Best practice guidance outlined by the Department of Health (2012) recommends the use of training diaries to log incremental progress through the setting of individualised goals for aerobic and strength (resistance) exercise training. As previously discussed, self-monitoring through diary keeping and goal setting are effective self-regulatory strategies for behaviour change. However, perceived self-efficacy is also an important construct here (Bandura, 1997) because research suggests that low self-efficacy for coping with exertional breathlessness is common in COPD (Wigal *et al.*, 1991). A recent review observed that pulmonary rehabilitation may actually increase motivation, self-efficacy for physical activity and functional capacity to support an active lifestyle in people with the condition (ZuWallack, 2009). In addition, pulmonary rehabilitation has been described as being instrumental in enhancing patients' participation in physical activity by improving their confidence to manage symptoms of breathlessness and by reducing their fear of exertional activity (Hogg *et al.*, 2012).

Box 10.1 Applying research in practice

People with COPD perceive ongoing, structured and socially supportive exercise opportunities to be important for maintaining an active lifestyle following pulmonary rehabilitation: a qualitative study (Hogg *et al.*, 2012)

This study explored the perceptions of people with COPD regarding maintaining an active lifestyle following participation in a pulmonary rehabilitation programme.

Focus groups were conducted with individuals with a diagnosis of COPD who had completed an 8-week pulmonary rehabilitation programme as an outpatient.

Ongoing peer and professional exercise support was perceived as fundamental for maintaining an active lifestyle after pulmonary rehabilitation. Participants valued the peer support found within pulmonary rehabilitation and expressed that this was an important factor for their continued participation in physical activity following a rehabilitation programme. Pulmonary rehabilitation was seen as a vehicle to facilitate greater participation in daily activities by improving self-confidence to manage breathlessness.

Applying this to Malcolm

Malcolm's capacity to become more physically active will be enhanced through participation in a pulmonary rehabilitation programme accessed through the NHS. The individualised exercise-training component of rehabilitation will improve and strengthen Malcolm's muscle function and enable him to self-manage acute episodes of breathlessness. The support gained from peers and professionals during the programme may help Malcolm to increase his daily activity level.

Interventions promoting smoking cessation

Quitting smoking is the most effective way to slow decline in lung function for people with COPD (ZuWallack, 2007). It is also the most cost-effective intervention and smokers with COPD should therefore be offered smoking cessation support as treatment for their disease (Hoogendoorn *et al.*, 2010). Health messages constructed around the concepts of lung health and lung age provide a positive way of expressing behaviour change messages and have demonstrated positive effects on smoking cessation in people with COPD (DoH, 2011). The concept of lung age is a psychological tool that shows smokers the apparent premature aging of their lungs due to their smoking behaviour (Morris and Temple, 1985). Promising findings from the Step2quit randomised controlled trial in the UK found that telling smokers their lung age was effective in promoting smoking cessation in this client group: 13.6 per cent of smokers who were told their lung age were not smoking at 12 months compared with 6.4 per cent who were not told their lung age (Parkes *et al.*, 2008). Interestingly, the act of simply telling people their lung age increased the likelihood of them stopping smoking irrespective of whether the lung age was within normal range. This study therefore gives support to the effective use of personal biomarker feedback to self-regulate behaviour, and strongly advocates the practice of giving patients their spirometric results expressed as lung age along with advice about the dangers of smoking and methods of quitting (Parkes *et al.*, 2008).

Applying this to Malcolm

Communicating Malcolm's spirometric results as 'lung age' may help him to quit smoking in the long term.

Community level interventions

COPD is largely caused by smoking, so interventions promoting smoking cessation at the community level have clear benefits to people with the condition. Policies that raise awareness of the dangers of second-hand smoke and legislation that restricts smoking in enclosed public spaces have been effective in altering people's attitudes towards the social acceptability of smoking. This shift in attitude may support the efforts of people with COPD who are attempting to quit because opportunities to smoke in public are reduced.

Physical activity is recognised as an important health behaviour in terms of benefits to quality of life and survival in people with COPD (Bourbeau, 2009). Public health campaigns that promote participation in physical activity at the community level are therefore important for this client group. Active transport schemes are a good example of how physical activity can be promoted within the community through engagement in walking and cycling initiatives. Integrating physical activity flexibly into daily routine in this way may be an appealing alternative to other structured forms of exercise, particularly for people with physical limitations associated with this complex health condition.

Applying this to Malcolm

The opportunity for Malcolm to smoke when he socialises locally with friends is now restricted by smoking legislation. These restrictions will support his attempts to quit smoking.

Malcolm can increase his daily activity by walking to and from the local shops rather than relying on his car as a mode of transport. Incorporating regular physical activity into his daily routine will gradually increase his exercise capacity in order to prevent further decline in lung function.

Working effectively with others

COPD care is delivered by a multi-disciplinary team and may include input from respiratory nurse specialists, physiotherapists, occupational therapists and dieticians (NICE, 2010). Although patients are generally cared for within primary care, acute exacerbations often require hospitalisation so a collaborative approach to disease management across the primary and secondary care sector is essential. Referral to a dietician is common for patients with moderate to severe COPD because this stage of the condition is associated with being underweight and having reduced muscle mass. Indeed, a UK based study identified that 23 per cent of subjects with COPD were classified as malnourished (Cochrane and Afolabi, 2004).

Nutritional management is an important aspect of care in this client group because weight loss is associated with decreased lung capacity, health status and increased morbidity (Houghton, 2008). The National Institute for Health and Clinical Excellence (NICE, 2010) guidelines for the management of COPD in adults suggests that nutritional supplements may be considered for individuals with a low BMI alongside regular exercise to increase muscle mass. As COPD progresses, breathlessness when eating may also restrict the amount a person can eat at one time so patients should be encouraged to adopt eating strategies to optimise their nutritional intake, such as eating frequent, small meals over the course of a day (Houghton, 2008).

Peer support is vital in motivating individuals to initiate and make sustained changes to their lifestyle (Matheson *et al.*, 2010). The efficacy of peer support to help people with COPD to stop smoking has been demonstrated by a recent buddy-led smoking cessation intervention (Cox, 2011). The Hope 2 Quit intervention harnessed the support of 'buddies' or expert patients with COPD who worked collaboratively with the multi-disciplinary team to design and deliver the smoking cessation intervention. The intervention was successful in supporting short- and long-term quit rates for those receiving buddy support. With a four-week quit rate of 81 per cent and a one-year quit rate of 50 per cent it is hard to ignore the impact that social support from buddies can achieve in this client group.

Applying this to Malcolm

Malcolm would benefit from dietetic advice and support because of his ongoing weight loss. This may include advice about eating strategies and dietary supplementation to optimise his nutritional status and increase his body weight and muscle mass.

A buddy scheme may provide Malcolm with the necessary social support to effectively quit smoking.

Conclusion

It is clear that the lifestyle choices we make can have a profound effect on our health over time. Rising prevalence rates for many of the chronic conditions that we see in the UK today suggest that lifestyle behaviours are significantly impacting on the health of the nation. These conditions tend to be progressive and long term, and when poorly managed can lead to further health problems and a reduced quality of life. Lifestyle interventions can be used effectively to manage conditions such as type 2 diabetes, CHD, COPD and depression. Health professionals must endeavour to work collaboratively with clients to promote health through behaviour change. There is evidence of a shift towards greater client autonomy whereby individuals are now encouraged to be active self-managers of their condition. This self-management often requires individuals to make and sustain multiple changes to their lifestyle. Behaviour change is never easy and challenges clearly exist for people with health limitations due to chronic illness. Nevertheless, psychological techniques for health behaviour change have been shown to be effective in improving health outcomes for people with specific conditions.

Key points

- Unhealthy lifestyles contribute to the high prevalence of chronic disorders in the UK.
- Positive and sustained changes to lifestyle can help manage these long-term health conditions.

- Self-regulatory techniques such as self-monitoring and goal setting are particularly effective in promoting behaviour change in clinical groups.
- Individuals are encouraged to be active self-managers of their condition.
- Multi-disciplinary teams are often involved in the care of people with ongoing health conditions.

Points for discussion

- How would you support an individual who is newly diagnosed with type 2 diabetes to self-manage their condition?
- Identify which self-regulatory strategies are important to support behaviour change in people with a long-term health condition. What are the relative benefits and limitations for each strategy you have identified?
- What factors do you need to consider when promoting a physically active lifestyle for individuals following a cardiac event?

Further resources

Diabetes UK: www.diabetes.org.uk
British Heart Foundation: www.bhf.org.uk
Mind, the mental health charity: www.mind.org.uk
Mental Health Foundation: www.mentalhealth.org.uk
British Lung Foundation: www.blf.org.uk

References

Introduction

Buck, D. and Frosini, F. (2012). *Clustering of Unhealthy Behaviours Over Time: Implications for Policy and Practice*. London: The Kings Fund.
Noordman, J., van der Weijden, T. and van Dulmen, S. (2012). Communication-related behavior change techniques used in face-to-face lifestyle interventions in primary care: a systematic review of the literature. *Patient Education and Counseling*, 89(2): 227–224.

Type 2 diabetes

Anderson, R.M. and Funnell, M.M. (2000). *The Art of Empowerment: Stories and Strategies for Diabetes Educators*. Cited in T. Deakin (2012). X-PERT structured education programmes improve control in diabetes. *Journal of Diabetes Nursing*, 16(7): 266–272
Bailey, C.J. (2011). The challenge of managing coexistent type 2 diabetes and obesity. *BMJ*: 342.

Baksi, A.K., Al-Mrayat, M., Hogan, D., Whittingstall, E., Wilson, P. and Wex, J. (2008). Peer advisers compared with specialist health professionals in delivering a training programme on self-management to people with diabetes: a randomized controlled trial. *Diabetic Medicine*, 25(9): 1076–1082.

Barrows, H.S. (1996). Problem-based learning in medicine and beyond. In T. Deakin (2012). X-PERT structured education programmes improve control in diabetes. *Journal of Diabetes Nursing*, 16(7): 266–272.

Brennan, A. (1996). Diabetes mellitus: biomedical health education/promotion approach. *British Journal of Nursing*, 5(17): 1060–1064.

Boothroyd, R.I. and Fisher, E.B. (2010). Peers for progress: promoting peer support for health around the world. *Family Practice*, 27(suppl 1): i62–i68.

Cade, J.E., Kirk, S.F.L., Nelson, P., Hollins, L., Deakin, T., Greenwood, D.C. and Harvey, E.L. (2009). Can peer educators influence healthy eating in people with diabetes? Results of a randomized controlled trial. *Diabetic Medicine*, 26(10):1048–1054.

Chudyk, A. and Petrella, R.J. (2011). Effects of exercise on cardiovascular risk factors in type 2 diabetes a meta-analysis. *Diabetes Care*, 34(5): 1228–1237.

Davies, M.J., Heller, S., Skinner, T.C., Campbell, M.J., Carey, M.E., Cradock, S.. Khunti, K. *et al.* (2008). Effectiveness of the diabetes education and self management for ongoing and newly diagnosed (DESMOND) programme for people with newly diagnosed type 2 diabetes: cluster randomised controlled trial. *BMJ*, 336(7642): 491–495.

Deakin, T.A. (2012). X-PERT structured education programmes improve control in diabetes. Journal of Diabetes Nursing, 16(7): 266–272.

Deakin, T.A., Cade, J.E., Williams, R. and Greenwood, D.C. (2006). Structured patient education: the Diabetes X-PERT Programme makes a difference. *Diabetic Medicine*, 23(9): 944–954.

Diabetes UK (2010). *Diabetes in the UK 2010: Key Statistics on Diabetes*. Available at: http://www.diabetes.org.uk/Documents/Reports/Diabetes_in_the_UK_2010.pdf (accessed 1 September 2012).

Department of Health (2001a). *National Service Framework for Diabetes*. London: Department of Health. Available at http://www.doh.gov.uk/nsf/diabetes/index.htm (accessed 1 September 2012).

——(2001b). *The Expert Patient*. London: Department of Health. Available at http://www.doh.gov.uk/cmo/ep-report.pdf (accessed 10 September 2012).

——(2009). *Change4Life*. London: Department of Health. Available at: www.dh.gov.uk/en/MediaCentre/Currentcampaigns/Change4Life/index.htm (accessed 18 April 2012).

Department of Health, Physical Activity, Health Improvement and Protection (2011). *Start Active, Stay Active*. London: Department of Health.

Duke, S.A., Colagiuri, S. and Colagiuri, R. (2009). Individual patient education for people with type 2 diabetes mellitus. *Cochrane Database Syst Rev*, 1(1).

Funnell, M.M. (2010). Peer-based behavioural strategies to improve chronic disease self-management and clinical outcomes: evidence, logistics, evaluation considerations and needs for future research. *Family Practice*, 27(suppl 1): i17–i22.

Gruber, K.J. (2008). Social support for exercise and dietary habits among college students. *Adolescence (San Diego): An International Quarterly Devoted to the Physiological, Psychological, Psychiatric, Sociological, and Educational Aspects of the Second Decade of Human Life*, 43(171): 557.

Healy, G.N., Wijndaele, K., Dunstan, D.W., Shaw, J.E., Salmon, J., Zimmet, P Z. and Owen, N. (2008). Objectively measured sedentary time, physical activity, and metabolic risk: the Australian Diabetes, Obesity and Lifestyle Study (AusDiab). *DiabetesCare*, 31(2): 369–371.

Healy, G.N., Dunstan, D.W., Salmon, J., Cerin, E., Shaw, J.E., Zimmet, P.Z. and Owen, N. (2008). Breaks in sedentary time beneficial associations with metabolic risk. *Diabetes Care*, 31(4): 661–666.

Jarvis, J., Skinner, T.C., Carey, M.E. and Davies, M.J. (2010). How can structured self-management patient education improve outcomes in people with type 2 diabetes? *Diabetes, Obesity and Metabolism*, 12(1): 12–19.

Kavookjian, J., Elswick, B.M. and Whetsel, T. (2007). Interventions for being active among individuals with diabetes: a systematic review of the literature. *The Diabetes Educator*, 33(6): 962–988.

Kirk, A., Barnett, J., Leese, G. and Mutrie, N. (2009). A randomized trial investigating the 12-month changes in physical activity and health outcomes following a physical activity consultation delivered by a person or in written form in type 2 diabetes: Time2Act. *Diabetic Medicine*, 26(3): 293–301.

Loveman, E., Frampton, G.K. and Clegg, A.J. (2008). The clinical effectiveness of diabetes education models for type 2 diabetes: a systematic review. *Health Technology Assessment*, 12(9): 1–136.

Marwick, T.H., Hordern, M.D., Miller, T., Chyun, D.A., Bertoni, A.G., Blumenthal, R. S. and Rocchini, A. (2009). Exercise training for type 2 diabetes mellitus impact on cardiovascular risk: a scientific statement from the American Heart Association. *Circulation*, 119(25): 3244–3262.

Nolan, C.J., Damm, P. and Prentki, M. (2011). Type 2 diabetes across generations: from pathophysiology to prevention and management. *Lancet*, 378(9786): 169–181.

Peel, E., Douglas, M., Parry, O. and Lawton, J. (2010). Type 2 diabetes and dog walking: patients' longitudinal perspectives about implementing and sustaining physical activity. *The British Journal of General Practice*, 60(577): 570.

Scheumer, M.T., Sieverding, P. and Shekelle, P.G. (2008). Delivery of genomic medicine for common chronic adult diseases. A systematic review. *Journal of American Medical Association*, 299(11): 1320–1334.

Smith, S. M., Paul, G., Kelly, A., Whitford, D.L., O'Shea, E. and O'Dowd, T. (2011). Peer support for patients with type 2 diabetes: cluster randomised controlled trial. *BMJ: British Medical Journal*, 342.

Steinsbekk, A., Rygg, L., Lisulo, M., Rise, M.B. and Fretheim, A. (2012). Group based diabetes self-management education compared to routine treatment for people with type 2 diabetes mellitus. A systematic review with meta-analysis. *BMC Health Services Research*, 12(1): 213.

Umpierre, D., Ribeiro, P.A., Kramer, C.K., Leitão, C.B., Zucatti, A.T., Azevedo, M.J. Schaan, B.D. et al. (2011). Physical activity advice only or structured exercise training and association with HbA1c Levels in type 2 diabetes: a systematic review and meta-analysis. *JAMA: The Journal of the American Medical Association*, 305(17): 1790–1799.

United Kingdom Prospective Diabetes Study (UKPDS) Group (1998). Intensive blood-glucose control with sulphonylureas or insulin compared with conventional treatment and risk of complications in patients with type 2 diabetes (UKPDS 33). *Lancet,* 352: 837–853.

Upton, D. and Thirlaway, K. (2010). *Promoting Healthy Behaviour.* London: Pearson.

van der Wulp, I., de Leeuw, J.R.J., Gorter, K.J. and Rutten, G.E.H.M. (2012). Effectiveness of peer-led self-management coaching for patients recently diagnosed with type 2 diabetes mellitus in primary care: a randomized controlled trial. *Diabetic Medicine*, 29(10): e390–e397.

Wei, M., Gibbons, L.W., Kampert, J.B., Nichaman, M.Z. and Blair, S. N. (2000). Low cardio respiratory fitness and physical inactivity as predictors of mortality in men with type 2 diabetes. *Annals of Internal Medicine*, 132(8): 605.

World Health Organization (2008). *Peer Support Programmes in Diabetes: Report of a WHO Consultation 5–7 November 2007*. Geneva: Switzerland: WHO.

Yates, T., Khunti, K., Troughton, J. and Davies, M. (2009). The role of physical activity in the management of type 2 diabetes mellitus. *Postgraduate Medical Journal*, 85(1001): 129–133.

Coronary heart disease

Artinian, N.T., Fletcher, G.F., Mozaffarian D., Kris-Etherton, P., Van Horn, L., Lichtenstein, A.H. *et al.* (2010). Interventions to promote physical activity and dietary lifestyle changes for cardiovascular risk factor reduction in adults. A scientific statement from the American Heart Association. *Circulation*, 122: 406–441

Barth, J., Schneider, S. and von Känel, R. (2010). Lack of social support in the etiology and the prognosis of coronary heart disease: a systematic review and meta-analysis. *Psychosomatic Medicine*, 72(3): 229–238.

Blumenthal, J.A., Babyak, M.A., Doraiswamy, P.M. *et al.* (2007). Exercise and pharmacotherapy in the treatment of major depressive disorder. *Psychosomatic Medicine*, 69(7): 587–596.

British Heart Foundation (2007). Cardiac rehabilitation...recovery or by-pass? *National Campaign for Cardiac Rehabilitation. The Evidence*. Available at: http://www.bhf.org. uk/publications/view-publication (accessed 20 September 2012).

——(2010). *Coronary Heart Disease Statistics 2010*. Available at: www.heartstats.org (accessed 20 September 2012).

——(2011). *The National Audit of Cardiac Rehabilitation. The Annual Statistical Report 2011*. Available at: http://www.bhf.org.uk/publications/view-publication (accessed 18 September 2012).

Burke, L.E., Sereika, S.M., Music, E., Warziski, M., Styn, M.A. and Stone, A. (2008). Using instrumented paper diaries to document self-monitoring patterns in weight-loss. *Contemporary Clinical Trials*, 29(2): 182–193.

Chow, C.K., Jolly, S., Rao-Melacini, P., Fox, K.A.A., Anand, S.S. and Yusuf, S. (2010). Association of diet, exercise, and smoking modification with risk of early cardiovascular events after acute coronary syndromes. *Circulation*, 121: 750–758.

Department of Health (2000). *National Service Framework for Coronary Heart Disease, 2000;* Chapter 7, Cardiac Rehabilitation. Available at: www.dh.gov.uk/assetRoot/04/05/75/24/04057524.pdf (accessed 15 September 2012).

——(2001). *Exercise Referral Systems: A National Quality Assurance Framework*. London: Department of Health.

Goldston, K. and Baillie, A.J. (2008). Depression and coronary heart disease: a review of the epidemiological evidence, explanatory mechanisms and management approaches. *Clinical Psychology Review*, 28: 288–306.

Goulding, L., Furze, G. and Birks, Y. (2010). Randomized controlled trials of interventions to change maladaptive illness beliefs in people with coronary heart disease: systematic review. *Journal of Advanced Nursing*, 66(5): 946–961.

Gulliksson, M., Burell, G., Vessby, B., Lundin, L., Toss, H. and Svardsudd, K. (2011). Randomized controlled trial of cognitive behavioural therapy vs. standard treatment to prevent recurrent cardiovascular events in patients with coronary heart disease. *Arch International Medicine*, 171(2): 134–140.

Held, C., Iqbal, R., Lear, S.A., Rosengren, A., Islam, S., Mathew, J. and Yusaf, S. (2012). Physical activity levels, ownership of goods promoting sedentary behaviour and risk of myocardial infarction: results of the INTERHEART study. *European Heart Journal*, 33: 452–466.

Heran, B., Chen, J.M.H., Ebrahi. S., Moxham, T., Oldridge, N., Rees, K., Thompson, D.R. and Taylor, R.S. (2011). Exercise-based cardiac rehabilitation for coronary heart disease. *Cochrane Database of Systematic Reviews*, 7. DOI: 10.1002/14651858.CD001800. pub2.

Janssen, V., De Gucht, V., Dusseldorp, E. and Maes, S. (2012). Lifestyle modification programmes for patients with coronary heart disease: a systematic review and meta-analysis of randomized controlled trials. *European Journal of Preventive Cardiology*. Online publication, 1–21

Jarrett, J., Woodcock, J., Griffiths, U.K., Chalabi, Z., Edwards, P., Roberts, I. and Haines, A. (2012). Effects of increasing active travel in urban England and Wales on costs to the National Health Service. *Lancet*, 379: 2198–205.

Lavie, C.J., Thomas, R.J., Squires, R.W., Allison, T.G. and Milani, R.V. (2009). Exercise training and cardiac rehabilitation in primary and secondary prevention of coronary heart disease. *Mayo Clinic Proceedings*, 84(4): 373–383.

Lett, H.S., Blumenthal, J.A., Babyak, M.A., Sherwood, A., Strauman, T., Robins, C. and Newman, M.F. (2004). Depression as a risk factor for coronary artery disease: evidence, mechanisms, and treatment. *Psychosomatic Medicine*, 66(3): 305–315.

Morrato, E.H., Hill, J.O., Wyatt, H.R., Ghushchyan, V. and Sullivan, P.W. (2007). Physical activity in US adults with diabetes and at risk for developing diabetes, 2003. *Diabetes Care*, 30(2): 203–209.

Mozaffarian, D., Wilson, P. and Kannel, W. (2008). Beyond established and novel risk factors: lifestyle risk factors for cardiovascular disease. *Circulation*, 117: 3031–3038.

NACR (2010). *British Heart Foundation. The National Audit of Cardiac Rehabilitation: Annual Statistical Report*. Available at: http://www.cardiacrehabilitation.org.uk/nacr/docs/2010.pdf (accessed 15 September 2012).

National Institute for Health and Clinical Excellence (NICE) (2007a). *Behaviour Change at Population, Community and Individual Level* [NICE public health guidance 6]. Available at: http://www.nice.org.uk/nicemedia/live/11868/37987/37987.pdf (accessed 5 October 2012).

——(2007b). *MI Secondary Prevention: NICE Clinical Guidance 48*. Available at: http://www.nice.org.uk/cg048 (accessed 23 September 2012).

Olivio, E.L., Dodson-Lavelle, B., Wren, A., Fang, Y., and Mehmet, C.O (2009). Feasibility and effectiveness of a brief meditation-based stress management intervention for patients diagnosed with or at risk for coronary heart disease: a pilot study. *Psychology, Health and Medicine*, 14(5): 513–523.

Riegel, B.J. (1993). Contributions to cardiac invalidism after acute myocardial infarction. *Coronary Artery Disease*, 4: 215–220.

Sniehotta, F., Gorski, C. and Araujo-Soares, V. (2010). Adoption of community-based cardiac rehabilitation programs and physical activity following phase III cardiac rehabilitation in Scotland: a prospective and predictive study. *Psychology and Health*, 25(7): 839–854.

Tierney, P., Hughes, C. and Hamilton, S. (2011). Promoting health behaviour change in the cardiac patient. *British Journal of Cardiac Nursing*, 6(3): 126–130.

Wellenius, G.A., Mukamal, K.J., Kulshreshtha, A., Asonganyi, S. and Mittleman, M.A. (2008). Depressive symptoms and the risk of atherosclerotic progression among patients with coronary artery bypass grafts. *Circulation*, 117(18): 2313–2319.

Whooley, M.A. (2006). Depression and cardiovascular disease: healing the broken-hearted. *JAMA*, 295(24): 2874–2881.

Whooley, M.A., de Jonge, P., Vittinghoff, E., Otte, C., Moos, R., Carney, R.M., Ali, S., Dowray, S., Na, B., Feldman, M.D., Schiller, N.B. and Browner, W.S. (2008). Depressive symptoms, health behaviours, and the risk of cardiovascular events in patients with coronary heart disease. *JAMA*, 300(20): 2379–2388.

Yusuf, S., Hawken, S., Ounpuu, S. *et al.* (2004). Effect of potentially modifiable risk factors associated with myocardial infarction in 52 countries (the INTERHEART Study): case-control study. *Lancet*, 364(9438): 937–952.

Depression

Azevedo Da Silva, M., Singh-Manoux, A., Brunner, E.J., Kaffashian, S., Shipley, M. J., Kivimäki, M. and Nabi, H. (2012). Bidirectional association between physical activity and symptoms of anxiety and depression: the Whitehall II study. *European Journal of Epidemiology*, 27: 537–546.

Barton, J. and Pretty, J. (2010). What is the best dose of nature and green exercise for improving mental health? A multi-study analysis. *Environmental Science & Technology*, 44(10): 3947–3955.

Cuijpers, P., Van Straten, A. and Warmerdam, L. (2007). Behavioral activation treatments of depression: a meta-analysis. *Clinical Psychology Review*, 27(3): 318–326.

Department of Health (2001). *Exercise Referral Systems: A National Quality Assurance Framework*. Available at: http://www.dh.gov.uk/en/Publicationsandstatistics/Publications/PublicationsPolicyAndGuidance/DH40096712001 (accessed 28 September 2012).

Forsyth, A., Deane, F.P. and Williams, P. (2009). Dietitians and exercise physiologists in primary care: lifestyle interventions for patients with depression and/or anxiety. *Journal of Allied Health*, 38(2): 63E–68E.

Jacka, F.N. and Berk, M. (2012). Depression, diet and exercise. *Medical Journal of Australia*, 10: 21.

Jacka, F.N., Mykletun, A., Berk, M., Bjelland, I. and Tell, G.S. (2011). The association between habitual diet quality and the common mental disorders in community-dwelling adults: the Hordaland Health Study. *Psychosomatic medicine*, 73(6): 483–490.

Kazantzis, N., Deane, F.P. and Ronan, K.R. (2000). Homework assignments in cognitive and behavioural therapy: a meta-analysis. *Clinical Psychology: Science and Practice*, 7(2): 189–202.

Mead, G.E., Morley, W., Campbell, P., Greig, C.A., McMurdo, M. and Lawlor, D.A. (2009). Exercise for depression. *Cochrane Database of Systematic Reviews*, Issue 3 (accessed 30 September 2012). DOI: 10.1002/14651858.CD004366.pub4.

Mead, N., Lester, H., Chew-Graham, C., Gask, L. and Bower, P. (2010). Effects of befriending on depressive symptoms and distress: systematic review and meta-analysis. *British Journal of Psychiatry*, 196(2): 96–110

Mental Health Foundation (2012). *Mental Health Statistics: Men and Women*. Available at: http://www.mentalhealth.org.uk/help-information/mental-health-statistics/men-women/?view=Standard (accessed 5 November 2012).

Mikolajczyk, R.T., El Ansari, W. and Maxwell, A.E. (2009). Food consumption frequency and perceived stress and depressive symptoms among students in three European countries. *Nutrition Journal*, 8(1): 31.

National Institute of Health and Clinical Excellence (NICE) (2004). *Depression: Management of Depression in Primary and Secondary Care. National Clinical Practice Guideline 23*. Available at: http://www.nice.org.uk/cg023 (accessed 14 November 2012).

——(2009). *The Treatment and Management of Depression in Adults. NICE Clinical Guideline 90*. Available at: http://www.nice.org.uk/nicemedia/live/12329/45888/45888. pdf (accessed 14 November 2012).

Pedersen, W. and von Soest, T. (2009). Smoking, nicotine dependence and mental health among young adults: a 13-year population-based longitudinal study. *Addiction*, 104(1): 129–137.

Prince, M., Patel, V., Saxena, S., Maj, M., Maselko, J., Phillips, M.R. and Rahman, A. (2007). No health without mental health. *Lancet*, 370(9590): 859–877.

Otto, M.W., Church, T.S., Craft, L.L., Greer, T.L., Smits, J.A. and Trivedi, M.H. (2007). Exercise for mood and anxiety disorders. *Primary Care Companion to the Journal of Clinical Psychiatry*, 9(4): 287–294.

Oddy, W.H., Robinson, M., Ambrosini, G.L., de Klerk, N.H., Beilin, L.J., Silburn, S.R., Stanley, F.J. *et al.* (2009). The association between dietary patterns and mental health in early adolescence. *Preventive Medicine*, 49(1): 39–44.

Rimer, J., Dwan, K., Lawlor, D.A., Greig, C.A., McMurdo, M., Morley, W. and Mead, G.E. (2012). Exercise for depression. *Cochrane Database Syst Rev*, 7.

Roshanaei-Moghaddam, B., Katon, W.J. and Russo, J. (2009).The longitudinal effects of depression on physical activity. *General Hospital Psychiatry*, 31(4): 306–315.

Sánchez-Villegas, A., Delgado-Rodriguez, M., Alonso, A., Schlatter, J., Lahortiga, F., Majem, L.S. and Martinez-Gonzalez, M.A. (2009). Association of the Mediterranean dietary pattern with the incidence of depression: the Seguimiento Universidad de Navarra/ University of Navarra follow-up (SUN) cohort. *Archives of General Psychiatry*, 66(10): 1090–1098.

Ströhle, A. (2009). Physical activity, exercise, depression and anxiety disorders. *Journal of Neural Transmission*, 116(6): 777–784.

Teychenne, M., Ball, K. and Salmon, J. (2008). Physical activity and likelihood of depression in adults: a review. *Preventive medicine*, 46(5): 397–411.

The Health & Social Care Information Centre (2009). *Adult Psychiatric Morbidity in England, Results of a Household Survey*. Available at: http://www.mind.org.uk/help/ research_and_policy/statistics_1_how_common_is_mental_distress#common (accessed 5 October 2012).

Tylee, A., Haddad, M., Barley, E., Ashworth, M., Brown, J., Chambers, J., Walters, P. *et al.* (2012). A pilot randomised controlled trial of personalised care for depressed patients with symptomatic coronary heart disease in South London general practices: the UPBEAT-UK RCT protocol and recruitment. *BMC Psychiatry*, 12(1): 58.

World Health Organization (2005). *Mental Health Facing the Challenges, Building Solutions*. Report from the WHO European Ministerial Conference. Copenhagen, Denmark: WHO Regional Office for Europe.

——(2010). *International Statistical Classification of Diseases and Related Health Problems 10th Revision (ICD-10)* Version for 2010. Chapter V Mental and behavioural disorders (F00–F99). Available at: http://apps.who.int/classifications/icd10/browse/2010/en#/ F30-F39 (accessed 1 November 2012).

COPD

Bandura, A. (1997). *Self-efficacy: The Exercise of Control*. New York: Freeman.

Bourbeau, J. (2009). Activities of life: the COPD patient. *COPD: Journal of Chronic Obstructive Pulmonary Disease*, 6(3): 192–200.

Cochrane, W.J. and Afolabi, O.A. (2004). Investigation into the nutritional status, dietary intake and smoking habits of patients with chronic obstructive pulmonary disease. *Journal of Human Nutrition and Dietetics*, 17(1): 3–11.

Cox, K. (2011). Smoking cessation buddies in COPD. *Nursing Times*, 107(44): 22.

Department of Health (2011). *A Strategic Approach to Prevention and Early Identification of COPD*. Available at http://www.improvement.nhs.uk (accessed 15 November 2012).

——(2012). *Service Specification. Pulmonary Rehabilitation Service*. London: Department of Health. Available at: www.dh.gov.uk/publications (accessed 25 November 2012).

Fromer, L. (2011). Diagnosing and treating COPD: understanding the challenges and finding solutions. *International Journal of General Medicine*, 4: 729–739.

Gruffydd-Jones, K. and Loveridge, C. (2011). The 2010 NICE COPD Guidelines: how do they compare with the GOLD guidelines? *Primary Care Respiratory Journal*, 20(2): 199–204.

Health and Safety Executive (2012). *Chronic Obstructive Pulmonary Disease (COPD)*. Available at: http://www.hse.gov.uk/statistics/index.htm (accessed 27 November 2012).

Hogg, L., Grant, A., Garrod, R. and Fiddler, H. (2012). People with COPD perceive ongoing, structured and socially supportive exercise opportunities to be important for maintaining an active lifestyle following pulmonary rehabilitation: a qualitative study. *Journal of Physiotherapy*, 58(3): 189–195.

Hoogendoorn, M., Feenstra, T.L., Hoogenveen, R.T. and Rutten-van Mölken, M.P. (2010). Long-term effectiveness and cost-effectiveness of smoking cessation interventions in patients with COPD. *Thorax*, 65(8): 711–718.

Houghton, L. (2008). The nutritional management of weight loss in COPD. *BPJ*, 15: 16–17.

IMPRESS (Improving and Integrating Respiratory Services, 2008). *Principles, Definitions and Standards for Pulmonary Rehabilitation*. Available at: http://www.impressresp.com/ServiceSpecifications/tabid/60/Default.aspx (accessed 20 November 2012).

Løkke, A., Lange, P., Scharling, H., Fabricius, P. and Vestbo, J. (2006). Developing COPD: a 25-year follow up study of the general population. *Thorax*, 61(11): 935–939.

Maltais, F., Bourbeau, J., Shapiro, S. *et al.* (2008). Effects of home-based pulmonary rehabilitation in patients with chronic obstructive pulmonary disease: a randomised trial. *Annals of International Medicine*, 149: 869–878.

Man, W., Kemp, P., Moxham, J. and Polkey, M. (2009). Skeletal muscle dysfunction in COPD: clinical and laboratory observations. *Clinical Science*, 117: 251–264.

Matheson, L., O'Connor, J., Cartwright, T., Blunt, C.H., Clow, A., Lee, C. and Elkin, S. (2010). P44 COPD patients derived benefits from attending PR: 'This has given me my life back'. *Thorax*, 65 (Suppl 4): A95–A95.

Morris, J.F. and Temple, W. (1985). Spirometric 'lung age' estimation for motivating smoking cessation. *Preventive Medicine*, 14: 655–662.

National Institute for Health and Clinical Excellence (NICE).(2010). *Chronic Obstructive Pulmonary Disease. Management of Chronic Obstructive Pulmonary Disease in Adults in Primary and Secondary Care. Clinical Guideline 101*. London (UK): National Institute for Health and Clinical Excellence (NICE).

O'Donnell, D.E., Hermandez, P., Kaplan, A. *et al.* (2008). Canadian Thoracic Society recommendations for management of chronic obstructive pulmonary disease – 2008 update – highlights for primary care. *Canadian Respiratory Journal*, 15 Supplement A: 1A–8A.

Parkes, G., Greenhalgh, T., Griffin, M. and Dent, R. (2008). Effect on smoking quit rate of telling patients their lung age: the Step2quit randomised controlled trial. *BMJ*, 336(7644): 598–600.

Price, D., Freeman, D., Cleland, J., Kaplan, A., and Cerasoli F. (2011). Earlier diagnosis and earlier treatment of COPD in primary care. *Primary Care Respiratory Journal*, 20(1): 15–22.

Rochester, C.L. (2003). Exercise training in chronic obstructive pulmonary disease. *Journal of Rehabilitation Research and Development*, 40(5): 59–80.

van Wetering, C.R., Van Nooten, F.E, Mol, S.J.M. *et al.* (2008). Systemic impairment in relation to disease burden in patients with moderate COPD eligible for a lifestyle program. *International Journal of COPD*, 3: 443–451.

van Wetering, C.R., Hoogendoorn, M., Mol, S.J.M., Rutten-van Molken, M.P.M. and Schols, A.M. (2010). Short and long-term efficacy of a community-based COPD management programme in less advanced COPD: a randomised controlled trial. *Thorax*, 65: 7–13.

Wigal, J.K., Creer, T.L. and Kotses, H. (1991). The COPD self-efficacy scale. *Chest*, 95: 1193–1196.

ZuWallack, R. (2007). How are you doing? What are you doing? Differing perspectives in the assessment of individuals with COPD. *COPD: Journal of Chronic Obstructive Pulmonary Disease*, 4: 293–297.

ZuWallack, R. L. (2009). How do we increase activity and participation in our patients? *Seminars in Respiratory and Critical Care Medicine*, 30(6): 708.

11 Special populations

Learning objectives

At the end of this chapter you will:
- be able to identify groups of individuals who may have specific health needs
- understand the challenges faced by healthcare professionals in working with these groups
- be able to identify and understand the use of psychology in promoting health to individual populations
- recognise how specific and community level interventions can help a range of individuals from across the population
- be able to appreciate how multidisciplinary teams can be effective in promoting health across the population.

Introduction

Hard to reach populations provide challenges for health professionals and the health service. As outlined in Chapter 3 health inequalities exist between a variety of groups and key to tackling, and reducing, these is to target the health behaviour of specific groups. This may encompass a whole swathe of individuals across from the population. Older people, drug addicts, people with learning disabilities and individuals in prison are all examples of distinct sections of the population, or as we have termed them 'Special Groups', that may require specific interventions. They are special groups since they require thought, application and commitment along with potentially special methods of support and intervention. In successfully reaching these groups it is imperative to understand what strategies towards health promotion are effective whilst understanding that this can be challenging, requiring a different skills set but ultimately it can be both rewarding and fruitful for all concerned.

In reaching these groups and attempting to maximise health status it is important that interventions adopt individualised strategies tailored towards the individual group's specific health needs. Adopting a 'blanket approach' to healthcare or health promotion is inappropriate given the variety of individuals within the population. For example, elderly individuals will have different views, opinions and needs to individuals within the prison population to those with a learning difficulty (and, of course, there may be a cross-over between all of these groups). In order to reach these populations, health promotion schemes need to take place in a variety of settings which may include nursing homes, prisons and other locations and require different and unique approaches.

The health needs of individuals vary according to a range of demographic factors (see, for example, Chapter 3) and these may be a consequence of a wealth of factors. Some health needs can be as a result of risky behaviours, for example those individuals who take drugs (including those in the prison population) may have impaired health. It goes without saying that individuals who engage in risky behaviours, for example taking illicit drugs, face potentially significant health risks – the drugs taken may not be controlled or supervised by professionals and those that are sold 'on the streets' are of variable quality, strength and origin. Alternatively, it may be because the environment is not conducive to positive health – living conditions may be harmful or cultural norms may influence behaviour negatively (e.g. in prison).

Assessing the needs of special populations

Health needs assessments are used as a methodical approach which aims to identify the health needs of specific and special groups such as those in prison, individuals with learning disabilities and the elderly. This chapter will consider several groups within the population and understand the specific health issues that arise from these groups, the skills needed to tackle them and the techniques that work best for health promotion in the specific groups. The groups presented in this chapter are, to a certain extent, randomly selected and there were a host of others we thought could have been included (e.g. pregnant women, teenagers). However, in the end we selected those in prison, those who take illicit drugs, those with a learning disability and those who are elderly. These groups were chosen to reflect the diversity of people with which professionals have to work, the specific issues of these populations and the range of skills needed by those trying to promote health.

Prison population

Case study

Julie is a 49-year-old woman who has been in and out of prisons all of her life. Most recently she has been recently released from a six-month prison sentence for shop lifting and resisting arrest. Her continued offences are as a result of her drug habit – she needs to steal in order to pay for the costs of the heroin. However, on this occasion, Julie has committed herself to stopping the drugs and has said that she never wants to return to prison again.

Julie's history is of previous significant social and psychological difficulties. As a child she suffered violence and abuse from her father (who was also a drug addict). As a result and in an attempt to hide visible bruises, Julie often skipped school throughout her childhood. She subsequently gained no qualifications, does not work. In addition, she would often shoplift from local shops and on occasions get caught. She also resorted to prostitution in order to obtain money and drugs.

When Julie was 21 she became pregnant and safely delivered a baby girl (although she was born pre-term and had to spend some months in a Special Baby Care Unit). Having a daughter made Julie change her ways and she became more responsible and tried to stay out of trouble, although with little success. Her criminal behaviour increased since her daughter moved out of the family home some eight years ago; Julie has resorted to her old ways and started taking drugs, shoplifting and prostitution again. As a result of this behaviour, Julie was sent back to prison.

Julie's daughter has recently given birth to a baby daughter and consequently, Julie wants to change her behaviour as she wants to be an active part of her granddaughter's life. She feels that she needs help and support while in prison to address several issues, including her mental health, the impact of her childhood and her drug taking in order to move forward with her life. This is important to her as she wants to be able to be a good Nan and role model for her new grandchild.

Introduction

There are currently an estimated 88,179 individuals in UK prisons (Berman, 2012). Healthcare within prisons has been previously criticised which has led to the reform of services for prisoners within the last two decades. This reform enabled the prison health services to be part of the NHS in 2006 and to be commissioned by local PCTs. In enabling this, healthcare and health promotion within prisons will be at the same standard as the general population.

Prisoners often express complex and diverse health needs with a high percentage of individuals smoking, taking drugs and having mental health problems (see Table 11.1). Research has also identified that these individuals are more likely to suffer with such problems to a greater extent in comparison to the rest of the population, with minority ethnic groups, women, young offenders and older inmates having the most diverse health needs of the entire prison population (Harris et al., 2007).

The prison population is a specific closed community; this in itself provides opportunities and challenges in delivering healthcare services and health promotion

Table 11.1 Prisoners suffering from anxiety and depression

	No anxiety and depression		Anxiety and depression	
	N	%	N	%
Male	1,004	77	299	23
Female	68	52	64	49
Total	1,072	75	363	25

Source: Ministry of Justice, 2012

(Table 11.2). It is important that initiatives are put in place that consider these and work at both an individual and community level within the prison in an attempt to improve health and well-being. In addition, the promotion of health within prisons will not only impact upon the prisoner but also their family and the prison staff.

Interventions to tackle the health of prisoners

When aiming to improve the health of prisoners and reduce the prevalence of risky behaviours it is important to consider the environment and personal factors that may contribute to the individual's health. In doing so, it is important that any intervention is based on multi-component models and uses both medical and psychological methods. This will endeavour not only to treat symptoms but to also change lifestyle behaviours for a lasting effect once the prisoner is released.

Table 11.2 Opportunities and challenges faced by health workers in prisons

Opportunities	Challenges
Provides access to individuals who would not consider healthcare and health promotion in the outside world.	Risky behaviours such as smoking and taking drugs can be more prevalent in prison due to boredom of inmates.
The complex health issues that prisoners possess make them a key target for health promotion.	The complex needs and variety of needs within each prison means healthcare staff need to have a vast knowledge base.
Provides a constant unchanging environment for the individual while tackling health issues. This environment might not have been possible outside of prison.	Constraints of the prison environment in providing healthcare.
Potentially, the prisoner will not be exposed to external cues that may trigger risky behaviour.	

Individual level interventions – individual prisoners

Prison healthy living centre

Conducted by the charity Rethink, healthy living centres provide a 12-week course for young offenders whilst they are in custody. The course aims to improve the general health and mental well-being of prisoners by providing them with the skills and the ability to understand the implications of their behaviour on their health and realise how they can make changes to their health behaviours.

The course which has been successfully undertaken at Swinfen Hall Prison takes a holistic approach and involves several aspects:

- regular physical exercise
- participation in education, working or training
- access to art and music
- anti-bullying strategies
- relationship and team building
- depression prevention
- cognitive behavioural therapies (CBT)
- spiritual reflection
- aromatherapy
- relaxation and meditation skills.

By considering theses aspects the offenders are encouraged to consider their motivation, potential barriers and also actions which will be needed in order for them to maintain good mental health.

This individual level intervention uses psychological based theory such as CBT. CBT emphasises the importance of internal thoughts on our behaviour and it is widely recognised that CBT can benefit individuals who suffer from mental health conditions. This therapy is recognised as being able to be adapted to the prison setting and can be used as an effective way of treating common mental health problems in prison (Warrilow, 2012). Many interventions within the prison setting use CBT for rehabilitation programs as it helps the individual resolve their personal problems, increase their self-efficacy and therefore helps achieve inner goals and expectations.

With the use of CBT prisoners can be made aware of the consequences of their behaviour and how this will affect their life and health. They learn to re-train the relationship between thoughts and behaviour (Figure 11.1). The importance of using psychological based models in the prison population can have many advantages, such as reducing crime rates (Home Office, 2002). Psychological models such as risk, need and responsivity, or 'RNR' can make valuable contributions to the understanding and management of criminal behaviour (Andrews and Bonta, 2010)

The importance of considering psychological variables in relation to health of the prison population, such as those acknowledged with in CBT, has been demonstrated. Much research has considered the link between health and psychological factors in the general population, however less is known about such relationships within the prison

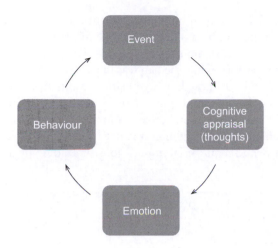

Figure 11.1 Basic Cognitive Behaviour Model

Source: http://www.rethink.org/how_we_can_help/news_and_media/national_press_releases/rethink
_prison_proje.html

community. Recent research has explored the relationship between the physical health of prisoners and optimism. In doing so, it was discovered that prisoners' optimism levels are related to physical health concerns – the higher the optimism the less physical health concerns (Heigel *et al.*, 2010). This highlights the importance of considering optimism as a psychological variable within interventions which aim to improve the health of prisoners.

Smoking in prisons

Within the United Kingdom prisoners can smoke within their own cell and inmates who smoke do not share cells with inmates who do smoke. There is a current debate as to whether to introduce a smoking ban in UK prisons. This would reflect current smoke-free legislation of young offender institutes within England who introduced the ban in 2007. Currently, prisons in the USA, Canada, Sweden, New Zealand and Isle of Man are all smoke free (ASH, 2010). It is believed that the introduction of smoke-free prisons would benefit in many ways:

- Help prisoners to quit
- Reduce exposure to second-hand smoke for inmates and prison officers
- Improve the health and safety within prisons by reducing the chances of fire breaking out
- Reduce costs.

As this is still a relatively new area of research, evaluation of total smoke-free legislation in prisons is scarce. Research conducted amongst prisoners who have been part of a smoke-free legislation provide both some promising and concerning results. A study conducted in the USA demonstrated both positive attitudinal and behavioural changes of inmates who had been part of a smoking ban while in prison (Thibodeau *et al.*, 2010), whereas, Lasnier *et al.* (2011) demonstrated less positive effects of a smoking ban, with inmates still reporting smoking while the ban was in place and also receiving no discipline for this behaviour if caught. Although many positive results from introducing this to the UK may be observed, the potential consequences also need to be considered. These consist of the possibility of disorder between inmates and the rise in the amount of contraband. The conflicting views highlight the need for future research which addresses the health, behavioural and managerial implications of abiding by a ban.

Applying this to Julie

As a result of her childhood experiences, Julie has a very negative view of herself and suffers from depression. Julie would benefit from undertaking CBT in an attempt to help her with the depression and understanding how her childhood experiences have impacted upon her behaviour.

Community level interventions – the prison as a whole

In 2002 it was considered necessary that a whole prison approach to health promotion in prisons was undertaken (Department of Health, 2002). The whole prison approach incorporated three main aims:

- Impact upon the mental, physical and social health of prisoners and staff
- Help to prevent any deterioration in prisoners' health while under custody or as a result of being in custody
- Help prisoners adopt healthy behaviours which can be translated to the community upon their release.

The issues to be addressed under this approach can vary from healthy eating to drug abuse and include a basis of five key areas (mental health promotion and well-being, smoking, healthy eating and nutrition, healthy lifestyles (including sex and relationships) and active living, and drug and other substance misuse). In implementing this approach, it is possible to address not only the prisoner's physical needs but also important psychological issues related to their behaviour. These can stem from classic behaviourism and can have implications for future behaviour. One such influence on behaviour is thought to be self-efficacy. Self-efficacy as previously outlined in Chapter 4 is the belief which individuals hold regarding their ability to carry out specific behaviours. This is thought to be an important factor to consider in relation to health behaviours (Posadzki *et al.*, 2010).

Recent research has supported the notion of self-efficacy amongst prisoners and concluded that the prison population has varying levels of self-efficacy in managing their health while in prison. In addition correlations were found between high levels of self-efficacy and the engagement in health promoting and health-monitoring behaviour (Loeb *et al.*, 2011). This research highlights the importance of considering self-efficacy in relation to the health of the prison population.

It is vital that inmates understand the importance of health and health management not only whilst in prison but also for the transference to the community setting upon release. Therefore, it may be necessary for prisons to consider assessing self-efficacy upon detention or using health related self-efficacy scales when attempting to tackle health issues. In applying a whole systems, community approach which acknowledges self-esteem it is possible that, conjointly, all the work will help to improve individuals' health related behaviour both inside and outside of prison.

A whole systems approach in prison is thought to be beneficial in creating a supportive environment for that specific behavioural change. A recent evaluation of a whole systems community approach towards oral health was undertaken in a Scottish prison. The project being evaluated (The Oral Health Improvement Project) aimed to influence knowledge, attitudes and behaviours in relation to oral health. It was also hoped that the project would not only benefit the inmates but also that it would transfer to the families of the inmates and the prison staff. Mixed results were seen and it was concluded some staff gained knowledge, whereas the prisoners were seen to gain knowledge and in addition, a change in attitude as a result of the intervention. However, this did not result in a change in oral health related behaviours (Akbar *et al.*, 2012). It is important that whole system approaches are developed, which result in behaviour change, if health is to be influenced.

Applying this to Julie

It is possible that Julie has low self-efficacy in relation to the ability to change her behaviour. In addition, there is a suggested link between low self-efficacy and depression. Therefore if Julie could work on improving her self-efficacy potential impacts could be seen upon her mental health.

Working effectively with others

To have a healthy prison a multidisciplinary team must be employed; this will enable all the health needs of the prisoners to be addressed in the best possible way. One way of bringing different agencies together to impact upon the health of prisoners is to conduct a healthcare needs assessment of the prison. As a result of this, various professionals, such as psychologists, GPs, nurses and healthcare staff, work effectively together to assess and impact upon health needs. In doing so, the implementation of new strategies to address health issues can be put in place (Marshall *et al.*, 2000). The fusion of care and custody can often be complex, with goals often being met by crossing professional boundaries, but through effective communication, an effective multidisciplinary relationship can ensure stability and suitable care for prisoners (Mullins, 2012).

Mentors

Mentoring can provide individuals who are either in prison or newly released with much needed support. This support could help impact upon crime rates, incarceration rates and health. Mentors can be used as a support mechanism in helping prisoners adapt to life back in the community whilst also providing support throughout the transition from prison to the community. The mentoring system has been set up in various areas within the UK and is thought to be invaluable in changing the lives of offenders. Currently, a review is being completed on the Peers in Prison Settings (PiPS) and, although the results appear promising, the results are yet to be published.

Nacro is the biggest crime reduction charity in the UK and provides support for vulnerable individuals who are likely to result to crime if unsupported. The service has several areas of focus including prevention, offender management and resettlement. In tackling these three main areas impacts are thought to be felt at both the individual and community level, such as reduced crime rates, the improved health and well-being of offenders and the general public (http://www.nacro.org.uk/).

Mentors can be from a public agency such as Nacro, a family member or a peer. In addition to providing general support for the individuals, mentors can also help to influence the cognitive processes of the individual. This can include impacting on personal attributes such as self-esteem and interpersonal traits which are thought to have contributed to the criminal behaviour.

Applying this to Julie

Julie would benefit from any health intervention within prison as she not only has psychological problems but she has never taken her health seriously which can have many implications. It is important that Julie changes her attitude towards her health and starts to attend regular health and dental check-ups if she is to have a healthy future with her daughter and grandchild.

Illicit drug use

Duane is a 20-year-old man who lives with his girlfriend in their shared flat. Currently he is working as a dustbin man for the local council. His parents had high hopes for him as he achieved 11 GCSEs at A* level. However, following this success he became more involved in cannabis (he had previously been involved in glue sniffing and some alcohol abuse) and was eventually expelled from school for attempting to sell cannabis to his peers. Since these early days at school he has always used cannabis, drinks alcohol regularly, is a heavy smoker and has also developed a habit for cocaine. Despite his assurances, his girlfriend feels that it does affect both his job and their social life. She has threatened to leave him and has given him a final ultimatum.

He has started acting strangely and is under investigation at work for some bizarre behaviour exhibited recently and for poor time keeping. However, Duane is finding it hard to deal with the pressures of working regularly and has started to increase his drug intake. Furthermore, he has started selling drugs at a local drug haunt as he is finding it difficult to fund his drug taking on his current salary. He goes down to the local pub most nights where he meets his mates before going back to either their flat or his own to take drugs into the early hours. Although this is a habit that Duane has tried to deal with on a number of occasions, he always seems to be drawn back to the same circle of friends and ends up on a downward spiral. His girlfriend has come to you in tears and wants support and advice – how can she help Duane?

Introduction

In a 2011/12 survey, some 36.5 per cent of the UK population reported having taken illegal drugs during their lifetime and almost three million people in the last year (Home Office, 2012). The amount of people aged between 16 and 24 years who had taken drugs in the last year was 19.3 per cent, the lowest level since measurement began in 1996. In addition, the use of Class A drugs in the last year among this same age group has remained stable since 1996 and stands at around 3 per cent. Other figures indicate that the most frequently used drug by adults is cannabis (Home Office, 2012).

Although drug use has either remained stable or decreased over the last years, there has been a reported rise in hospital admissions in England as a result of drug poisoning in the last 10 years, with figures rising by 100 per cent (see Table 11.3). In addition, it is also estimated that the highest number of drug related hospital admissions in 2011/12 was seen in the 25–34 age group and almost three times as many males were admitted to hospital with drug related mental health or behavioural disorder than females (Health and Social Care Information Centre, 2012).

Table 11.3 Drug poisoning hospital related admissions

Year	Total
2000/2001	25,683
2001/2002	28,063
2002/2003	31,490
2003/2004	34,957
2004/2005	35,737
2005/2006	38,005
2006/2007	38,170
2007/2008	40,421
2008/2009	42,170
2009/2010	44,585
2010/2011	51,353
2011/2012	57,733

Source: Health and Social Care Information Centre, 2011

It goes without saying that individuals who take illicit drugs face potentially significant health risks – the drugs taken are often not controlled or supervised by professionals and those that are sold 'on the streets' are of variable quality, strength and origin. As well as the immediate health risks, drugs can also lead to long-term addiction, health damage and potentially death.

Drug-related deaths often attract a great deal of political and media attention. The Office for National Statistics (ONS) produces mortality statistics for drug-related deaths based upon information on death certificates (see Table 11.4), and these indicate over 2,600 deaths related to substance misuse in the UK during 2011.

These deaths are, of course, relatively low and significantly less than those caused by either alcohol or smoking (see Chapters 7 and 8). Nonetheless, they are avoidable and significant to individual families and friends. Obviously, the consequences of substance misuse are not restricted to death, and there may be an impact on health that differs dependent on the drugs being used (see Table 11.5). However, what is clear is that all illicit drug use is associated with significant morbidity.

In addition to the link between substance use, mortality and morbidity, it is also important to recognise the relationship between illicit drug use and other risky health behaviours. For example, associations have been identified between drug use and risky sexual behaviours (Broman, 2007). Consequently it is understood that drug use can have a negative effect on the cessation of additional risky behaviours, such as smoking (Stapleton *et al.*, 2009). Acknowledging the associations between drug use and other risky health behaviours provides complex challenges when not only aiming to reduce drug use but other risky behaviours too.

Table 11.4 Number of deaths related to substance misuse in England and Wales (as recorded on death certificate)

Drug	Deaths
Heroin and morphine	596
Methadone	486
Cocaine (including crack)	112
All amphetamines	62
(of which MDMA/ecstasy)	13
Cannabis	7
Gamma-hydroxybutyrate (GHB)	20
BZP/TFMPP	2
Mephedrone	6
All benzodiazepines	293
Zopiclone/Zolpidem	71
All antidepressants	393
Antipsychotics	104
Paracetamol (including compound formulations)	199
Codeine (non-compound formulation)	88
Dihydrocodeine (non-compound formulation)	109
Helium	42
Tramadol	154

Source: Deaths related to drug poisoning in England and Wales, 2010 (ONS, 2011)

Table 11.5 Illicit drug use and health consequences

Drug	Consequences
Heroin and morphine	Short-term effects include a surge of euphoria followed by alternately wakeful and drowsy states and cloudy mental functioning. Associated with fatal overdose and, particularly in users who inject the drug, infectious diseases such as HIV/AIDS and hepatitis
Cocaine (including crack)	A powerfully addictive drug, cocaine usually makes the user feel euphoric and energetic. Common health effects include heart attacks, respiratory failure, strokes and seizures. Large amounts can cause bizarre and violent behaviour. In rare cases, sudden death can occur on the first use of cocaine or unexpectedly thereafter

Drug	Consequences
Club drugs (the most common club drugs include GHB, Rohypnol, ketamine, methamphetamine)	Chronic use of MDMA may lead to changes in brain function. GHB abuse can cause coma and seizures. High doses of ketamine can cause delirium, amnesia and other problems. Mixed with alcohol, Rohypnol can incapacitate users and cause amnesia
Cannabis	Short-term effects include memory and learning problems, distorted perception, and difficulty thinking and solving problems
LSD	Unpredictable psychological effects. With large enough doses, users experience delusions and visual hallucinations. Physical effects include increased body temperature, heart rate and blood pressure; sleeplessness; and loss of appetite
Ecstasy	Short-term effects include feelings of mental stimulation, emotional warmth, enhanced sensory perception and increased physical energy. Adverse health effects can include nausea, chills, sweating, teeth clenching, muscle cramping and blurred vision
PCP/Phencyclidine	Many PCP users are brought to emergency rooms because of overdose or because of the drug's unpleasant psychological effects. In a hospital or detention setting, people high on PCP often become violent or suicidal

Interventions to reduce illicit drug use and subsequent risky health behaviours

The UK Government's Drug Strategy 2010 is built upon the previous strategies and focuses on 'reducing the harms caused by drug misuse … and offer every support for people to choose recovery as an achievable way out of dependency' (HM Government, 2010). In achieving this three main areas will be tackled:

- Reducing demand
- Restricting supply
- Building recovery in communities.

Consequently, the strategy is aimed at reducing the prevalence of drugs on our streets and reducing the number of current drug users by the use of effective treatment and support in a whole systems approach. Although a whole systems approach is adopted, the relationship between drug use and other risky health behaviours is not addressed. When considering treatments it can also be considered important to address other risky health behaviours to either stop or prevent the uptake of them. The following sections of this chapter will address how interventions can be used with individuals that take drugs to ensure other health behaviours are not concomitantly increased.

Assessment of drug use

The most effective way of assessing a potential client is through an interview (or self-administered tool). Although several such questionnaires are available, the CAGE questionnaire (Ewing, 1984) is the most practical for healthcare professionals to use as a screening tool. CAGE is a mnemonic that asks about attempts to Cut down on drinking, Annoyance with criticisms about drinking, Guilt about drinking and using alcohol as an Eye-opener.

The CAGE questionnaire consists of four questions that probe the respondent's *own feelings* regarding their drinking habits to make a diagnosis. The health practitioner asks the respondent if they have ever *felt* that they should cut down on the amount they regularly drink, or been annoyed by other people's criticisms of their drinking habits, or felt guilty about how much they drink or have felt the need to have a drink first thing in the morning to face the day. Each question carries a score of '0' for 'no' and '1' for 'yes' as an answer. A total score of '2' or more is considered clinically significant and worthy of further investigation.

Although initially designed for alcohol (as you can tell), it has been adapted for use with other drugs (see Table 11.6) and individuals with substance abuse (Couwenbergh *et al.*, 2009). As this tool can be used with both drug and alcohol concerns, it provides a useful tool when considering other risky behaviours which may increase or develop when drug use and abuse is being addressed. The questionnaire takes approximately one minute to complete and can act as a screening tool to ensure that the healthcare professional is prompted to look further.

The normal cut-off for the CAGE is two positive answers, although if one is positively responded to then this may suggest the healthcare professional should look further.

The CAGE questionnaire does not differentiate between current and former problems, and it is more accurate in detecting alcoholism than problem drinking. However, it is reported as being 60–90 per cent sensitive when two or more questions are positive and 40–60 per cent specific for excluding substance abuse (Mersy, 2003).

Table 11.6 CAGE questions Adapted to Include Drugs (CAGE-AID)

1.	Have you ever felt you ought to cut down on your drinking or drug use?
2.	Have people annoyed you by criticising your drinking or drug use?
3.	Have you felt bad or guilty about your drinking or drug use?
4.	Have you ever had a drink or used drugs first thing in the morning to steady your nerves or to get rid of a hangover (eye-opener)?

Source: Brown and Rounds, 1995

An even shorter questionnaire (if you should need one) is the conjoint screening test that involves only two questions:

- 'In the past year, have you ever drunk or used drugs more than you meant to?' and
- 'Have you felt you wanted or needed to cut down on your drinking or drug use in the past year?'

Brown et al., 2001

At least one positive response detects current substance use disorders with nearly 80 per cent sensitivity and specificity.

If the patient denies use, you can acknowledge the wise choice that they have made by abstaining from drugs. However, it is necessary to continue to screen, ideally at each encounter. In some situations, patients may deny use, but a constellation of signs and symptoms suggests abuse. In this case, it may be prudent to re-screen frequently or conduct specific blood/urine/hair testing.

Individual level interventions

Stages of Change model

On an individual basis, if a patient has shared with you that they are abusing illicit drugs (after you have *asked* them) but are not ready to take the next step of comprehensive assessment and treatment through a professional programme, then it is useful to turn to the Stages of Change model (SoC) developed by Prochaska *et al.* (1992). As discussed in previous chapters (for example, how the SoC can be applied to smoking interventions in Chapter 8), the five stages of change can be used to guide both the patient and the practitioner and these will be discussed in the intervention section after we have first explored why people actually take drugs. It is useful in both the *Assessment* and the *Advice* section. Although this model has been discussed extensively elsewhere in this book, it is worth re-capping this and demonstrating how it can be applied to drug misuse:

1. *Pre-contemplation:* The patient is not considering change during the pre-contemplation stage.

    - They do not believe it is necessary.
    - They do not know or understand the risks involved.
    - They have tried many times to quit without success, so they give up and don't want to try again.
    - They have gone through withdrawal before and are fearful of the process or effects on their body.
    - They feel strongly that no one is going to tell them what to do with their body.
    - They have a mental illness and do not have a good grasp of what using drugs and alcohol means, even when information is given to them.

- They have family members or partners whom they depend on who use. They may not contemplate changing when everyone else continues to use.

The individual in pre-contemplation may present as resistant, reluctant, resigned or rationalising (see Table 11.7).

Table 11.7 Elements of pre-contemplation phase and healthcare professional response

Presents as:	What the patient is saying:	Healthcare professional response:
Resistant	Don't tell me what to do	Work with the resistance. Avoid confrontation by giving facts about what drugs and alcohol will do to them. Ask what they know about the effects; ask permission to share what you know, and then ask their opinion of the information. This often leads to a reduced level of resistance and allows for a more open dialogue.
Reluctant	I don't want to change; there are reasons	Empathise with the real or possible results of changing (for example, if their partner left). It is possible to give strong medical advice to change and still be empathetic to possible negative outcomes to changing. Guide them to problem-solving.
Resigned	I can't change, I've tried	Instil hope and explore barriers to change. Increase self-efficacy and confidence. Provide small steps with achievable goals.
Rationalising	I don't use that much	Decrease discussion. Listen rather than responding to the rationalisation. Respond to them by empathising and reframing their comments to address the conflict of wanting to be healthy and not knowing whether 'using' is really causing harm.

2. *Contemplation:* The patient is ambivalent about changing their behaviour. They can think of the positive reasons to change but are also very aware of the negative sides of change. In this stage it is important to provide the health benefits of changing their behaviour (as discussed earlier in the chapter). There is a need to help the patient explore goals for health, and problem-solve how to deal with the negative aspects of abstinence.

3. *Preparation:* They are exploring options to assist their process of change. They may be experimenting by cutting down or have been able to quit for one or more days. Although their ambivalence is lessening, it is still present and may increase when they are challenged by those around them, triggered by the environment, or are under other types of stress they have handled by using in the past. The healthcare professional should be acknowledging the individual's strengths in reaching this stage but at the same time anticipate problems and pitfalls to changing, and assist the patient in generating their own plan for obtaining abstinence. Problem-solve with them regarding barriers to success.

4. *Action:* The patient has stopped using drugs and/or alcohol and their success needs to be celebrated. Offer to be available for assistance if they feel that they want to use drugs/alcohol again.

5. *Relapse:* Relapse is common and should not be thought of as failure, but as part of the recovery process. At this stage the healthcare professional needs to discuss triggers, stressors and social pressures that may lead to relapse and help the patient plan for them. At future visits, if relapse has occurred, guide the patient towards identifying what steps they used to quit before. Offer hope and encouragement, and allow the patient to explore the negative side of quitting and what they can do to deal with those issues. Offer to help find resources to help the patient return to abstinence.

Applying this to Duane

Duane is at the pre-contemplation stage of change and is presenting himself as resigned. Therefore, it is important that his self-efficacy and confidence are improved along with discussing any barriers which are impacting upon behaviour change. In addition it is also important that Duane is made aware of the consequences of all of his risky health behaviours including drug taking, smoking and drinking alcohol. This is a good opportunity for the health professional to monitor the impact of any change in Duane's drug taking behaviour upon his other risky behaviours such as smoking. It is important to be aware that as Duane ceases taking drugs, other risky health behaviours may be undertaken and increased.

One of the most important things that an individual healthcare professional can do for somebody who is abusing drugs is to provide some information and education. Although it is a safe assumption that most individuals will have some knowledge of the effects of alcohol and other drugs, it is important to assess this. Ask the patient what they know and then fill in the missing pieces and clarify misconceptions. This is an excellent opportunity to educate the patient about adverse effects of alcohol/drugs and any other risky health behaviours and the benefits of stopping them at any time.

A number of cognitive behavioural approaches have developed an evidence base for treating substance misuse and these include interventions such as those described in further detail below.

Contingency management therapies

Contingency management is one form of behavioural therapy in which patients receive incentives for achieving specific behavioural goals. These approaches are based on operant conditioning whereby appropriate behaviour is rewarded with positive consequences and therefore more likely to be repeated. Contingency management can be applied to any behaviour which is needed to be changed, from drug use to smoking and alcohol use (e.g. Volpp et al., 2009). These forms of intervention have particularly strong and robust empirical support (Dutra et al., 2008). For example, Petry et al. (2011) demonstrated the efficacy of earning chances to win prizes to adherence to the intervention in addition to longer abstinence rates.

There are, of course, some limitations to contingency management interventions. For example, the effects of the intervention tend to reduce after the contingencies are reduced. Second, not all users of illicit drugs are responsive to contingency management and there is consequently a need to explore individual differences in responses to behavioural treatment. For example, differences in effectiveness of contingency management between younger and older groups of drug addicts have been discovered (Weiss and Petry, 2011).

Cognitive behaviour and skills training therapies

Cognitive behaviour approaches, such as relapse prevention, are grounded in social learning theories and principles of operant conditioning. A number of meta-analyses and literature reviews have established the value of cognitive behavioural approaches in drug-using populations (e.g. Lee and Rawson, 2008).

Motivational interviewing

Motivational interviewing approaches have strong empirical support for use in treating alcohol users and smokers (see Chapters 7 and 8). Marijuana-dependent adults who received motivational interviewing had significant reductions in marijuana use, compared to a delayed-treatment control group (Stephens et al., 2000). In a study on

Table 11.8 A brief summary of the main psychological therapies used in treating substance misuse

Behavioural therapy (BT)	A structured therapy focusing on changing behaviour and the environmental factors that trigger maladaptive behaviour. *Includes:*
Cue exposure treatment (CET)	A structured treatment involving exposure to drug-related cues that have been associated with past drug use without consumption of the drug. This is intended to lead to a reduction (or habituation) of reactivity to drug cues and hence to a reduced likelihood of relapse.
Community reinforcement approach (CRA)	A behavioural approach that focuses on what the client finds rewarding in their social, occupational and recreational life. It aims to help them change their lifestyle and social environment to support long-term changes in behaviour whereby using substances is less rewarding than not using them.
Contingency management (CM)	Also known as voucher-based therapy, this aims to encourage adaptive behaviour by rewarding the client for attaining agreed goals (e.g. no use of illicit drugs as checked by urine screens) and not rewarding them when these goals are unmet (e.g. illicit drug use). Vouchers can usually be exchanged for consumer goods.
Cognitive therapy (CT)	A structured therapy using cognitive techniques (e.g. challenging a person's negative thoughts) and behavioural techniques (e.g. behavioural experiments; activity planning) to change maladaptive thoughts and beliefs. *Includes:*
Cognitive behavioural therapy (CBT)	A combination of both cognitive and behavioural therapies.
Relapse prevention (RP)	Uses several CBT strategies to enhance the client's self-control and prevent relapse. It highlights problems that the client may face and develops strategies they can use to deal with high-risk situations.
Motivational interviewing (MI)	A focused approach aiming to enhance motivation for changing substance use by exploring and resolving the individual's ambivalence about change.
Motivational enhancement therapy (MET)	A brief intervention based on MI which also incorporates a 'check-up' assessment and feedback.

Table 11.8 *continued*

Twelve-step approaches	Interventions used by self-help organisations like Alcoholics Anonymous. They are based on a philosophy that adopts an illness model and sees substance use as stemming from an innate vulnerability. An individual must acknowledge their addiction and the harm it has caused to themselves and others; they must also accept their lack of control over use and thus the only acceptable goal is abstinence.
Other approaches	The involvement of partners and family through marital and family therapy builds on the known social context of substance use. There are also various forms of counselling, group therapy and milieu therapy.

heavy cocaine users, motivational intervention was shown to reduce days of cocaine use by 30 per cent, even amongst those who were not actively seeking help (Brown University, 2009), therefore illustrating the potential benefits of using this treatment with individuals who undertake multiple risky health behaviours as the approach is adaptive to other behaviours. However, the research has not always been positive and equivocal results have been found. For example, Miller *et al.* (2003) did not support the efficacy of motivational interviewing. McCambridge *et al.* (2008) found no differences in outcome between motivational interviewing and simply offering drug information and advice amongst over 300 adolescents.

The National Institute for Health and Clinical Excellence (NICE, 2007) issued guidelines on psychosocial interventions for drug misuse. They made recommendations for the use of psychosocial interventions in the treatment of people who misuse opioids, stimulants and cannabis in the healthcare and criminal justice systems. There were several key priorities for implementation:

- *Brief interventions:* Opportunistic brief interventions focused on motivation should be offered to people in limited contact with drug services (for example, those attending a needle and syringe exchange or primary care settings) if concerns about drug misuse are identified by the service user or staff member.
- *Self-help:* Staff should routinely provide people who misuse drugs with information about self-help groups. These groups should normally be based on 12-step principles.
- *Contingency management:* Drug services should introduce contingency management programmes. The programme should offer incentives (usually vouchers that can be exchanged for goods or services of the service user's choice, or privileges such as take-home methadone doses) contingent on each presentation of a drug-negative test (for example, free from cocaine or non-prescribed opioids).
- *Contingency management to improve physical healthcare:* For people at risk of physical health problems (including transmittable diseases) resulting from their drug misuse, material incentives (for example, shopping vouchers of up to £10 in value) should be considered to encourage harm reduction.

Community level interventions

The Theory of Planned Behaviour

The Theory of Planned Behaviour (TBP) and Theory of Reasoned Action (TRA) have been applied to the use of illicit drugs, as have other such models. The Theory of Reasoned Action proposes that an individual's substance abuse behaviours are based on intentions, which in turn are determined by attitudes and perceived social norms regarding substance use (see Chapter 4). Furthermore, the TRA suggests that attitudes are determined by perceived costs and benefits and the affective value placed on those consequences (Petraitis et al., 1995). Intervention campaigns that have targeted key TRA variables have proven successful in preventing substance use (Flynn et al., 1994). On this basis, media campaigns have been developed that influence attitudes and perceived norms regarding substance misuse.

Such approaches have used psychological models in a social marketing context and it is worth exploring the social marketing techniques that have been used for illicit drug taking. Social marketing is the application of commercial sector marketing tools to the resolution of a number of social and health problems. The idea dates back to 1951 when Wiebe asked the question 'Can brotherhood be sold like soap?' (Wiebe, 1951/1952). Social marketing thinking is now located at the centre of many government health improvement programmes, including reducing illicit drug use. A distinguishing feature of social marketing is that it goes beyond mere education and awareness raising and focuses instead on behaviour. Although outcomes have traditionally been conceptualised in terms of behaviour change, more recent work has expanded this conceptualisation to include the prevention of certain behaviours such as the use of illicit substances (Andreasen, 2006).

'FRANK'

The UK's attempt at reducing drug taking through social marketing is 'Project FRANK' which has been widely advertised both through traditional media and using the more informal advanced methods preferred by the target audience (i.e. teenagers). The state of evaluation of such prevention programmes is currently 'very poor' (McGrath et al., 2006). Although no formal evaluation of the FRANK programme's effectiveness of drug reduction has been published, Sumnall and Bellis (2007) suggest that it may be little different from the other social marketing campaigns in the US and UK. Although there is evidence that FRANK is well known, the overall impact on drug taking appears more limited.

Moreover, Sumnall and Bellis (2007) suggest that such campaigns may have a negative impact on health. They imply that since the campaigns regularly suggest that taking cannabis results in mental health difficulties and affect the 'brain' or 'mind' (see Table 8.6), individuals may begin to believe that they are experiencing such effects. Consequently, Sumnall and Bellis (2007) suggest that cannabis users may suffer 'amotivation, memory loss or even paranoia, not as a direct result of the drug, but through psychological mechanisms induced through high-profile social-marketing campaigns that effectively "sell" such negative effects'. Although there is no clear evidence of such at the moment, it is obviously important for policy makers and healthcare professionals to be aware of such concerns so that they can deal appropriately with any such cases on an individual basis.

Community level interventions aimed at reducing and preventing the uptake of drug use focus predominantly on these aspects and do not consider the implications of other risky behaviours when promoting behaviour change. It may be considered necessary for such campaigns to acknowledge the potential relationship between risky behaviours. In providing such information to the public it will potentially enable individuals to not replace their drug taking behaviour with a different risky behaviour but to reduce the prevalence of the risky behaviour in question.

Applying this to Duane

Community level campaigns can make Duane more aware of the potential health consequences of his drug taking habits. In addition they could help him realise that he needs some help with his risky health behaviours.

Working effectively with others

Couples and family treatments

The defining feature of couples and family treatments is that they treat drug-using individuals in the context of family and social systems in which substance use may develop or be maintained. The engagement of the individual's social networks in treatment can be a powerful predictor of change, and thus the inclusion of family members in treatment may be helpful in reducing attrition (particularly among adolescents) and addressing multiple problem areas (Liddle *et al.*, 2001) (see Box 11.1). Reviews of such treatments, including meta-analyses, have indicated that these approaches are effective (e.g. Deas and Thomas, 2001). The Department of Education reported that intensive, multi-agency family interventions resulted in 597 families no longer being involved in substance misuse, a 50 per cent success rate (Dixon *et al.*, 2010).

When abstinence is not possible, harm reduction assists a patient to take steps to reduce use and harm to themselves. Strategies for preventing further harm may include:

- Evaluate and refer for any underlying problems e.g. alcohol use.
- Encourage the patient to keep track of substance use.
- Decrease use:
  - Reduce dosage and frequency of use.

- Recommend reducing their use by one half each day; if this is not possible, any decrease in use is beneficial.
- Intersperse use with periods of abstinence.
- Use a safer route of drug administration.
- Find a substitute for the substance e.g. a prescribed, safer alternative (methadone).
- Avoid friends who use.

Whichever method is used, it is important to be constantly vigilant to ensure there is no relapse. Relapse prevention, is often based on psychological principles (Marlatt and Donovan, 2005). Relapse prevention is a treatment intervention designed to teach clients a wide range of cognitive and behavioural coping skills to avoid or deal with a brief return to substance use (lapse), or a protracted return to previous levels of use (relapse), following a period of moderation or abstinence.

Box 11.1 Applying research in practice

A longitudinal analysis of some risk and protective factors in marijuana use by adolescents receiving child welfare services (Cheng and Lo, 2011)

This study sought to examine risk and protective factors in marijuana use by adolescents involved in child welfare services. Records of 1,797 adolescents were extracted from the National Survey of Child and Adolescent Well-Being data set.

In total the results identified that 1 out of 10 adolescents reported using marijuana in the past 30 days. Adolescents' likelihood of being a current marijuana user increased with prior lifetime use of the drug. The findings also demonstrated that among adolescents, parental monitoring and closeness to parents, engagement with school environment, and out of home services deterred current marijuana use.

Applying this to Duane

It is important that Duane's girlfriend gets involved with any methods that are used to help Duane to stop using drugs. This will provide him with the support that he will need.

Learning disabilities

Case study

Sean is a 33-year-old man who has Down's syndrome. His mother and father are now elderly and he lives in sheltered housing with a warden. Although this is the case, he is very independent and likes to go to the shops and take care of himself. He does all of his own shopping, cleaning and general household jobs.

Sean is hard of hearing and has a heart complaint which requires regular medication and monitoring. Although Sean is very independent, he does occasionally forget to take his medication and attend his check-ups at the hospital. He is also classed as obese and does not eat a healthy diet.

His parents are getting increasingly worried that Sean needs support to help him with day-to-day activities as each time they visit him his flat appears ill kept. They are also concerned about his health as he has admitted to not taking his medicine regularly. His parents are too old and frail to take on the role themselves even though they want to support him. His parents have come to you to get some support for Sean which will put their minds at ease as they will know that he is looking after himself properly.

Introduction

It is estimated that there are over 1,190,000 individuals living in England who have learning disabilities (see Table 11.9; Emerson *et al.*, 2011). It is well recognised that individuals who have learning disabilities suffer from poorer health (Disability Rights Commission, 2006). As a result, such individuals are expected to have a reduced life expectancy by up to 25 years (Emerson *et al.*, 2011). In part this is due to difficulties in identifying ill health among people with learning disabilities, and gaining timely access to appropriate services (Emerson et al, 2011; Turner, 2013). As a consequence of this, it was suggested that annual health checks for people with learning disabilities living in England be introduced (Disabilities Rights Commission, 2006).

Table 11.9 Estimated number of individuals with learning disabilities by gender

Age	Male	Female	Total
0–17	180,487	105,818	286,305
18–80+	529,507	375,249	904,756

Source: Adapted from Emerson *et al.*, 2011

In addition to individuals with learning disabilities having poorer health, it is also thought that an estimated only 21 per cent of individuals are known to learning disabilities services. It goes without saying that if such individuals do not make themselves known they will not be able to have the help and assistance that they may need. This fact alone can impact upon the health outcomes of individuals with learning disabilities.

Emerson and Baines (2010) identified the factors which contribute to health inequalities for people with learning disabilities. They are thought to be:

1. The increased risk to the exposure of social factors which affect our health (social determinates of health) such as unemployment and poorer living conditions.
2. The increased risk of developing genetically based health problems which are linked to the learning disability.
3. Communication difficulties including poor communication skills.
4. Poor understanding and adherence to healthy lifestyle guidelines
5. Problems in accessing healthcare and high quality healthcare.

In an attempt to improve the health of individuals with learning disabilities, it is important to understand an individual's views and barriers towards health services alongside the impacts of interventions or polices. Codling and Macdonald (2011) suggested that the impact of health education was minimal in people with learning disabilities. The authors suggested that although health education was effective, the transfer of this knowledge to an individual's own health was more problematic.

Interventions to improve the health of individuals with learning disabilities

Government policies have acknowledged the importance of providing a fair society for individuals with learning disabilities. Each of the four UK countries has its own policies on how the needs of people with learning disabilities should be met. These policies describe a holistic approach for supporting people with learning disabilities to reach their potential and take their place in the community.

The policies aim to improve quality of life and are based on broad themes:

*   citizenship
*   empowerment
*   having choices and making decisions
*   having the same opportunities as other people
*   having the same rights as other people
*   social inclusion.

The UK policies on people with learning disabilities are:

England: Department of Health (2009) *Valuing People Now: A New Three-year Strategy for People with Learning Disabilities.*

Northern Ireland: Department of Health and Social Security (2005) *Equal Lives: Review of Policy and Services for People with a Learning Disability in Northern Ireland.*

Scotland: Scottish Executive (2000) *The Same as You: A Review of Services for People with Learning Disability.*

Wales: Learning Disability Advisory Group (2001) *Fulfilling the Promises: Report of the Learning Disability Advisory Group.*

Each policy addresses health needs in various ways, but focuses on similar issues:

- Promoting collaborative working
- Access to general health services with specialist support
- General healthcare staff to receive specialist training
- Registration with their GPs
- Offering personalised healthcare plan with, in England and Northern Ireland, a specialised health action plan
- Regular health checks
- Accessible health promotion materials.

This will enable such individuals to have the same opportunities as all other individuals in society. In reflection of this it could be assumed that the health of this population will benefit as government targets are worked towards. This assumption is, of course, optimistic.

Individual level interventions

Health checks

The recommendation for annual health checks for individuals with learning disabilities was made in 2006. It is suggested that these health checks benefit the individual in two ways: first in the detection of new health concerns and second they result in actions to address health needs (Robertson *et al.*, 2010). Although these consultations are potentially beneficial the uptake of them is seen to be less than 50 per cent (Emerson *et al.*, 2011). In attempting to improve the health of individuals with learning disabilities and reduce health inequalities in this group it is important that more is done to encourage the uptake of this service. Research should consider the effectiveness of the promotion of such services in an attempt to increase attendance.

Social learning theory

As previously mentioned in chapters throughout this book, social learning theory can play a part in improving the health of individuals irrespective of whether the individual has a learning disability or not. In people with a learning disability, it is important that the carers and family surrounding the individual model healthy lifestyle behaviours in a positive way. It is suggested that modelling these behaviours can impact upon behaviour change (Shoneye, 2012).

Mentors have been shown to be effective in influencing the lives of the mentees in many settings such as foster care (Ahrens *et al.*, 2008). It is suggested that matching personality traits of individuals with learning disabilities to their mentor enhances the success of the mentor in changing or influencing behaviour (Glomb *et al.*, 2006). Mentors could be used to apply the social learning theory to health and health related behaviours for individuals with learning disabilities. This could help promote healthy lifestyles at an individual level.

Person-centred planning

This approach takes a bottom-up approach by putting control with the individual. It enables the patient or client to address the needs they feel are important to them. Person-centred planning has been shown to be effective not only enabling such individuals to undertake more activities but to also enhance their individual characteristics such as self-esteem (Wigham *et al.*, 2008). In terms of health promotion and improving the health of individuals with learning disabilities, it could be suggested that taking an individual stance on health outcomes may be appropriate. Carers and families can work with the individuals in developing a person-centred planning approach to their health which could include goal setting.

Applying this to Sean

Sean could benefit from having some support to help him in his daily activities. A mentor could help to devise a health action plan and encourage him to have healthy lifestyle behaviours.

Community level interventions

Well-being

It has been suggested that in an attempt to improve the health of individuals with learning disabilities it is necessary to move away from traditional health promotion to a promotion of well-being (Hall, 2010). In doing so, it is suggested that direct and indirect implications on health could be seen. For example, if health promotion for this group took the stance of advertising activity groups, such as swimming groups, several health benefits would be seen from both a physical and psychological stance.

Learning disability community nurses

Learning disability community nurses provide a vast range of services from health checks to health advice and promotion. It is their role to ensure individuals with learning difficulties within their community receive all the healthcare they need. They also can assist with routine screening (e.g. health checks) with this population.

Applying this to Sean

Sean could make use of local support groups for individuals with learning disabilities. These will not only help with improving his weight and overall fitness but will improve his self-esteem.

Working effectively with others

This population is considered to be more vulnerable than most, therefore it is important that health and well-being is effectively addressed, whether this be supporting individuals with learning disabilities within the community or successfully promoting healthy behaviours. There are various professionals who can provide on-going support for these individuals in terms of health and well-being. These may be part of multidisciplinary teams such as:

Community learning disability team

This service is multidisciplinary and consists of a variety of professionals including:

- Doctors
- Psychologists
- Occupational therapists
- Nurses
- Dieticians
- Physiotherapists
- Speech and language therapists.

By providing access to these professionals, individuals with learning disabilities can receive the best possible support in order to live an independent, healthy life. The approach takes the individual through an assessment to discover their needs and then provides the required treatment and support. As the approach is multidisciplinary it enables the individual to gain access to any service which they may need whether it is for a physical or mental health problem.

Social workers

Social workers have a wide range of skills and can provide advice on health related issues in addition to general support. They aim to impact upon the general well-being of specific groups within the community such as those with learning disabilities. After undertaking an assessment, the social worker can work with the individual and their family to suggest services or organisations which may be of use.

Applying this to Sean

It may be an appropriate time for Sean's parents to arrange an assessment with the community learning disability team. This will enable Sean to get all the help and support he needs to remain independent.

Turner and Robinson (2010) stressed the importance of working in partnerships for people with learning disabilities and highlighted the importance of working with:

- the Learning Disability Partnership Board
- self-advocates
- the family carers group
- public health
- social care providers
- local involvement networks (LINks).

Older age

Case study

Emma is an 86-year-old woman who currently lives in a semi-detached house in a small village. She has two children who are in their 60s and her husband of 65 years has recently died as a result of a stroke.

Now that Emma lives alone, her children are becoming increasingly worried for her health and safety around the house. They have set a downstairs bedroom up for her so she doesn't have to climb the stairs, which she now finds nearly impossible. Emma's mobility has rapidly declined and she now uses a Zimmer frame in the house and an electric wheelchair when she goes out. In addition, her confidence in her ability to go out of the house and even just into her garden has also declined. As she now lives alone she is worried that she could fall whilst in the garden and there would be nobody to help her up.

Emma and her late husband had always been sociable people who regularly met with friends, went on holiday and attended their local bowls club. However, since Emma's husband passed away and her mobility has deteriorated she is less able to see her friends and spends a lot of time on her own at home. Her children are worried about her and would like some advice on how they can improve her health and social life.

Introduction

The UK is an ageing population, with the number of individuals aged over 85 in the UK continually rising. Since 1981, the number of individuals in this age bracket has risen by 0.8 million to 1.4 million (ONS, 2011a). In addition, over 16 per cent of the population is over the age of 65 (ONS, 2012). The rise in this population provides challenges for the health service and government from both an equality and financial point of view.

The Office for National Statistics reported that the leading cause of death in individuals aged over 65 is coronary heart disease (ONS, 2011b) with influenza, pneumonia and dementia also being cited as common causes of death. As people are now living longer it is even more important to have effective health promotion strategies that address the health issues which are most prominent in this population. It is essential that effective health promotion methods are used which acknowledge both the physical and psychological needs of this particular group. Interventions and policies should target this specific group in addition to the whole population in an attempt to increase all of society's healthy living years. This will ensure productive and healthy years in later life for all.

Interventions to improve the health of the elderly

Many interventions which target the elderly have been shown to be effective (Beswick et al., 2008). If interventions are seen to be effective in improving the health and well-being of the elderly then knock-on effects can be seen in relation to nursing home admissions, hospital admissions and individual well-being. Below, different types of interventions will be identified and explored.

Individual level interventions

Falls prevention

A large proportion of individuals aged over 65 suffer from falls. These can have serious health implications such as broken and fractured bones and even mortality.

This not only has implications for the individual's health and well-being but also for the economy through hospital and NHS expenditure. Falls present a significant public health concerns almost a third of those aged over 65 who live in the community fall at least once a year with this figure rising to 45 per cent for people aged 80 and over (Department for Work and Pensions). Suffering a hip fracture (fractured neck of femur) is one of the most serious consequences of a fall, with a mortality rate of 30 per cent within a year of the fall and subsequent fracture amongst older people. It is for these reasons that interventions for fall preventions are of upmost importance within the elderly.

A Cochrane review (Gillespie *et al.*, 2007) considered the effectiveness of fall prevention interventions and concluded that benefits can be seen from these interventions. The interventions which were considered most beneficial were those which addressed various risk factors and which were multidisciplinary in nature. In addition, benefits were seen from working on muscle strength and balance techniques. One form of exercise which has become increasingly popular with the older generation is Tai Chi. This form of exercise involves slow movements which build muscle and aids balancing techniques. Participating in this form of exercise is thought to have implications on the amount of falls an individual will suffer, by reducing the occurrence (Schleicher *et al.*, 2012).

In addition to interventions which address the prevention of falls from a physical stance, it's also important to address the psychological components that can contribute to falls and the fear of falling. As highlighted elsewhere, Cognitive Behavioural Therapy (CBT) can be effective in treating not only psychological issues but also lifestyle behaviours. As CBT addresses the cognitive thought processes associated with a behaviour it can be considered useful for addressing fear of falling in this population. Interventions which combine both physical and psychological therapy have been shown to be effective in not only preventing falls but also improving quality of life (Tzu-Ting *et al.*, 2011).

Fall assessments

In addition to interventions being rolled out it is also necessary that effective assessments are undertaken to consider the individuals risk of suffering a fall. The National Institute for Clinical Excellence (NICE, 2004) state that every individual aged 65 or older who is in contact with a health professional should have an assessment performed on them. Tools have also been developed which are thought to successfully impact upon the individual and enable fall prevention strategies to be put in place before the incident happens (Robertson *et al.*, 2012).

Applying this to Emma

As Emma is worried about falling in her home and garden it is necessary to undertake a falls and risk assessment in her home. This will enable any potential risks to be identified and dealt with. In turn, this could help improve Emma's confidence and reduce her fear of falling.

Community level interventions

Public services

In attempting to reduce the prevalence of falls, the local council can ensure that public services are kept in the best condition and are easily accessible to the older population. This could include ensuring that roads and footpaths are in good condition and are level and transport services available as well as taking measures to ensure the elderly feel safe in their community. An example of one of these measures is the introduction of tilting buses. These buses are able to lower the step up to the bus to make it more accessible for the elderly and individuals who use wheelchairs.

Day centres

These are used as a means of providing social and general support for the elderly in addition to providing breaks for careers and family members. The centres can provide a range of activities such as art, craft, games and physical exercise sessions. In addition to providing social activities, the majority of them also provide the elderly with a meal. In supplying such facilities, the older generation will potentially benefit in both a physical and psychological way.

Physical health can be improved by the activities undertaken, for example, exercise classes to improve muscle strength. Psychological health can be influenced by the social aspect of the event in addition to the mental stimulation of the brain through games and activities. From a psychological stance, it is thought that the participation in such games and activities is associated with improved subjective well-being, for example (Jenkins, 2011). Overall, the sessions provide a vast range of stimulation which may not have otherwise been possible.

In addition to these benefits, this time can also be used to educate participants on health awareness and general well-being. Sessions could be used to inform the elderly of any help and resources that may be of benefit to them. Conjointly day centres can contribute towards the health and well-being of the individuals and can be a useful means of health promotion.

Emma would benefit from finding a local day centre which she could attend once a week. This would provide her with the opportunity to interact and meet new people as she spends a lot of her time by herself.

Working effectively with others

NHS falls clinic

Parts of the UK have specific NHS falls clinics. These clinics are made up of a multidisciplinary team who work with the individual to assess, advise and rehabilitate them either after a fall or with the intention of preventing a fall. The team work with the individual to understand why they are suffering from falls and how they can prevent them. This can have long-term implications on their health and independence, alongside reducing admissions to Accident and Emergency departments. The team of professionals can involve:

- Nurses
- Occupational therapists
- Physiotherapists
- Fall consultants
- Doctors
- Therapists.

Fall clinics are evident in many countries and have been evaluated to determinate their effectiveness. It can be suggested such clinics are successful in preventing falls and injuries related to the falls, in addition to improving balance, strength and confidence (Hill *et al.*, 2008).

Home fire and safety visits

In an attempt to improve the health and safety of the older generation, elderly people are entitled to a free home fire and safety visit by the fire service. They will assess the individual's home and suggest any ways in which it can be made a safer environment. This may mean installing smoke alarms or pointing out any potential fire hazards.

Gym sessions/personal trainers

As seen in the healthy eating chapter, personal trainers can provide a valuable service for the whole population. Elderly people can have many benefits from exercise sessions; as previously mentioned this can include strengthening muscles and improving posture which can have implications on fall rates etc. (Karinkanta *et al.*, 2009). Once again, in addition to the physical benefits, it is also suggested that benefits can be seen in relation to the individual's psychological well-being as a result of exercise. Undertaking gym sessions at either an individual or group level can provide a good opportunity to improve and influence the health and well-being of the older generation.

Applying this to Emma

It could be suggested that Emma may benefit from some form of light physical exercise/training. This could work on strengthening her muscles which could impact on her ability to carry out day-to-day activities.

Conclusion

Individual segments of the population provide challenges for healthcare professionals due to the complex needs of individual groups. This chapter has considered some of the ways in which the health promotion can be conducted effectively to promote change in a small review of different segments of the population. It is apparent, of course, that different groups will not only have different health needs but will also require different approaches and different methods of engaging with them.

Key points

- It is essential to adapt health interventions in order to make them effective for all members of the population.
- Understanding the impact of psychological variables within these populations is important in the development and implementation of interventions.
- CBT is a useful tool for behaviour change, especially for the psychological issues.
- Working with offenders in prisons offers advantages (e.g. easy access) and disadvantages (e.g. constraints of the environment) when attempting behaviour change.
- Illicit drug use has increased over the recent period and brings with it a range of potential health concerns.

- Applying the Stages of Change model and/or motivational interviewing can bring about change to illicit drug use.
- Social marketing programmes for reducing illicit drug use show variable success rates.
- People with learning disabilities have specific health concerns and have greater health issues than others.
- Improving access and availability of health check-ups for people with a disability would prove beneficial.
- Working with the elderly to prevent falls can prove beneficial overall for the individual.
- Multi-faceted and multidisciplinary approaches to falls prevention in the elderly can be very effective.

Points for discussion

- Critically discuss the arguments for and against health promotion in the prison setting.
- What health promotion could be given to the elderly in day centres?
- Consider the advantages and disadvantages of targeting special groups in health promotion.
- What psychological variables do you consider to be important in health promotion within special groups?

Further resources

Talk to Frank – Advice on drugs http://www.talktofrank.com
Improving health and lives: Learning disability observatory http://www.improving healthandlives.org.uk
Age UK http://www.ageuk.org.uk

References

Prison population

Akbar, T., Turner, T., Themessl-Huber, M. and Freeman, R. (2012). *The Evaluation of HMP Shotts' Oral Health Improvement Project*. Available at: http://www.sps.gov.uk (accessed 30 March 2012).

Andreasen, A.R. (ed.) (2006). *Social Marketing in the 21st Century*. London: Sage.

Andrews, D.A. and Bonta, J. (2010). Rehabilitating criminal justice policy and practice. *Psychology, Public Policy, and Law*, 16(1): 39–55.

ASH. (2010). *Smokefree Prisons*. London: ASH.

Berman, G. (2012). *Prison Population Statistics*. Available at www.parliament.uk/briefing-papers/sn04334.pdf (accessed 6 January 2013).

Department of Health. (2002). *Health-promoting Prisons: A Shared Approach*. London: Department of Health.

Harris, F., Hek, G. and Condon, L. (2007). Health needs of prisoners in England and Wales: the implications for prison healthcare of gender, age and ethnicity. *Health & Social Care in the Community*, 15(1): 56–66.

Heigel, C., Stuewig, J. and Tangney, J. (2010). Self-reported physical health of inmates: impact of incarceration and relation to optimism. *Journal of Correctional Health Care*, 16(2): 106–116.

Home Office (2002). *Crime in England and Wales 2001/2002*. Available at http://www.homeoffice.gov.uk/rds/index.htm (accessed 5 May 2012).

Lasnier, B., Cantinotti, M., Guyon, L., Royer, A., Brochu, S. and Chayer, L. (2011). Implementing an indoor smoking ban in prison: enforcement issues and effects on tobacco use, exposure to second-hand smoke and health of inmates. *Canadian Journal of Public Health*, 102(4): 249–253.

Loeb, S. J., Steffensmeier, D. and Kassab, C. (2011). Predictors of self-efficacy and self-rated health for older male inmates. *Journal of Advanced Nursing*, 67(4): 811–820.

Marshall, T., Simpson, S. and Stevens, A. (2000). *Toolkit for Health Care Needs Assessment in Prisons*. Birmingham: Department of Public Health & Epidemiology.

Ministry of Justice (2010). *Population in Custody Monthly Tables August 2010 England and Wales Statistics Bulletin*. London: Ministry of Justice.

Mullins, J. (2012). A multidisciplinary approach to mental health care for prisoners. *Mental Health Practice*, 15(10): 30.

Posadzki, P., Stockl, A., Musonda, P. and Tsouroufli, M. (2010). A mixed-method approach to sense of coherence, health behaviours, self-efficacy and optimism: towards the operationalization of positive health attitudes. *Scandinavian Journal of Psychology*, 51(3): 246–252.

Thibodeau, L., Jorenby, D.E., Seal, D.W., Su-Young, K. and Sosman, J. M. (2010). Prerelease intent predicts smoking behaviour postrelease following a prison smoking ban. *Nicotine & Tobacco Research*, 12(2): 152–158.

Turner, S. (2013). Improving the uptake of health checks for adults with learning disabilities. *Evidence into Practice Report 6*. London: Department of Health.

Warrilow, A. (2012). Improving the mental health care of prisoners. *Mental Health Practice*, 15(8): 20–24.

Illicit drug use

Broman, C. L. (2007). Race, drug use and risky sexual behaviour. *College Student Journal*, 41(4): 999–1010.

Brown, R.L. and Rounds, L.A. (1995). Conjoint screening questionnaires for alcohol and drug abuse. *Wisconsin Medical Journal*, 94: 135–140.

Brown, R.L., Leonard, T., Saunders, L.A. and Papasouliotis, O.A. (2001). A two item conjoint screen for alcohol and other drug problems. *Journal of the American Board of Family Practice*, 14: 95–106.

Brown University (2009) *Brief Motivational Intervention Reduces Drug Use in Community-based Heavy Cocaine Users*. Wiley Online Library: Wiley Periodicals, Inc.

Couwenbergh, C., van der Gaag, R.J., Koeter, M., De Ruiter, C. and Van den Brink, W. (2009). Screening for substance abuse among adolescents validity of the CAGE-AID in youth mental health care. *Substance Use & Misuse*, 44(6): 823–834.

Cheng, T. and Lo, C. (2011). A longitudinal analysis of some risk and protective factors in marijuana use by adolescents receiving child welfare services. *Children & Youth Services Review*, 33(9): 1667–1672.

Deas, D. and Thomas, S.E. (2001). An overview of controlled studies of adolescent substance abuse treatment. *American Journal of Addiction*, 10(2): 178–189.

Dixon, J., Schneider, V., Lloyd, C., Reeves, A., White, C., Tomaszewski, W., Green, R. and Ireland, E. (2010). *Monitoring and Evaluation of Family Interventions: Information on Families Supported to March 2010* (Research report DFE-RR044). London: DfE (online). Available: http://publications.education.gov.uk/eOrderingDownload/DFE-RR044.pdf (accessed November, 2010).

Dutra, L., Stathopoulou, G., Basden, S., Leyro, T., Powers, M. and Otto, M. (2008). A meta-analytic review of psychosocial interventions for substance use disorders. *American Journal of Psychiatry* (serial online), 165(2):179–187. Available from: Academic Search Complete, Ipswich, MA (accessed 18 July 2012).

Ewing, J.A. (1984). Detecting alcoholism: the CAGE questionnaire. *Journal of the American Medical Association*, 252: 1905–1907.

Flynn, B.S., Worden, J.K., Secker-Walker, R.H., Pirie, P.L. Badger, G.J., Carpenter, J.H. and Geller, B.M. (1994). Mass-media and school interventions for cigarette smoking prevention: effects 2 years after completion. *American Journal of Public Health*, 84: 1148–1150.

Health and Social Care Information Centre (2012). *Statistics on Drugs Misuse: England*. London: HM Government.

Home Office (2012). *Drug Misuse Declared: Findings from the 2011/12 Crime Survey for England and Wales*. Available at http://www.homeoffice.gov.uk/publications/science-research-statistics/research-statistics/crime-research/drugs-misuse-dec-1112/drugs-misuse-dec-1112-pdf?view=Binary (accessed 6 January 2013)

HM Government (2010). *Drug Strategy 2010: Reducing Demand, Restricting Supply, Building Recovery: Supporting People to Live a Drug Free Life*. Available at: http://www.homeoffice.gov.uk/publications/alcohol-drugs/drugs/drug-strategy/drug-strategy-2010?view=Binary (accessed 7 April 2012).

Lee, N.K. and Rawson, R.A. (2008). A systematic review of cognitive and behavioural therapies for methamphetamine dependence. *Drug & Alcohol Review*, 27(3): 309–317.

Liddle, H.A., Dakof, G.A., Parker, K., Diamond, G.S., Barrett, K. and Tejeda, M. (2001). Multidimensional family therapy for adolescent drug abuse: Results of a randomized clinical trial. *The American Journal of Drug and Alcohol Abuse*, 27: 651–688.

Marlatt, G.A. and Donovan, D.M. (eds) (2005). *Relapse Prevention: Maintenance Strategies in the Treatment of Addictive Behaviours*, 2nd edn. New York: Guilford Press.

McCambridge, J., Slym, R.L. and Strang, J. (2008). Randomized controlled trial of motivational interviewing compared with drug information and advice for early intervention among young cannabis users. *Addiction* 103(11): 1809–1809.

Mersy, D.J. (2003). Recognition of alcohol and substance abuse. *American Family Physician*, 67: 1529–1532.

McGrath, Y.T., Sumnall, H.R., McVeigh, J. *et al*. (2006). *Review of Grey Literature on Drug Prevention among Young People*. London: NICE.

Miller, W.R., Yahne, C.E. and Tonigan, J.S. (2003). Motivational interviewing in drug abuse services: a randomized trial. *Journal of Consulting and Clinical Psychology*, 71: 754–763.

National Institute for Health and Clinical Excellence (NICE). (2007). *Drug Misuse: Psychosocial Interventions*. London: NICE.

Office for National Statistics (ONS). (2011). *Deaths Related to Drug Poisoning in England and Wales, 2010*. London: ONS.

Petraitis, J., Flay, B.R., and Miller, T.Q. (1995). Reviewing theories of adolescent substance use: organising piece in the puzzle. *Psychological Bulletin,* 117: 67–86.

Petry, N.M., Weinstock, J. and Alessi, S.M. (2011). A randomized trial of contingency management delivered in the context of group counselling. *Journal of Consulting and Clinical Psychology*, 79(5): 686–696.

Prochaska, J.O., DiClemente, C.C. and Norcross, J.C. (1992). In search of how people change: applications to addictive behaviours. *American Psychologist,* 47: 1102–1114.

Stapleton, J.A., Keaney, F. and Sutherland, G. (2009). Illicit drug use as a predictor of smoking cessation treatment outcome. *Nicotine & Tobacco Research*, 11(6): 685–689.

Stephens, R.S., Roffman, R.A. and Curtain, L. (2000). Comparison of extended versus brief treatments for marijuana use. *Journal of Consulting and Clinical Psychology,* 68: 898–908.

Sumnall, H.R. and Bellis, M.A. (2007). Can health campaigns make people ill? The iatrogenic potential of population-based cannabis prevention. *Journal of Epidemiology and Community Health,* 61: 930–931.

Volpp, K.G., Troxel, A.B., Pauly, M.V., Glick, H.A., Puig, A., Asch, D.A. and Audrain-McGovern, J. *et al.* (2009). A randomized, controlled trial of financial incentives for smoking cessation. *New England Journal Of Medicine*, 360(7): 699–709.

Weiss, L.M. and Petry, N.M. (2011). Interaction effects of age and contingency management treatments in cocaine-dependent outpatients. *Experimental and Clinical Psychopharmacology*, 19(2): 173–181.

Wiebe, G.D. (1951–1952). Merchandising commodities and citizenship on television. *Public Opinion Quarterly,* 15: 679–91.

Learning disabilities

Ahrens, K., DuBois, D., Richardson, L., Fan, M. and Lozano, P. (2008). Youth in foster care with adult mentors during adolescence have improved adult outcomes. *Paediatrics*, 121(2): e246–e252.

Codling, M. and Macdonald, N. (2011). Sustainability of health promotion for people with learning disabilities. *Nursing Standard*, 25(22): 42–47.

Department of Health (2009). *Valuing People Now: A New Three-year Strategy for Learning Disabilities.* London: Department of Health.

Department of Health and Social Security (2005). *Equal Lives: Review of Policy and Services for People with a Learning Disability in Northern Ireland.* Dublin: DHSS.

Disability Rights Commission (2006) *Equal Treatment: Closing the Gap.* Stratford upon Avon: Disability Rights Commission.

Emerson, E. and Baines, S. (2010). *Health Inequalities and People with Learning Disabilities in the UK.* Stockton on Tees: Improving Health and Lives: Learning Disabilities Observatory.

Emerson, E., Copeland, A. and Glover, G. (2011). *The Uptake of Health Checks for Adults with Learning Disabilities: 2008/9 to 2010/11.* Stockton on Tees: Improving Health and Lives: Learning Disabilities Observatory.

Glomb, N.K., Buckley, L.D., Minskoff, E.D. and Rogers, S. (2006). The learning leaders mentoring program for children with ADHD and learning disabilities. *Preventing School Failure*, 50(4): 31–35.

Hall, E. (2010). Spaces of wellbeing for people with learning disabilities. *Scottish Geographical Journal*, 126(4): 275–284.

Learning Disability Advisory Group (2001). *Fulfilling the Promises: Report of the Learning Disability Advisory Group*. Cardiff: Welsh Assembly Government.

Robertson, J., Roberts, H. and Emerson, E. (2010). *Health Checks for People with Learning Disabilities: Systematic Review of Impact*. Durham: Improving Health and Lives: Learning Disability Observatory.

Scottish Executive (2000). *The Same as You: A Review of Services for People with Learning Disability*. Edinburgh: Scottish Executive.

Shoneye, C. (2012). Prevention and treatment of obesity in adults with learning disabilities. *Learning Disability Practice*, 15(3), 32–37.

Turner, S. and Robinson, C. (2010) *Health Inequalities and People with Learning Disabilities in the UK: Implications and Actions for Commissioners*. Lancaster: Learning Disability Observatory.

Wigham, S., Robertson, J., Emerson, E., Hatton, C., Elliott, J., McIntosh, B., Joyce, T. *et al.* (2008). Reported goal setting and benefits of person centred planning for people with intellectual disabilities. *Journal of Intellectual Disabilities*, 12(2): 143–152.

Older age

Beswick, A., Rees, K., Dieppe, P., Ayis, S., Gooberman-Hill, R., Horwood, J. and Ebrahim, S. (2008). Complex interventions to improve physical function and maintain independent living in elderly people: a systematic review and meta-analysis. *Lancet*, 371(9614): 725–735.

Gillespie, L.D., Gillespie, W.J., Robertson, M.C., Lamb, S.E., Cumming, R.G. and Rowe, B.H. (2007). Interventions for preventing falls in elderly people (Review). *Cochrane Library*, 11: 1–289.

Hill, K.D., Moore, K.J., Dorevitch, M.I. and Day, L.M. (2008). Effectiveness of falls clinics: an evaluation of outcomes and client adherence to recommended interventions. *Journal of the American Geriatrics Society*, 56(4): 600–608.

Jenkins, A. (2011). Participation in learning and wellbeing among older adults. *International Journal of Lifelong Education*, 30(3): 403–420.

Karinkanta, S., Heinonen, A., Sievänen, H., Uusi-Rasi, K., Fogelholm, M. and Kannus, P. (2009). Maintenance of exercise-induced benefits in physical functioning and bone among elderly women. *Osteoporosis International*, 20(4): 665–674.

National Institute for Clinical Excellence (NICE). (2004). *Clinical Practice Guideline for the Assessment and Prevention of Falls in Older People*. Clinical Guideline No. 21. London: NICE.

Office for National Statistics (ONS). (2011a). *Annual Mid-year Population Estimates, 2010*. London: ONS. Available from http://www.ons.gov.uk/ons/rel/pop-estimate/population-estimates-for-uk--england-and-wales--scotland-and-northern-ireland/mid-2010-population-estimates/index.html (accessed 4 May 2012).

——(2011b). *Leading Causes of Death in England and Wales, 2009*. London: ONS. Available from http://www.ons.gov.uk/ons/dcp171780_239682.pdf (accessed 4 May 2012).

——(2012). 2011 *Census – Population and Household Estimates for England and Wales, March 2011*. London: ONS. Available from http://www.ons.gov.uk/ons/dcp171778_270487.pdf (accessed 4 May 2012).

Robertson, K., Logan, P., Ward, M., Pollard, J., Gordon, A., Williams, W. and Watson, J. (2012). Thinking falls – taking action: a falls prevention tool for care homes. *British Journal of Community Nursing*, 17(5): 206–209.

Schleicher, M.M., Wedam, L. and Wu, G. (2012). Review of Tai Chi as an effective exercise on falls prevention in elderly. *Research in Sports Medicine*, 20(1): 37–58.

Tzu-Ting, H., Lin-Hui, Y. and Chia-Yih, L. (2011). Reducing the fear of falling among community-dwelling elderly adults through cognitive-behavioural strategies and intense Tai Chi exercise: a randomized controlled trial. *Journal of Advanced Nursing*, 67(5): 961–971.

12 Conclusion

Learning objectives

At the end of this chapter you will:
- appreciate the differences between an interventionist and a libertarian approach to health promotion
- understand the current public health policy
- recognise the practitioner role in behavioural change
- recognise the difficulties faced by individuals attempting to change
- have considered future directions for health promotion.

Sex, food, drink and smoking: either an enjoyable night out or a potential time bomb, depending on your perspective. This book has addressed these behaviours (and drugs and lack of exercise) from a psychological perspective – exploring how psychology can explain such behaviours and how it can be used to modify unsafe practices. This does not mean that we, or other promoters of healthy lifestyle, should be labelled as kill-joys or party poopers. It just means that we advocate changing lifestyle for the better, to improve health and to promote life expectancy: you cannot enjoy yourself if you are dead from coronary heart disease, lung cancer or some other 'lifestyle disease'.

This concluding chapter will explore the role of psychological interventions within a political and social context. Although the techniques, research and evidence we have presented within this book will be of use to the individual healthcare professional, it is important that the policy framework is recognised. Whilst it is beyond the scope of this text to explore all of these elements and there are other books that take a more socio-political perspective on lifestyle (e.g. Thirlaway and Upton, 2009), it is essential that the healthcare professional appreciates the context in which they work. Consequently, this chapter will outline the lifestyle policy in the UK since the 1990s and how this impacts on the ethics of intervention and individual practice.

Health professionals promoting evidence-based strategies (and we have tried to concentrate on these research or evidence-based methods) for lifestyle change face criticism and competition from many sources, many of whom base their critiques and alternative solutions on personal experience. For example, Janet Street-Porter in the *Independent on Sunday* (2008a) claimed that 'Obesity is a result of wilful self-abuse' rather than offering any coherent psychological explanation. Similarly, as we pointed out at the outset of this text, Rod Liddle in the *Sunday Times* suggested that: 'Most obesity is a consequence of stupidity and indolence and not of some genetic affliction. It is a lifestyle choice which people would be less inclined to adopt if they knew we all hated them for it' (Liddle, 2008).

Such columnists are often opposed to any strategy that limits personal choice and have accused the government of building a 'nanny state'. However, Janet Street-Porter had changed her mind a month later and was proposing rationing of sugar, chocolate, fats and salt (Street-Porter, 2008b). Janet-Street Porter has also thrown her oar into the debate about how to curb drinking. She confidently stated, in direct contradiction to the actual research evidence (Room 2004; Meng *et al.*, 2012; Purshouse *et al.*, 2010), that: 'there is absolutely no evidence that making drink more expensive will have any effect on the number of people getting slaughtered night after night' (Street-Porter, 2008c). It is the job of columnists like Janet Street-Porter and Rod Liddle to write controversial text, so we can take some of their comments with a pinch of salt (although no more than 6g per day). Of course, it is encouraging that lifestyle diseases and lifestyle behaviours are finally getting media coverage and that the health problems that arise from unsafe sex, binge drinking and so on are front-page news. It was not long ago that Harrabin *et al.* (2003) were voicing concern at the media's lack of interest in lifestyle diseases. What is concerning, however, is that everybody now sees themselves as an expert on lifestyle, and alongside the columnists creating controversy are a plethora of lay persons offering health and lifestyle advice that ranges from the ill-advised to the positively dangerous. Consequently, this text sets out to offer fundamentally sensible advice based on psychological principles supported by consistent and high-quality research.

Of course, the healthcare professional does not operate within a vacuum – and there is a need for the healthcare professional to appreciate the socio-economic and policy environment in which their practice occurs. Prevention of lifestyle diseases through promoting healthy lifestyle choices has been a central tenet of health policy in the UK since 1999 (Department of Health, 1999). The government faces two interrelated challenges. First, they need to change the established lifestyle habits of the current generation of adults, and second, they need to prevent the next generation of adults establishing similar or worse lifestyle habits. Lifestyle policy in the UK addresses these two issues, firstly by attempting to modify cultural norms. For example, in an attempt to promote sensible drinking the policy has been to shape the environment – to change the cultural norms to one of sensible and safe drinking rather than one characterised by binge drinking (HM Government, 2007). However, what has to be recognised is that this will be a long and generational process: 'cultures exist where being active or eating "healthy" foods are not top priorities' (Jones *et al.*, 2007, p. 38). Furthermore, it is important to appreciate that culture is difficult to change, especially if people do not have the resources to change: 'the behaviour of these individuals may be the most difficult to modify due to both the difficulties in reaching them and overcoming their norms' (Jones *et al.*, 2007, p. 38) irrespective of the amount of facilities and support available to them. As Alan Johnson (the UK's then current Health Secretary) stated: 'The causes of poor health are not so much about the choices people make, *but the choices they are able to make*' (Johnson, 2009).

Changing cultural norms could both establish healthy lifestyle habits from the outset and make it easier for individuals to change established unhealthy lifestyles, and there would no longer be a need for this book. Lifestyle policy clearly aims to direct cultural trends (HM Government, 2007; Department of Health, 1999; Jones *et al.*, 2007) but is itself a product of our history and culture. For instance, there is no clear scientific rationale for a drug like cannabis to be illegal whilst a drug like alcohol is not. Alcohol is an integral part of our history and culture and banning it in Britain has never been considered a viable response to the problems that arise from drinking. The opening statement of 'Safe. Sensible. Social' (HM Government, 2007) makes it clear that alcohol is seen as a primarily positive aspect of society despite the severe behavioural and health consequences. The same document goes on to report that 'Alcohol can play an important and positive role in British culture' (HM Government, 2007).

A population-level approach to public health interventions has always been assumed to be the most cost-effective and efficient way to produce behavioural change. It is cheaper and can get the message to a greater number of individuals than the clinical measures ever can, and it will result (hopefully) in the development of cultural changes. The most significant population-level smoking intervention in recent years has been legislation to restrict smoking in public places. Since March 2006 in Scotland, April 2007 in Northern Ireland and Wales, and July 2007 in England, all public places and workplaces have been smoke free. The introduction of this change was not particularly controversial – the proportion of the population supporting such a change was high. Of course, commentators such as Rod Liddle have argued strongly against the ban. For example, when commenting on the smoking ban introduced by Sir Liam Donaldson, the Chief Medical Officer:

> Sir Liam is the chap who believes today's unjust and draconian smoking ban is 'only a start' and wishes to pursue smokers into the family home. Despite evidence to the contrary, Donaldson believes passive smoking kills millions of people; but then his career has been built upon scaring people.
>
> Liddle, 2007

However, it appears that this 'draconian ban' has already reduced the number of heart attacks in the UK. Indeed, this legislation has resulted in substantial population health gain, including reductions in workplace exposure to second-hand smoke (SHS: Semple *et al.*, 2010), increased smoking quit rates (Hackshaw *et al.*, 2010) and decreased hospital admissions for acute myocardial infarction (Sims *et al.*, 2010; Mackay *et al.*, 2010) along with improvements in childhood asthma rates (Millett *et al.*, 2013). It may be draconian but it is clearly effective, and more effective than decades of anti-smoking promotion activities (Pell and Haw, 2009).

An interesting perspective and debate was raised by the Nuffield Council on Bioethics (2007) who argued that public health policies should be about enforcement. They proposed an 'intervention ladder' as a useful way of conceptualising public health interventions and their impact on an individual's choice (see Table 9.1). In the case of smoking, how does this fit into the ladder? It can be seen that currently the government 'guides by disincentives' and 'restricts choice' to a certain extent. The ban on smoking in public places is significant as it is the first legislative attempt to alter lifestyle choices made by governments for many years. However, surely it can be argued that the government should totally eliminate choice, i.e. we should ban smoking. On the one hand, smoking is a behaviour which is avoidable – society and civilisation would not suffer considerably if it was banned across the country. Certainly, the Nuffield Council on Bioethics (2007) would argue that this would be important and that enforcement should be used and this curtailment of individual freedom would be ethically justified. Their argument concerns proportionality – can the enforcement benefits outweigh the interference in people's lives? Smoking is a dangerous lifestyle behaviour that has its roots in social, physiological and psychological elements. Its dangers are obvious to most and it can kill not only the individual but the innocent bystander. Is this sufficient to 'eliminate choice' (to use the phrasing of the Nuffield Council, aka 'ban', 'coerce' or 'outlaw')? Obviously, libertarians would argue that smoking is a right of the individual and if individuals want to choose this behaviour then this is their right. Consequently, it is up to health promoters, health psychologists and healthcare professionals to promote smoking cessation and not to severely curtail our freedoms. An editorial in *The Times* (13 November 2007) argues that 'John Stuart Mill held that the only justification for state coercion was to prevent harm, or "evil", being done to others. It is a stretch to say that … smoking at home meets this definition.' However, others have argued that the ladder provides an ethical framework for public health interventions which can be applied to other lifestyle behaviours such as alcohol use and poor diet (Walton and Megwasser, 2012).

Laws that eliminate or restrict lifestyle choices are generally in place to protect others from harm, not the individuals themselves. Consequently, people can no longer smoke in a public place in order to protect others, and driving under the influence of alcohol is illegal. Critics of such interventionist policies (including Janet Street-Porter, Dominic Lawson and Rod Liddle) have argued that such measures are 'nanny state-ist' (Jochelson, 2006) and an unnecessary intrusion into people's personal lives. The current government, and the official opposition, distance themselves from such interventionist attitudes, although the current health secretary did teasingly ask 'is it too great a leap to assume that what works today for smoking will also work for obesity, or for that matter alcohol?' (Johnson, 2009). However, this debate about the limits to state freedom and public health is not new. Libertarians have long argued that minimal state intervention is the way to protect individual freedom. For example, a commentator suggested that the original Public Health Act of 1848 was 'paternalistic' and 'despotic' and 'a little dirt and freedom' was 'more desirable than no dirt at all and slavery' (Porter, 1999).

From the other end of the intervention ladder (Table 12.1) the government remains committed to a policy of guiding choice, despite the irrefutable evidence across all lifestyle behaviours that educational and risk communication messages do not have any significant effect on lifestyle choices (Floyd *et al.*, 2000; Milne *et al.*, 2000; Blue, 2007; Ruiter, 2004; Taubman Ben-Ari and Findler, 2005). Attempts to develop a culture of sensible drinking have been a dismal failure and young women are actually drinking more than ever. However, cultural norms can be modified; drink-driving is no longer

Table 12.1 The intervention ladder

Level	Description	Example
Eliminate choice	Introduce laws that entirely eliminate choice	Compulsory isolation of those with an infectious disorder
Restrict choice	Introduce laws that restrict the options available to people	Remove unhealthy foods from shops
Guide through disincentives	Introduce financial or other disincentives to influence behaviour	Increase taxes on cigarettes
Guide through incentives	Introduce financial or other incentives to influence people's behaviour	Tax breaks for bicycle purchases
Guide choices	Change the default policy	Change the standard side dish from chips to salad
Enable choice	Help individuals to change their behaviour	Free stop-smoking programmes
Provide information	Inform and educate public	Encourage people to eat five portions of fruit/veg a day
Do nothing	Or monitor situation	

Source: Nuffield Council on Bioethics, 2007

considered an acceptable behaviour and drink-related road accidents have been reduced. Smoking in public places is no longer acceptable and the move to this position was not nearly as contentious as was feared (ONS, 2005). However, all these cultural shifts have been supported by clear legislation; it is unlikely that health promotion alone will change lifestyle culture.

In the context of this social and policy background, the healthcare practitioner has to promote healthy behaviour and behaviour change. The government has set many targets around reducing the incidence of lifestyle diseases and their main strategy to achieve these goals is to increase healthy and decrease unhealthy lifestyle choices. However, although the healthcare professional has a fundamental role, they are not the only one that has a responsibility for improving health and behavioural choices. For example, in the alcohol policy document 'Safe. Sensible. Social' (HM Government, 2007), virtually all public servants – the police, local authorities, the NHS, schools, voluntary organisations – are tasked with delivering the government's strategy. Furthermore, the government also identifies the alcohol industry and the wider business industry, the media and local communities as having a role to play in delivering their strategy. However, who is to deliver the behavioural change component of this strategy, which receives scant attention in the document but has the clearest evidence-base as to its efficacy, is not addressed (Moyer *et al.*, 2002; Mulvihill *et al.*, 2005; Poikolainen, 1999; Williams *et al.*, 2007). Similarly, various public servants and businesses are involved in the promotion of healthy eating and physical activity but the central question of who should deliver the essential behavioural change component of the strategy remains unclear.

Of course, the principal candidates for the delivery of behavioural change interventions are primary care practitioners: general practitioners, practice nurses, health visitors and other associated healthcare professionals (Ashenden *et al.*, 1997). Primary care has been central in the delivery of individual lifestyle advice for some time, and there is conflicting evidence about whether merely advising patients to change their lifestyle can lead to lifestyle change (Ashenden *et al.*, 1997; Moyer *et al.*, 2002). However, it is clear that a psychologically based intervention is more likely to be successful (Moyer *et al.*, 2002; Biddle *et al.*, 1997) and that appropriate training can provide primary care professionals with the skills necessary to change behaviour (e.g. Simkin-Silverman and Wing, 1997). To give healthcare professionals the best chance of delivering psychologically based lifestyle interventions they will need more than a copy of this book. Here we simply introduce the key concepts and ideas. Healthcare professionals will need training and resources if they are to deliver the changes in behaviour that governments are looking for.

In order to deliver effective preventative lifestyle interventions, health practitioners will need a range of resources and skills. First, they will need to be able to measure current lifestyle behaviours quickly and reliably and to recognise individuals who have severe problems that need referral to a specialist. Within each of the chapters we have presented information on how to assess, and there may be many such techniques. Importantly, the individual healthcare professional needs to be able to recognise the limits of their expertise and refer on as appropriate. So, for example, they need to be able to recognise the difference between substance use, misuse and addiction and refer on for specialist help as appropriate.

Health professionals who wish to enable the patients they work with to change their lifestyle first and foremost need to recognise that simply providing people with information about the risks of unhealthy lifestyles will not result in lifestyle change. If health professionals wish to encourage lifestyle change they should be looking to increase self-motivation, increase self-regulatory skills, set achievable goals and increase self-efficacy in their clients. Although reading this text has been a start, it is not a finishing point: there are additional seminars, courses and resources available that healthcare professionals need to make use of.

We are at a turning point in health promotion. The ineffectiveness of the previous decades of educational interventions is irrefutable and policy makers and health professionals are both starting to recognise the importance of psychological processes in lifestyle change (Thirlaway and Upton, 2009). Fortunately, psychology is a discipline with a strong record of high-quality research and we are already in a position to provide evidence-based advice about appropriate psychological interventions. Lifestyle behaviours are extremely varied but nevertheless the same psychological constructs are relevant to promoting change in them all. The potential opportunity to develop training and protocols for interventions that can be applied across all lifestyle behaviours should not be ignored.

Conclusion

This final chapter has attempted to pull together the material presented throughout this text within a social and policy context. It is important that the healthcare professional recognises the key role of public policy in the promotion of healthy lifestyle and their individual practice. The chapter stresses the tension between the libertarian perspective currently predominant in our society and the evidence that a more interventionist approach to public health policy can have a significant impact on health and well-being.

Motivation and self-efficacy have been established as key cognitive factors in successful lifestyle change. For now, the healthcare professional needs to maximise intervention-based knowledge and to develop and enhance self-efficacy as a key route for lifestyle change. However, we need to explore further the role of non-cognitive factors such as habitual responses and enjoyment in the establishment of lifestyle choices. We need to develop research protocols, evidence-based interventions and strategies that can extend our understanding and implementation of successful lifestyle change. People do not usually make initial lifestyle choices based on future health implications and by the time they wish to protect their health they need to overcome well-established bad habits. Ultimately we hope that the material in this text becomes redundant and the focus alters from changing unhealthy behaviours to maintaining healthy ones.

Summary points

- Everyone is an expert on lifestyle change and often advice is based on personal experience of change rather than research evidence.
- There is a tension between libertarian and interventionist approaches to public health.
- Restricting lifestyle choices through legislation can play an important role in changing cultural norms and individual behaviour and in improving long-term health.
- Healthcare professionals have a key role in promoting behaviour change.
- A psychological approach to lifestyle change can play a central role in the development of a healthy society.

References

Ashenden, R., Silagy, C. and Weller, D. (1997). A systematic review of the effectiveness of promoting lifestyle change in general practice. *Family Practice*, 14: 160–174.

A Sugared Pill: The Nuffield Council Tries, But Fails, to Justify The Nanny State (2007). *The Times*, 13 November. Available at: http://www.timesonline.co.uk/tol/comment/leading_article/article2859367.ece (accessed 23 September 2009).

Biddle, S., Edmunds, L., Bowler, I. and Killoran, A. (1997). Physical activity promotion through primary health care in England. *British Journal of General Practice*, 47(419): 367–369.

Blue, C.L. (2007). Does the theory of planned behaviour identify diabetes-related cognitions for intention to be physically active and eat a healthy diet? *Public Health Nursing*, 24(2): 141–150.

Department of Health (DoH). (1999). *Saving Lives: Our Healthier Nation*. London: The Stationery Office.

Floyd, D.L., Prentice-Dunn, S. and Rogers, R.W. (2000). A meta-analysis of protection motivation theory. *Journal of Applied Social Psychology*, 30: 407–429.

Hackshaw, L., McEwen, A., West, R. and Bauld, L. (2010). Quit attempts in response to smoke-free legislation in England. *Tobacco Control*, 19(2): 160–164

Harrabin, R., Coote, A. and Allen, J. (2003). *Health in the News: Risk, Reporting and Media Influence*. London: King's Fund.

HM Government. (2007). *Safe, Sensible, Social. The Next Steps in the National Alcohol Strategy*. London: Department of Health and The Home Office.

Jochelson, K. (2006). Nanny or steward? The role of government in public health. *Public Health*, 120: 1149–1155.

Johnson, A. (2009). *Nanny State, Nudge State or No State?* Royal Society of Arts, London, 19 March.

Jones, A., Bentham, G., Foster, C., Hillsdon, M. and Panter, J. (2007). *Tackling Obesities: Future Choices – Obesogenic Environments – Evidence Review*. London: Foresight.

Liddle, R. (2007). So that's his real NHS priority – a £2 billion stealth cut in England. *Sunday Times*, 1 July.

——(2008). Laugh at lard butts – but just remember Fatty Fritz lives longer. *Sunday Times*, 27 January.

Mackay, D.F., Irfan, M.O., Haw, S., Pell, J.P. (2010). Meta-analysis of the effect of comprehensive smoke-free legislation on acute coronary events. *Heart*, 96(19): 1525–1530

Meng, Y., Hill-McManus, D., Brennan, A. and Meier, P. (2012). *Model-based Appraisal of Alcohol Minimum Pricing and Off-licensed Trade Discount Bans in Scotland using the Sheffield Alcohol Policy Model (v.2): Second Update Based on Newly Available Data*. University of Sheffield: ScHARR.

Millett, C., Lee, J.T., Laverty, A.A., Glantz, S.A. and Majeed, A. (2013). Hospital admissions for childhood asthma after smoke-free legislation in England. Pediatrics, 131(2): e495–e501.

Milne, S., Sheeran, P. and Orbell, S. (2000). Prediction and intervention in health-related behaviour: a meta review of protection motivation theory. *Journal of Applied Social Psychology*, 30, 106–143.

Moyer, A., Finney, J.W., Swearingen, E. and Vergun, P. (2002). Brief interventions for alcohol problems: a meta-analytic review of controlled investigations in treatment seeking and non-treatment seeking populations. *Addiction*, 97: 279–292.

Mulvihill, C., Taylor, L., Waller, S., Naidoo, B. and Thom, B. (2005). *Prevention and Reduction of Alcohol Misuse: Evidence Briefing*, 2nd edn. London: Health Development Agency.

Nuffield Council on Bioethics (2007). *Public Health Ethical Issues*. London: Nuffield Council. Available at: www.nuffieldbioethics.org (accessed 23 September 2011).

Office for National Statistics (ONS). (2005). *Smoking-related Behaviour and Attitudes, 2005*. London: HMSO.

Pell, J.P. and Haw, S. (2009). The triumph of national smoke free legislation. *Heart*, 95: 1377–1380.

Poikolainen, K. (1999). Effectiveness of brief interventions to reduce alcohol intake in primary care populations: a meta analysis. *Preventative Medicine*, 28: 503–509.

Porter, D. (1999). *Health, Civilisation and the State. A History of Public Health from Ancient to Modern Times*. London: Routledge.

Purshouse, R.C., Meier, P.S., Brennan, A., Taylor, K.B. and Rafia, R. (2010) Estimated effect of alcohol pricing policies on health and health economic outcomes in England: an epidemiological model. *Lancet*, 375(9723): 1355–1364.

Room, R. (2004). Disabling the public interest: alcohol strategies and policies for England. *Addiction*, 99: 1083–1089.

Ruiter, R.A.C. (2004). *Effecten van angstaanjagende tv-spotjes [Effects of fear-arousing TV commercials]. Final report*. Maastricht, Netherlands: Maastricht University, Department of Experimental Psychology.

Semple, S., van Tongeren, M., Galea, K.S. *et al.* (2010) UK smoke-free legislation: changes in PM2.5 concentrations in bars in Scotland, England, and Wales. *The Annals of Occupational Hygiene*, 54(3): 272–280

Simkin-Silverman, L.R. and Wing, R.R. (1997). Management of obesity in primary care. *Obesity Research*, 5: 603–612

Sims, M., Maxwell, R., Bauld, L. and Gilmore, A. (2010) Short term impact of smoke-free legislation in England: retrospective analysis of hospital admissions for myocardial infarction. *British Medical Journal*, 340: c2161.

Street-Porter, J. (2008a). Let the adult fatties eat themselves to death. The kids we can save. *Independent on Sunday*, 27 January.

——(2008b). A return to the ration book is the answer to obesity. *Independent on Sunday*, 24 February.

——(2008c). Don't blame it on the young, we're a nation of boozers. *Independent on Sunday*, 24 February.

Taubman Ben-Ari, O. and Findler, L. (2005). Proximal and distal effects of mortality salience on willingness to engage in health promoting behavior along the life span. *Psychology & Health*, 20: 303–318.

Thirlaway, K. and Upton, D. (2009). *The Psychology of Lifestyle: Promoting Healthy Behaviour*. London: Routledge.

Walton, M. and Megwasser, E. (2012). An ethical evaluation of evidence: a stewardship approach to public health policy. *Public Health Ethics*, 5(1): 16–21.

Williams, E.C., Horton, N.J., Samet, J.H. and Saitz, R. (2007). Do brief measures of readiness to change predict alcohol consumption and consequences in primary care patients with unhealthy alcohol use? *Alcoholism: Clinical and Experimental Research*, 31: 428–435.

Index

Locators in **bold** refer to figures/diagrams

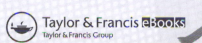